**W9-CPO-177**

PROCEEDINGS OF THE
SIXTH BERKELEY SYMPOSIUM

Volume IV

8m 2/21/73 /3.r

PROCEEDINGS *of the* SIXTH BERKELEY SYMPOSIUM ON MATHEMATICAL STATISTICS AND PROBABILITY

Held at the Statistical Laboratory
University of California
June 21–July 18, 1970
April 9–12, 1971
June 16–21, 1971
July 19–22, 1971

with the support of
University of California
National Science Foundation
National Institutes of Health
Air Force Office of Scientific Research
Army Research Office
Office of Naval Research

VOLUME IV

BIOLOGY AND HEALTH

June 16–21, 1971

EDITED BY LUCIEN M. LE CAM,
JERZY NEYMAN, AND ELIZABETH L. SCOTT

UNIVERSITY OF CALIFORNIA PRESS
BERKELEY AND LOS ANGELES
1972

UNIVERSITY OF CALIFORNIA PRESS
BERKELEY AND LOS ANGELES
CALIFORNIA

CAMBRIDGE UNIVERSITY PRESS
LONDON, ENGLAND

COPYRIGHT © 1972, BY
THE REGENTS OF THE UNIVERSITY OF CALIFORNIA

The United States Government and its offices, agents, and employees, acting within the scope of their duties, may reproduce, publish, and use this material in whole or in part for governmental purposes without payment of royalties thereon or therefor. The publication or republication by the government either separately or in a public document of any material in which copyright subsists shall not be taken to cause any abridgment or annulment of the copyright or to authorize any use or appropriation of such copyright material without the consent of the copyright proprietor.

ISBN: 0-520-02187-8

LIBRARY OF CONGRESS CATALOG CARD NUMBER: 49-8189

PRINTED IN THE UNITED STATES OF AMERICA

CONTENTS OF PROCEEDINGS
VOLUMES I, II, III,
IV, V, AND VI

Volume I—Theory of Statistics

General Theory

R. J. BERAN, Upper and lower risks and minimax procedures. C. R. BLYTH and D. M. ROBERTS, On inequalities of Cramér-Rao type and admissibility proofs. J. OOSTERHOFF and W. R. VAN ZWET, The likelihood ratio test for the multinomial distribution. W. E. STRAWDERMAN, On the existence of proper Bayes minimax estimators of the mean of a multivariate normal distribution.

Sequential Analysis

P. J. BICKEL and J. YAHAV, On the Wiener process approximation to Bayesian sequential testing problems. YU. V. LINNIK and I. V. ROMANOVSKY, Some new results in sequential estimation theory. R. MILLER, Sequential rank tests—one sample case. R. A. WIJSMAN, Examples of exponentially bounded stopping time of invariant sequential probability ratio tests when the model may be false.

Asymptotic Theory

R. R. BAHADUR and M. RAGHAVACHARI, Some asymptotic properties of likelihood ratios on general sample spaces. D. M. CHIBISOV, On the normal approximation for a certain class of statistics. J. HÁJEK, Local asymptotic minimax and admissibility in estimation. R. A. JOHNSON and G. G. ROUSSAS, Applications of contiguity to multiparameter hypotheses testing. J. KIEFER, Iterated logarithm analogues for sample quantiles when $p_n \downarrow 0$. L. LE CAM, Limits of experiments. M. D. PERLMAN, On the strong consistency of approximate maximum likelihood estimators. P. SWITZER, Efficiency robustness of estimators.

Nonparametric Procedures

R. E. BARLOW and K. A. DOKSUM, Isotonic tests for convex orderings. Z. W. BIRNBAUM, Asymptotically distribution free statistics similar to Student's t. K. A. DOKSUM, Decision theory for some nonparametric models. J. M. HAMMERSLEY, A few seedlings of research. A. W. MARSHALL and F. PROSCHAN, Classes of distributions applicable in replacement with renewal theory implications. R. PYKE, Spacings revisited. H. RUBIN, On large sample properties of certain nonparametric procedures. I. R. SAVAGE and J. SETHURAMAN, Asymptotic distribution of the log likelihood ratio based on ranks in the two sample problem. I. VINCZE, On some results and problems in connection with statistics of the Kolmogorov-Smirnov type.

Regression Analysis

T. W. ANDERSON, Efficient estimation of regression coefficients in time series. D. R. BRILLINGER, The spectral analysis of stationary interval functions. H. BÜHLMANN, Credibility procedures. W. G. COCHRAN, Some effects of errors of measurement on linear regression. L. J. GLESER and I. OLKIN, Estimation for a regression model with an unknown covariance matrix. J. M. HOEM, On the statistical theory of analytic graduation.

v

Multivariate Analysis

C. R. RAO and S. K. MITRA, Generalized inverse of a matrix and its applications. H. CHERNOFF, Metric considerations in cluster analysis. F. N. DAVID, Measurement of diversity. L. A. GOODMAN, Some multiplicative models for the analysis of cross classified data. T. ORCHARD and M. A. WOODBURY, A missing information principle: theory and applications. M. SOBEL and G. H. WEISS, Recent results on using the play the winner sampling rule with binomial selection problems. M. ZELEN, Exact significance tests for contingency tables imbedded in a 2^n classification.

Volume II—Probability Theory

Introduction

J. L. DOOB, William Feller 1906–1970. M. KAC, William Feller, *in memoriam*. L. K. SCHMETTERER, Alfréd Rényi, *in memoriam*.

Measure Theory

D. W. MÜLLER, Randomness and extrapolation. R. M. BLUMENTHAL and H. H. CORSON, On continuous collections of measures. G. DEBREU and D. SCHMEIDLER, The Radon-Nikodým derivative of a correspondence. R. DUDLEY, A counterexample on measurable processes. Z. FROLÍK, Projective limits of measure spaces. W. HILDENBRAND, Metric measure spaces of economic agents. C. IONESCU TULCEA, Liftings commuting with translations. J. H. B. KEMPERMAN, On a class of moment problems. D. MAHARAM, Consistent extensions of linear functionals and of probability measures. H. ROSENTHAL, On the span in L^p of sequences of independent random variables. L. K. SCHMETTERER, On Poisson laws and related questions. M. L. STRAF, Weak convergence of stochastic processes with several parameters.

Inequalities

D. L. BURKHOLDER, B. J. DAVIS, and R. F. GUNDY, Integral inequalities for convex functions of operators on martingales. S. DAS GUPTA, M. L. EATON, I. OLKIN, M. PERLMAN, L. J. SAVAGE, and M. SOBEL, Inequalities on the probability content of convex regions for elliptically contoured distributions.

Combinatorial Analysis

P. DOUBILET, G.-C. ROTA, and R. STANLEY, On the foundations of combinatorial theory, VI: the idea of generating function.

Ergodic Theory

S. KAKUTANI, Strictly ergodic symbolic dynamical systems. W. KRIEGER, On unique ergodicity. D. S. ORNSTEIN, On the root problem in ergodic theory.

Gaussian Processes

J. FELDMAN, Sets of boundedness and continuity for the canonical normal process. A. M. GARSIA, Continuity properties of Gaussian processes with multidimensional time parameter. G. KALLIANPUR and M. NADKARNI, Supports of Gaussian measures. R. Š. LIPTSER and A. M. SHIRYAYEV, Statistics of conditionally Gaussian random sequences. M. B. MARCUS and L. A. SHEPP, Sample behavior of Gaussian processes. S. OREY, Growth rate of certain Gaussian processes.

Central Limit Theorem

R. N. BHATTACHARYA, Recent results on refinements of the central limit theorem. R. F. COGBURN, The central limit theorem for Markov processes. A. DVORETZKY,

Asymptotic normality of sums of dependent random variables. B. V. GNEDENKO, Limit theorems for sums of a random number of positive independent random variables. M. ROSENBLATT, Central limit theorem for stationary processes. V. V. SAZONOV, On a bound for the rate of convergence in the multidimensional central limit theorem. C. STEIN, A bound for the error in the normal approximation to the distribution of a sum of dependent random variables.

Volume III—Probability Theory

Passage Problems

Yu. K. BELYAYEV, Point processes and first passage problems. A. A. BOROVKOV, Limit theorems for random walks with boundaries. N. C. JAIN and W. E. PRUITT, The range of random walk. H. ROBBINS and D. SIEGMUND, On the law of the iterated logarithm for maxima and minima. A. D. SOLOVIEV, Asymptotic distribution of the moment of first crossing of a high level by a birth and death process.

Markov Processes—Potential Theory

R. G. AZENCOTT and P. CARTIER, Martin boundaries of random walks on locally compact groups. J. L. DOOB, The structure of a Markov chain. S. PORT and C. STONE, Classical potential theory and Brownian motion. S. PORT and C. STONE, Logarithmic potentials and planar Brownian motion. K. SATO, Potential operators for Markov processes.

Markov Processes—Trajectories—Functionals

R. GETOOR, Approximations of continuous additive functionals. K. ITÔ, Poisson point processes attached to Markov processes. J. F. C. KINGMAN, Regenerative phenomena and the characterization of Markov transition probabilities. E. J. McSHANE, Stochastic differential equations and models of random processes. P. A. MEYER, R. SMYTHE, and J. WALSH, Birth and death of Markov processes. P. W. MILLAR, Stochastic integrals and processes with stationary independent increments. D. W. STROOCK and S. R. S. VARADHAN, On the support of diffusion processes with applications to the strong maximum principle. D. W. STROOCK and S. R. S. VARADHAN, Diffusion processes.

Point Processes, Branching Processes

R. V. AMBARTSUMIAN, On random fields of segments and random mosaic on a plane. H. SOLOMON and P. C. C. WANG, Nonhomogeneous Poisson fields of random lines with applications to traffic flow. D. R. COX and P. A. W. LEWIS, Multivariate point processes. M. R. LEADBETTER, On basic results of point process theory. W. J. BÜHLER, The distribution of generations and other aspects of the family structure of branching processes. P. S PURI, A method for studying the integral functionals of stochastic processes with applications: III. W. A. O'N. WAUGH, Uses of the sojourn time series for the Markovian birth process. J. GANI, First emptiness problems in queueing, storage, and traffic theory. H. E. DANIELS, Kuhn-Grün type approximations for polymer chain distributions. L. KATZ and M. SOBEL. Coverage of generalized chess boards by randomly placed rooks. R. HOLLEY, Pressure and Helmholtz free energy in a dynamic model of a lattice gas. D. MOLLISON, The rate of spatial propagation of simple epidemics. W. H. OLSON and V. R. R. UPPULURI, Asymptotic distribution of eigenvalues or random matrices.

Information and Control

R. S. BUCY, A priori bounds for the Riccati equation. T. FERGUSON, Lose a dollar or double your fortune. H. J. KUSHNER, Necessary conditions for discrete parameter stochastic optimization problems. P. VARAIYA, Differential games. E. C. POSNER and E. R. RODEMICH, Epsilon entropy of probability distributions.

Volume IV—Biology and Health

Clinical Trials and Sequential Procedures

B. W. BROWN, Statistical aspects of clinical trials. D. KODLIN and M. F. COLLEN, Automated diagnosis in multiphasic screening. W. F. TAYLOR and P. O'BRIEN, Some practical problems in clinical trials. D. DARLING, When is a fixed number of observations optimal? H. ROBBINS and D. SIEGMUND, On a class of stopping rules for testing parametric hypotheses. B. J. FLEHINGER and T. A. LOUIS, Sequential medical trials with data dependent treatment allocation. D. HOEL and M. SOBEL, Comparisons of sequential procedures for selecting the best binomial population.

Population Studies and Branching Processes

H. WEINER, Critical age dependent branching processes. S. KARLIN and J. McGREGOR, Equilibria for genetic systems with weak interaction. N. KEYFITZ, The mathematics of sex and marriage. F. N. DAVID, Measurement of diversity: multiple cell contents. W. A. O'N. WAUGH, Models and approximations for synchronous cellular growth. G. L. YANG and C. L. CHIANG, A time dependent simple stochastic epidemic. D. FEARN, Galton-Watson processes with generation dependence. J. KLOTZ, Markov chain clustering of births by sex.

Biostatistics

C. L. CHIANG, An equality in stochastic processes. M. TARTER and S. RAMAN, A systematic approach to graphical methods in biometry. F. N. DAVID, Applications of Neyman's $C(\alpha)$ techniques. P. S. PURI and S. SENTURIA, On a mathematical theory of quantal response assays. G. M. SOUTHWARD and J. R. VAN RYZIN, Estimating the mean of a random binomial parameter.

Cellular Phenomena and Carcinogenesis

P. CLIFFORD, Nonthreshold models of the survival of bacteria after irradiation. M. R. WHITE, Studies of the mechanism of induction of pulmonary adenomas in mice. C. GUILLIER, Evaluation of the internal exposure due to various administered dosages of urethane to mice.

Psychological Aspects of Observational Studies

I. R. SAVAGE and M. WEBSTER, Source of evaluations reformulated and analyzed. J. YERUSHALMY, Self-selection—a major problem in observational studies.

Volume V—Darwinian, Neo-Darwinian, and Non-Darwinian Evolution

Darwinian and Non-Darwinian Evolution Theory

J. F. CROW, Darwinian and non-Darwinian evolution. G. L. STEBBINS and R. C. LEWONTIN, Comparative evolution at the levels of molecules, organisms, and populations. M. KIMURA and T. OHTA, Population genetics, molecular biometry, and evolution. J. L. KING, The role of mutation in evolution.

DNA, RNA, Amino acid Sequences

T. H. JUKES, Comparison of polypeptide sequences. R. J. MacINTYRE, Studies of enzyme evolution by subunit hybridization. H. VOGEL and E. ZUCKERKANDL, The evolution of polarity relations in globins. H. VOGEL, Two dimensional analysis of polarity changes in globin and cytochrome c. D. KOHNE, J. CHISCON, and B. HOYER, Evolution of mammalian DNA.

Population Studies and Evolution

F. AYALA, Darwinian *versus* non-Darwinian evolution in natural populations of *Drosophila*. R. W. ALLARD and A. L. KAHLER, Patterns of molecular variation in plant populations. W. BODMER and L. CAVALLI-SFORZA, Variation in fitness and molecular evolution.

Role of Theory in Evolutionary Studies

L. L. GATLIN, Evolutionary indices. T. A. REICHERT, The amount of information stored in proteins and other short biological code sequences. R. BELLMAN, Hierarchies of control processes and the evolution of consciousness. R. HOLMQUIST, Theoretical foundations of paleogenetics. W. J. EWENS, Statistical aspects of the non-Darwinian theory.

Volume VI—Effects of Pollution on Health

Programs and Studies of Governmental Agencies

J. R. GOLDSMITH, Statistical problems and strategies in environmental epidemiology. J. V. BEHAR, Application of computer simulation techniques to problems in air pollution. J. R. TOTTER, Research programs of the Atomic Energy Commission's Division of Biology and Medicine relevant to problems of health and pollution. J. F. FINKLEA, M. F. CRANMER, D. I. HAMMER, L. J. McCABE, V. A. NEWILL, and C. M. SHY, Health intelligence for environmental protection: a demanding challenge. W. B. RIGGAN, D. I. HAMMER, J. F. FINKLEA, V. HASSELBLAD, C. R. SHARP, R. M. BURTON, and C. M. SHY, CHESS, a community health and environmental surveillance system. W. C. NELSON, V. HASSELBLAD, and G. R. LOWRIMORE, Statistical aspects of a community health and environmental surveillance system. M. G. SIRKEN, Survey strategies for estimating rare health attributes.

Radiation and Health Controversy

E. J. STERNGLASS, Environmental radiation and human health. M. H. DeGROOT, Statistical studies of the effect of low level radiation from nuclear reactors on human health. J. W. GOFMAN and A. R. TAMPLIN, Epidemiologic studies of carcinogenesis by ionizing radiation. E. A. TOMPKINS, P. M. HAMILTON, and D. A. HOFFMAN, Infant mortality around three nuclear power reactors. V. L. SAILOR, Population exposure to radiation: natural and man-made. H. W. PATTERSON and R. H. THOMAS, Radiation and risk—the source data. E. LANDAU, Radiation and infant mortality—some hazards of methodology.

Problems of Monitoring

E. B. HOOK, Monitoring human birth defects: methods and strategies. G. D. FRIEDMAN and M. F. COLLEN, A method for monitoring adverse drug reactions. A. D. KEITH, Chemical induction of mutagenesis and carcinogenesis. M. C. CLARK, D. GOODMAN, and A. C. WILSON, The biochemical approach to mutation monitoring in man. F. S. GOULDING, X-ray fluorescence—an improved analytical tool for trace element studies. R. E. BARLOW, Averaging time and maxima for air pollution concentrations.

Pollutants in Food Chains

R. W. RISEBROUGH, Effects of environmental pollutants upon animals other than man. H. L. ROSENTHAL, Implications of environmental strontium 90 accumulation in teeth and bone of children. T. D. STERLING, Problems in determining if a commonly used herbicide (2,4,5-T) has an effect on human health. B. E. VAUGHAN, Ecological and environmental problems in the application of biomathematics.

Ecological Studies

W. R. GAFFEY, Possible manifestations of worsening environmental pollution. R. W. GILL, Effects of toxicity on ecosystems. H. B. MESSINGER, Demographic data for local areas. W. WINKELSTEIN, Utility or futility of ordinary mortality statistics in the study of air pollution effects.

Skeletal Plans for a Comprehensive Health-Pollution Study, Discussion and Epilogue

J. R. GOLDSMITH, Skeletal plan for a comprehensive epidemiologic study of pollution: effects of exposure on growth and development of children. A. C. HEXTER, Skeletal plan for a study of daily mortality. J. NEYMAN, Skeletal plan for a comprehensive statistical health-pollution study. H. K. URY, Some skeletal plans for studying health effects of air pollution. E. L. SCOTT, Summary of Panel Discussion. J. NEYMAN, Epilogue of the health-pollution conference.

PREFACE

Berkeley Symposia on Mathematical Statistics and Probability have been held at five year intervals since 1945, with the Sixth Symposium marking a quarter of a century of this activity. The purpose of the Symposia is to promote research and to record in the *Proceedings* the contemporary trends in thought and effort. The subjects covered in the Berkeley statistical Symposia range from pure theory of probability through theory of statistics to a variety of fields of applications of these two mathematical disciplines. The fields selected are those that appear especially important either as a source of novel statistical and probabilistic problems or because of their broad interdisciplinary character combined with particular significance to the society at large. A wide field of application traditionally represented at the Berkeley Symposia is the field of biology and health problems. Physical sciences, including astronomy, physics, and meteorology are also frequently represented. Volume 5 of the *Proceedings* of the Fifth Symposium was entirely given to weather modification.

With the help of advisory committees and of particular scholars, the participants of the Berkeley Symposia are recruited from all countries of the world, hopefully to include representatives of all significant schools of thought. In order to stimulate fruitful crossfertilization of ideas, efforts are made for the symposia to last somewhat longer than ordinary scholarly meetings, up to six weeks during which days with scholarly sessions are combined with excursions to the mountains and other social events. The record shows that, not infrequently, novel ideas are born at just such occasions.

According to the original plans, the entire Sixth Berkeley Symposium was to be held during the summer of 1970, with the generous support of the University of California, through an allocation from the Russell S. Springer Memorial Foundation, of the National Science Foundation, of the National Institutes of Health, of the Office of Naval Research, of the Army Research Office, and of the Air Force Office of Scientific Research. This help is most gratefully acknowledged. Certain circumstances prevented the Biology-Health Section from being held in 1970 and the meeting held in that year, from June 21 to July 18, was concerned with mathematical domains of probability and statistics. The papers presented at that time, and also some that were sent in by the individuals who were not able to attend personally, fill the first three volumes of these *Proceedings.* Volume 1 is given to theory of statistics and Volumes 2 and 3 to the rapidly developing theory of probability.

The Biology-Health Section of the Sixth Symposium had to be postponed to 1971. Every postponement of a scholarly meeting involves a disruption of the plans and all kinds of difficulties. Such disruption and difficulties certainly occurred in the present case. As originally planned, the Biology-Health Section of the Sixth Symposium was to be comparable to that of the Fifth, the *Proceedings* of which extended close to 1,000 pages in print. This is much larger than

Volume 4 of the present *Proceedings* that summarizes the Biology-Health Section held from June 16 to 21, 1971. However, the losses suffered in some respects have been compensated by gains in others. Those gains are reflected in Volumes 5 and 6 of these *Proceedings*.

During the fall of 1970 we became much impressed by the development and rapid growth of a new field of biological studies which includes the areas known as "non-Darwinian" and "neo-Darwinian" studies of evolution. These are studies based on the structure of macromolecules present in many now living species and performing in them similar functions. One example is the hemoglobin molecule, carried by all mammals as well as by fish. The differences among the homologous macromolecules in different species are usually ascribed to mutations that are in some sense inconsequential, and are supposed to occur more or less at a uniform rate. The number of differences between any two species is indicative of the time that elapsed from the moment of separation from the presumed common ancestor. The probabilistic-statistical problems involved in such studies include the estimation of philogenetic trees of several species and, in particular, the estimation of the time since two species separated from their ancestor.

It was found that, with only a few exceptions, mathematical statisticians are not familiar with the new domain and that, at the same time, a great many biologists make strong efforts to treat the statistical problems themselves. A joint meeting of biologists and statisticians was clearly indicated and a separate conference, especially given to novel studies of evolution, was held from April 9 to 12, as part of the Biology-Health Section of the Sixth Berkeley Symposium. It is summarized in Volume 5 of these *Proceedings*. Somewhat unexpectedly, it appeared that the new field of studies of evolution involves controversies that are just as sharp as those that occasionally enliven the meetings of mathematical statisticians . . .

We were introduced to problems of evolution treated on the level of macromolecules by Professor T. H. Jukes, V. N. Sarich, and A. C. Wilson. Their very interesting seminar talks and later their advice on the organization of the conference on evolution are highly appreciated.

While studies of evolution involve observational research, particularly that concerned with the relation between classical population genetics and novel findings on the level of molecular biology, the whole domain is clearly conceptual. Contrary to this, the third part of the Biology-Health Section of the Sixth Symposium was totally given to observational studies in a domain of great importance to society at large and of great public interest.

The domain in question, a highly controversial domain, is that of the relation between environmental pollution and human health. The growing population in the United States and in other countries needs more electric power, more automobiles, and other products. The relevant industries are eager to satisfy these needs. However, the expanded industrial activity, unavoidably conducted with an eye on costs, leads to pollution of the environment. The controversies at public hearings, in the daily press, and in scholarly publications center around the question whether the currently adopted standards of safety are sufficient or not. The volume of research, largely statistical, surrounding this question is immense. The intention that the *Proceedings* provide a cross section of contemporary statistical work dictated the organization of a special conference entirely given to the problem of health and pollution. This conference, held from July 19 to 22, is summarized in Volume 6 of these *Proceedings*. In organizing the conference we benefitted greatly from the advice of Dr. S. W. Greenhouse of the National Institutes of Health, of Professor B. Greenberg of Chapel Hill, North Carolina, and of Drs. J. M. Hollander and H. W. Patterson of the Berkeley Lawrence Laboratory.

The first purpose of the Health-Pollution Conference was to take stock of the studies already performed. The second and the ultimate purpose was to see whether a novel statistical study is called for, hopefully more comprehensive and more reliable than those already completed. With this in mind, invitations to the conference were issued to Federal and State governmental agencies concerned with health and pollution, to authoritative scholarly institutions, and to a number of particular individual scholars known to have worked on one or another aspect of this problem.

As a special stimulus for thought on the entire problem of pollution and health, its present state and the future, the invitations to the conference were formulated to include a call for submission of skeletal plans for a fresh comprehensive statistical study, capable of separating the effects of particular pollutants. Four such plans were submitted and they are published in Volume 6.

All the participants had complete freedom of expression, both in their prepared papers and in their contributions to the discussion. Thus it is likely that the goal of providing a realistic cross section of contemporary statistical research on the problem is reasonably approached. Also it is not unlikely that the present state of knowledge on human health and pollution, and the scholarly level of the substantive studies prepared are fairly reflected in these *Proceedings*.

In addition to funds provided by the University of California and the National Institutes of Health, the Health-Pollution Conference was organized using a grant from the Atomic Energy Commission, Division of Biology and Medicine. This help is gratefully acknowledged.

The organization and the running of three distinct scholarly meetings, one in April, another in June, and the third in July 1971, each attended by some 100 to more than 300 participants, would not have been possible without the willing, efficient, and cheerful help and cooperation of the staff of the Department of Statistics and the Statistical Laboratory. Our most hearty thanks go to our successive "ministers of finance," Mrs. Barbara Gaugl and Mrs. Freddie Ruhl. who watched the sinking balances and surveyed the legality of proposed expenditures, some appropriate under one grant and not under another, etc. In addition to financial matters, Mrs. Gaugl supervised the local arrangements for scholarly sessions, for several social events and for servicing the participants. In this she was efficiently helped by Mrs. Dominique Cooke, by Miss Judy Whipple and by a number of volunteers from among the graduate students in the Department. Mrs. Cooke and Miss Whipple had their own very important domain of activities: to keep straight the correspondence and the files. Coming in addition to the ordinary university business, this was no mean job and the performance of the two ladies is highly appreciated.

All the above refers to the early part of the year 1971 and up to the end of the conferences. Then the manuscripts of the papers to be published in the *Proceedings* started to arrive, totalling 1849 typewritten pages, not counting figures and numerical tables. This marked a new phase of the job in which we enjoyed the cooperation of another group of persons, who prepared the material for the printers. At the time, the team of editors, Miss Carol Conti, Mrs. Margaret Darland, and Miss Jean Kettler, under the able guidance of Mrs. Virginia Thompson and supervised by Professor LeCam, Chairman of the Organizing Committee, worked assiduously on proofs of papers in Volumes 1, 2 and 3. The arrival of the material for Volumes 4, 5, and 6, unavoidably involving some correspondence with the authors and conferences at the University Press, created heavy burden. We are very grateful to the four ladies whose cooperation has been inspiring to us.

Last but not least, our hearty thanks to the University of California Press, Mr. August Frugé and his colleagues for their help, cooperation and also their patience when confronted with piles of manuscripts which we hoped to see published both excellently as in the past quarter of a century and "right away, yesterday!"

J. Neyman   E. L. Scott   L. Le Cam (Chm.)

CONTENTS

Clinical Trials and Sequential Procedures

B. W. BROWN—Statistical Aspects of Clinical Trials . . .   1

D. KODLIN and M. F. COLLEN—Automated Diagnosis in Multiphasic Screening   15

W. F. TAYLOR and P. O'BRIEN—Some Practical Problems in Clinical Trials   25

D. DARLING—When Is a Fixed Number of Observations Optimal?   33

H. ROBBINS and D. SIEGMUND—On a Class of Stopping Rules for Testing Parametric Hypotheses   37

B. J. FLEHINGER and T. A. LOUIS—Sequential Medical Trials with Data Dependent Treatment Allocation   43

D. HOEL and M. SOBEL—Comparisons of Sequential Procedures for Selecting the Best Binomial Population   53

Population Studies and Branching Processes

H. WEINER—Critical Age Dependent Branching Processes . .   71

S. KARLIN and J. McGREGOR—Equilibria for Genetic Systems with Weak Interaction   79

N. KEYFITZ—The Mathematics of Sex and Marriage . . .   89

F. N. DAVID—Measurement of Diversity: Multiple Cell Contents   109

W. A. O'N. WAUGH—Models and Approximations for Synchronous Cellular Growth   137

G. L. YANG and C. L. CHIANG—A Time Dependent Simple Stochastic Epidemic   147

D. FEARN—Galton-Watson Processes with Generation Dependence   159

J. KLOTZ—Markov Chain Clustering of Births by Sex . . .   173

Biostatistics

C. L. CHIANG—An Equality in Stochastic Processes 187

M. TARTER and S. RAMAN—A Systematic Approach to Graphical Methods in Biometry 199

F. N. DAVID—Applications of Neyman's $C(\alpha)$ Technique . . 223

P. S. PURI and S. SENTURIA—On a Mathematical Theory of Quantal Response Assays 231

G. M. SOUTHWARD and J. R. VAN RYZIN—Estimating the Mean of a Random Binomial Parameter 249

Cellular Phenomena and Carcinogenesis

P. CLIFFORD—Nonthreshold Models of the Survival of Bacteria after Irradiation 265

M. R. WHITE—Studies of the Mechanism of Induction of Pulmonary Adenomas in Mice 287

C. GUILLIER—Evaluation of the Internal Exposure Due to Various Administered Dosages of Urethane to Mice . . . 309

Psychological Aspects of Observational Studies

I. R. SAVAGE and M. WEBSTER—Source of Evaluations Reformulated and Analyzed 317

J. YERUSHALMY—Self-selection—a Major Problem in Observational Studies 329

STATISTICAL ASPECTS
OF CLINICAL TRIALS

BYRON WM. BROWN, JR.
STANFORD UNIVERSITY

1. Introduction

My object in this lecture will be to give an overview of the statistical aspects of current clinical trial methodology, including a very brief history, my view of current practice, recent relevant statistical developments, and areas that need further statistical research.

My primary concern will be clinical experiments, though I will have some comments on other types of study of clinical data also.

Of course, the idea of trying out a new treatment and then comparing the results with past experience with other remedies is natural. Insistence on some systematic attempt to assure a *controlled* comparison of treatment effects is a recent development. Scattered reports of controlled studies have appeared in the literature only within the last few hundred years. The idea of *random* allocation of treatments to experimental units, in agricultural science, originated with Fisher [30] and gained acceptance in agriculture through the work of such men as Yates and Snedecor [51]. My impression is that agricultural scientists now accept the ideas of randomization, experimental design, and statistical evaluation as essential to sure and orderly scientific progress.

These experimental principles were introduced into clinical medicine in the post World War II period by Hill [36], [37] and taken up by Mainland [43], Lasagna [41], and others. In recent years Cornfield [18] and Armitage [4] have played important roles in encouraging further development of the methodology for planning and evaluating clinical experiments.

2. Present practice

Clinical trial methodology, employing concurrent controls, randomization, and the blindfold technique, has had a great impact on medical scientists. Hundreds of valid medical experiments have been completed and currently it can safely be said that the method is accepted and in use by at least some investigators in every medical specialty. However, it must be quickly added that in many fields, such as surgery, randomized clinical trials are still rare. In fact, there are influential and fluent clinical scientists who enthusiastically point out the difficulties and publicly ponder the usefulness of the experimental approach in clinical

1

medicine. Some, indeed, are opposed to the whole idea of using the patient as an experimental subject.

Although randomized, even blindfold, trials have been used in many types of clinical investigation, the methodology has taken hold and been accepted as standard experimental technique only in the evaluation of drugs and immunizing agents. This is due in large part to the greater ease of application of the techniques in this field as contrasted with applications in surgery or radiation therapy, for example. In the United States, pressures from the Federal granting agencies, particularly the National Heart and Lung Institute, and from the Food and Drug Administration [2], as the regulatory body for approval of drugs for marketing, have hastened the use, if not the acceptance, of clinical trial methodology for the evaluation of drugs.

Even in clinical investigations of the efficacy of drugs the methodology is far from uniformly well accepted and practiced. The National Cancer Institute strongly encourages the use of randomized clinical trials in the evaluation of cancer treatments, yet in a recent meeting on the design of clinical studies in cancer, well known scientists raised their voices on each side of the issue. Chalmers [15] has recently reviewed the clinical cancer research literature and he states that only about 20 per cent of the clinical studies, reported in abstracts submitted in 1965–1970 to the American Association for Cancer Research, could be considered controlled experiments. Among this 20 per cent, only a portion would be randomized or double blind. Chalmers [14] has reported also that a recent survey of clinical trial abstracts submitted to an annual meeting of the American Gastroenterological Association revealed only 4.5 per cent contained evidence of adequate techniques to minimize investigator bias.

At the present time there are important clinical trials under way in areas of critical importance to the public health. A diet-heart study in Minnesota has most of the patients in the state mental institutions on double blind, randomly assigned normal or low fat diets; the purpose is to determine long term effects of low fat diet in preventing heart disease. The Coronary Drug Project [21] has thousands of men on randomly assigned drugs, including placebo, in order to discover which of the drugs are effective in preventing coronary heart disease. The UGDP (University Group Diabetes Program [40]), a study now in its 11th year of followup, has been a landmark in clinical research in diabetes. This study has shed new light on the use of insulin in diabetes therapy and has raised disturbing questions about the efficacy, and even the safety, of oral hypoglycemic substitutes for insulin in mild forms of diabetes.

Today analgesic agents and other psychoactive drugs used by the anesthetist and the psychiatrist are routinely evaluated in double blind, randomized experiments. The same is true of the study of antibiotics, and research in these fields is marked by sure and steady progress.

A new aspect of modern clinical research is the cooperative study, a study in which investigators from several hospitals or clinics follow the same study protocol and pool their results to obtain a definitive answer more quickly than any one investigator could obtain alone with his limited supply of appropriate patients. These cooperative studies have become more and more common as medical investigators have begun to ask more subtle questions requiring larger sample sizes. The Coronary Drug Project [21], the Veterans Administration study of prostate cancer [55], and the University Group Diabetes Project [40] are good examples of current cooperative studies.

In any review of current clinical study methodology, it is important to mention the growing concern for information on the risk of side effects, especially those of relatively low incidence, associated with medical treatments. Sometimes these risks are uncovered in randomized trials carried out to evaluate efficacy, as in the VA and CDP trials (mentioned above) which disclosed that estrogen causes heart attacks. Most investigators feel that a randomized clinical trial, purposely designed to study an imputed side effect, would be unethical. This is one reason for the lack of experimental data on the carcinogenic effects of birth control pills, the risk of liver damage caused by the anesthetic agent, Halothane, and the various lethal effects attributed to smoking. Of course, a second very good reason for not studying low incidence side effects experimentally is the tremendous cost and effort involved in detecting the very small differences in rates involved.

3. Current statistical problems and recent work in the design of clinical trials

The objection most often raised to the randomized clinical trial is the ethical question of withholding from a patient by random choice what appears to be a new and better treatment, or, conversely, randomly assigning him to a new treatment, carrying unknown hazards, when he could be given the more familiar and reliable standard treatment. The most common rejoinder by clinicians and statisticians alike is that they would not randomize unless the competing treatments were preferred equally. To me, this has always seemed to be an evasion of a real issue. Taking all current information on the treatments into account, and taking into account specific information on the given patient, cases of absolutely equal preference for competing treatments would be rare. Indeed, this is why so many clinical scientists object so strenuously to the randomized trial. The issue must be met squarely in terms of prior probabilities, risks to the patient, counterbalancing benefits the patient derives from being in a carefully executed and generously staffed clinical experiment, and possibly the moral obligation of the patient to add a little information for the benefit of his fellow man when the added risk he might incur is small. Only when statisticians help to formalize this ethical dilemma in a simple and convincing way, for some real situations, only then, will we have helped the clinician and consulting statistician out of their dilemma, so that they can deal honestly with themselves, if not with the patients.

The organization and management of a clinical trial, especially a cooperative trial, are very important and there are some good guides on the design of a clinical trial. The writings of Hill [37], Mainland [43], and Feinstein [27], and the books edited by Witts [56], and by Hill [35], would be extremely helpful to anyone who is designing a clinical study; the UGDP [40] and CDP [21] trials are models of organization and management for a cooperative trial.

It is always tempting to "use the patient as his own control," as the clinical scientist puts it. Oftentimes the patient can be given one treatment, later "crossed over" to the other treatment, and his response to therapy can be measured in each time period. This kind of design is used in allergy experiments, for example, and in other chronic diseases such as arthritis. Cochran and Cox [16], and D. R. Cox [22] discuss these designs. Most discussions assume the first treatment has no residual effects in the second period, but Grizzle [32] and others have discussed the difficulties of handling residual treatment effects. The design and analysis become complicated, however, and they often depend on the assumption of additive residual effects. The current tendency in practice seems to be to avoid the crossover where possible, even at the expense of necessarily larger sample size, because of the difficulties in interpreting crossover results.

In the case of completely randomized experiments, where the patients come to the physician and are admitted to the study one at a time, there is always a worry about lack of balance in numbers of patients assigned to the several treatments, as the trial subjects accumulate. This is even more important when the patients are blocked by type, and balance within each block is important. The method of pseudorandomization by alternating patients or admitting patients to one treatment or another on alternate days has long been discredited, after some unfortunate experiences. The usual method of assuring balance today is to randomize within groups of six or eight or ten patients arriving one after the other at the clinic, without disclosing the group size to the investigators who admit the patients to the study. Efron [26] has investigated this strategy and compared it to the completely randomized design and to what he calls the biased coin design. The latter design assigns the next treatment with an assignment probability that varies so as to tend to even the cases assigned to the several treatments at each step. Efron compares the designs with regard to susceptibility to several sources of bias, but he comes to no conclusions concerning the design of choice. Stigler [54] has also considered methods of eliminating or minimizing bias in randomized experiments.

Selection of patients is a question in any clinical trial. It is obvious that there is a distinct advantage in selecting patients who are moderately ill where this is possible, because severely ill patients won't respond to either treatment, and mildly ill patients will respond to any treatment. However, the clinical scientist, and especially the practicing physician, are leery of any selection of patients. Results are most credible to them when the experimental patients resemble their own patient population. This is partly due to an attitude developed in evaluating uncontrolled studies, where comparability with other sets of data was essential, and partly due to a valid concern for the degree to which the results of a randomized experiment can be generalized to other experimental units.

The specification of sample size for planning purposes, before a trial is started, is a common problem to the biostatistician. Often he can use tables for the power of the two sample binomial test or two sample t test, as found in Owen [48], Schneiderman [50], Dixon and Massey [23], Snedecor and Cochran [52], or Mainland [43]. However, special problems arise in the planning of clinical trials. In particular, the endpoint or measurement made in the clinical trial is often a matter of *when* an event occurs (that is, a waiting time, perhaps to death) rather than *if* the event occurs. Since the patients are admitted to the study at varying times and the observations are terminated at a common time, namely, at the calendar time cutoff date for the study, the data present a problem in waiting time distributions, with censoring at a different time for each patient. Ederer [24] has presented a table that allows a computation of required number of patients, assuming an exponential waiting time distribution, a given patient admission rate, an estimate of the survival rate, and a specification of the desired standard error for the estimate of survival rate at a given time. Pasternack and Gilbert [49] have carried this work further and present some tables that are useful in planning.

A committee of the National Heart and Lung Institute [1] has presented tables of required sample size for the special clinical trials (for example, diet-heart trials) in which the treatment is not expected to take effect for some time after the commencement of therapy and there is a certain attrition on drop-out rate for patients during followup. Halperin, Rogot, Gurian, and Ederer [33] present the details of this work. A committee of the American Heart Association [11] has presented sample sizes for the same sort of clinical trial, ignoring the factors of delay time and dropout rate, and concentrating on the problem of the effect on required sample size of unreliability in the judgment of cause of death. Both of these papers are rather specific to the diet-heart question, though the results are of some general use.

Of course, the fact that patients are usually admitted to a clinical trial sequentially, and slowly enough to permit rather frequent, if not continuous, analysis of the data, suggests that sequential stopping rules for clinical trials would be most appropriate. The first to point this out seems to have been Bross [8], who published some truncated sequential plans for the one sample binomial case. He proposed that the patients be paired as they were admitted to the study, each pair being declared a win or loss for a given treatment, this Bernoulli variable furnishing the sequential data for the test. Armitage's book [4], contains a rather complete exposition of sequential analysis applied to clinical trials, and he presents plans for the case of a single Bernoulli variable, and also a normally distributed variable. Armitage also suggested a way of handling the analysis of exponential variables observed in survival time studies.

Miller [45] has recently published sequential plans for nonparametric sequential analysis, especially well suited to clinical trial application. The Miller plans are based on Monte Carlo sampling results and his work is concerned with the one sample case, so that pairing of patients is required. The procedure is based on the one sample signed rank statistic and the limits are set at a fixed multiple of the conditional standard deviation of the statistic, so as to control the probability of going out of limits at any point from sample size one to a preassigned truncation point. Gehan [63] has developed a two sample procedure for variable censoring times, typical of clinical trial time data, based on a generalization of the Wilcoxon statistic. Efron [25] proposed modifications of the procedure that increase its power for certain alternatives. Breslow [7] has generalized the Gehan procedure to the case of more than two treatments under trial.

The statisticians for the UGDP (Meinert, Knatterud, and Canner) also used Monte Carlo sampling to develop a sequential plan for monitoring the diabetics in that clinical trial. However, they used as their waiting time distribution function the survival function defined by *U.S. Life Tables*. They assigned each patient in the trial the expected survival function appropriate for his age and sex at entry into the trial.

Anscombe [3], in his review of Armitage's book, was quite critical of the whole idea of looking on the clinical trial as a hypothesis testing situation. Anscombe's arguments are quite Bayesian in flavor and reminiscent of Fisher's criticism [29] of the Neyman-Pearson view of inference. Most statisticians today who are involved in the planning and evaluation of clinical trials would sympathize with Anscombe's views. Though they may use Neyman-Pearson theory to calculate a required trial size or to set up sequential limits for the trial, acceptance-rejection rules are not taken to be hard and fast. The data are continually scrutinized, analyzed in ways unanticipated at the start of the trial, and analyzed in the light of new information on additional ancillary variables, as the number of patients increases and makes such analyses possible.

Armitage himself was the first to suggest the adaptation of some work by Maurice [44] as a new and more practical way of calculating the required size of a clinical trial. The idea was to estimate the total number N of patients to be treated by one of two treatments, it being unknown which of the two treatments was better. A clinical trial with n patients per treatment was to be carried out, in order to decide on the better treatment, and the remaining $N - 2n$ patients would be treated with the chosen treatment. How large should the trial be, that is, what is the optimal choice of n? Colton [17] pursued the problem at the suggestion of Armitage, for the normal case, sigma known, with loss function equal to the difference in means for each use of the inferior treatment. He looked at the unknown difference between treatments from both a minimax and a Bayesian point of view. Colton obtained some interesting results, the most surprising of which was that the optimum clinical trial size in certain circumstances might be as much as ⅓ of all patients to be treated, even when the total number of patients to be treated N was very large. Canner [13] pursued these ideas for the Bernoulli case, obtaining results similar to Colton's, and with additional results that demonstrated that the optimal sample size n did not depend very strongly on the total population size N. For example, in the case of uniform prior distributions Canner showed that the estimate of N could be off by a factor of two without serious increase in the loss function. Canner also investigated the required trial size when the cost of clinical trial observations was added to the cost of treatment failures.

The results of Colton and Canner are really single stage solutions to the two arm bandit problem. Colton has published two stage results also. The underlying dilemma here is that of allowing a clinical trial to go on when the evidence is mounting in favor of one of the treatments. Cornfield, Halperin, and Greenhouse [20], Zelen [60], and Sobel and Weiss [53], have explored variations of a more radical solution, the play the winner strategy, where the next patient is assigned the treatment given the last patient if the last treatment was a "success"; otherwise, the alternate treatment is given. The play the winner strategy has the obvious advantage of tending to assign the better treatment to more of the patients and it does this more successfully than its competitors in a variety of circumstances. However, the strategy has practical difficulties for the clinical trial situation in that the outcome for the last patient is not often known at the time the next patient comes in; and more serious, the method of assignment, even if done on a random basis with varying probabilities causes difficulties in assuring the unbiasedness or blindfold aspect of the trial. A further difficulty that I have experienced is that the clinical scientist who can convince himself that random allocation with equal probabilities for the several treatments is ethical, cannot bring himself to allocate with unequal probabilities or to play the winner. In fact, when I suggested the strategy to some eminent clinical colleagues, they regarded it as a quite incredible proposal.

With regard to planning clinical trials, it should be mentioned that there are efforts among clinicians to work out the rationale for a trial design in terms of underlying mechanisms for the specific disease of interest. In leukemia, there are efforts to understand how the disease develops and how it reacts to chemotherapy and radiotherapy, and to choose therapy strategies accordingly. The clinical pharmacologist in general is concerned with the appropriate dose levels, times of administration and route of administration, with regard to the bio-availability of the drug with various strategies. The statisticians must also concern themselves with these facets of design; and, as this type of approach becomes more formal, statisticians find themselves acting as mathematical biologists, mapping out plans, even simulating the clinical trial itself. An example is Bross's mathematical modeling work [9] purporting to show that a proposed clinical trial in breast cancer would be futile.

4. Analysis of clinical trial data

Biostatisticians are familiar with the computer and usually have programming and computing resources available to them. The computer has produced an extraordinary revolution in the routine analyses that are done on data from clinical trials. I have already mentioned sequential analysis since it is so closely tied to planning as well as analysis; most of the work of Armitage, Miller, Meinert, Knatterud, Canner, Zelen, and Sobel in deriving and evaluating sequential strategies depended to some extent on the use of computers.

Computers have made possible complex analyses of the typical waiting time data with varying censoring points so familiar in clinical trials. The actuarial methods like that of Berkson and Gage [5] using grouped data, can now be carried out easily without grouping, as suggested by Kaplan and Meier [38]. Furthermore, the analysis can be carried out each time a patient is seen again or a new death or other event is reported, by adding the new observation to the computer file, updating the file, and printing out the new survival curve, with confidence band. Gehan [31] has proposed methods for obtaining estimates of the hazard function or the force of mortality function and the density function, as well as the survival function, using actuarial methods, though these are not popular yet.

In the early fifties, Littell [42] proposed a maximum likelihood method for estimating an exponential survival function using typically censored clinical trial data. Now, with the aid of the computer, much more general parametric models are used and the estimates and standard errors are easily obtained. The generalizations go in several directions—the hazard function may be taken to be an appropriate function of time, linear or exponential, for example. Competing risk models may be used, with each risk a function of time. In particular, competing risks that are linear functions of time yield a convenient and useful model because the sum of the risks will also be linear in time.

Zelen and Feigl [61] and Zippin and Armitage [62] have furnished good examples of efforts to allow the hazard function to be dependent on ancillary variables, yet another avenue for the use of the computer that allows fuller exploration of the data. The work of Boag [6] and Berkson and Gage [64] and, more recently, the work of Haybittle [34] illustrate another approach to the formulation of parametric models for survivorship that are tailor made for specific diseases and treatment comparisons. The Berkson and Gage model, for example, allowed a cure rate following surgery, with the cured and noncured patients following different survival functions following surgery.

These efforts to extend classical significance testing and estimation to more satisfying models that allow for more realistic changes in the force of mortality, and the use of ancillary information, have been extremely important. However, more fundamental changes in methods of analysis have come about through the use of the computer in the evaluation of clinical trial data. First, along with the use of more complex models has come a heavier use of the likelihood function or likelihood contours, though such analyses are still not common in clinical journals. Second, permutation tests are coming into use. Third, Bayesian and semi-Bayesian procedures are coming into play, with Cornfield as a principal exponent [18], [19]. An example is the Cornfield approach [40] used in the UGDP report on the effects of Tolbutamide. Cornfield computes the ratio of the likelihood for the null hypothesis to the average likelihood over a set of alternatives, where the averaging function is specified beforehand or else determined from the data by minimization. He calls these ratios relative betting odds (RBO's). Another example of Bayesian techniques applied to a set of clinical trial data can be found in a paper by Novick and Grizzle [47].

A fourth development or set of developments is typified by the reports on the Halothane Study [12]. This study was not a randomized clinical trial, but a comparison of the mortality results for persons getting Halothane as a general anesthetic at surgery *versus* those getting other agents. A number of statistical procedures were developed for adjusting for many ancillary variables as covariates, in comparing death rates. The procedures developed in the Halothane Study for handling large numbers of covariates in samples of modest size, are being applied to current randomized clinical trials.

5. Future statistical research and development

There are many areas in the statistical methodology for clinical trials that need the attention of the statistician.

5.1. Some specific examples of dilemmas in choice of scientific strategy should be studied formally, with the object of shedding some light on the question of when a randomized clinical *experiment* is indicated, as opposed to a retrospective or prospective study. The factors of cost, the possibilities of bias, the ethics and the question of scientific credibility should all be considered in a mathematical formulation of the problem.

5.2. Tables of sample size requirements should be generated that apply to the types of situation encountered in clinical trials, including varying forms of hazard function, patient accrual rates, and dropout rates.

5.3. The whole question of stopping rules should be considered with regard to the credibility of the final report. What does influence the scientific audience with regard to the way in which the decision to stop is made? What should influence them? How should the decision rule be reported?

5.4. The adjustment of results for a multitude of baseline variables, or covariates, must be considered. We need more methodological development and a closer look at the methods already developed such as those reported in the Halothane Study, but consideration of the interpretation of results is even more important. Can one test the validity of the randomization itself by checking the multitude of baseline variables? How should one adjust for carrying out a multitude of *a priori* and *a posteriori* inferences on the same set of data, and how should one report the results?

5.5. Methodology should be laid down for looking at the likelihood function for many parameters, and both statisticians and medical scientists must become practiced in looking at such presentations and interpreting them.

5.6. The clinical trial must not be regarded only as a tool for isolated experiments. It must be adapted to routine operations of the clinic or hospital, as an accepted part of normal practice. Kiresuk, Salasin and Sherman have reported

[39] that at the Hennepin County Mental Health Center in Minneapolis, every patient coming to the Center is given a standard workup. Objectives of therapy are set, followup plans are laid, and possible forms of treatment are listed (day clinic, group therapy, drugs, and so forth) by an Intake Committee. If several methods of treatment are thought to be feasible, the patient is randomly allocated to one of the competing treatments. Thus, clinical experimentation with systematic followup becomes a part of routine medical practice. Statisticians must work with the clinician to see that this kind of automatically evolving and improving system becomes the rule. Such a system will involve new concepts in clinical trial management, in statistical analysis, monitoring and decision making.

5.7.   These days we are concerned with health care systems and the quality of medical care. Again the statistician must consider adaptation of the clinical trial methodology to this area. If it is unethical to choose a treatment for one patient on the basis of unscientifically collected data, then it must be all the more unethical to change a whole health care system on the basis of intuition and opinion. Shouldn't we argue for clinical experiments, using hospitals, clinics, communities, and physicians, as the experimental units? The methodology needs development but the need is clear. Moses and Mosteller [46], for example, several years ago called for a study of the reason for the large variations in death rate, from hospital to hospital, found in the Halothane Study. Investigation of this question is under way, under the sponsorship of the National Academy of Science, and financed in part by the NIH. Certainly any proposals for change in hospitals that come out of this study must be checked experimentally in a randomized "clinical trial" of hospitals before they are implemented on the thousands of hospitals in this country.

6. Summary

In summary, I would call for joint efforts of all interested statisticians to do what they can to find out what the specific methodological problems are in clinical medicine and health care systems, to encourage strongly and enthusiastically the wise use of well tested statistical procedures on these questions, and to develop and demonstrate the use of new procedures where these are needed to communicate results and measure the credibility of scientific conclusions.

REFERENCES

[1] E. H. AHRENS, JR., "Mass field trials of the diet-heart question (their significance, timeliness, feasibility and applicability)," *American Heart Association Monograph Number 28*, 1969.

[2] C. ANELLO, "FDA principles on clinical investigations," *FDA Papers*, Vol. 4, No. 5 (1970), pp. 14–15.

[3] F. J. ANSCOMBE, "Sequential medical trials," *J. Amer. Statist. Assoc.*, Vol. 58 (1963), pp. 365–383.

[4] P. ARMITAGE, *Sequential Medical Trials*, Oxford, Blackwell Scientific Publications, 1960.

[5] J. BERKSON and R. P. GAGE, "Calculation of survival rates for cancer," *Proceedings of the Staff Meetings of the Mayo Clinic*, Vol. 25 (1950), pp. 270–286.

[6] J. W. BOAG, "Maximum likelihood estimates of the proportion of patients cured by cancer therapy," *J. Roy. Statist. Soc. Ser. B*, Vol. 11 (1949), pp. 15–53.

[7] N. BRESLOW, "A generalized Kruskal-Wallis test for comparing K samples subject to unequal patterns of censorship," *Biometrika*, Vol. 57 (1970), pp. 579–594.

[8] I. BROSS, "Two choice selection," *J. Amer. Statist. Assoc.*, Vol. 45 (1950), pp. 530–540.

[9] ———, "Scientific strategies for deep models in the growth and spread of human cancer," Symposium on the Statistical Aspects of Protocol Design, San Juan, Puerto Rico, December, 1970. Available through the Clinical Investigations Branch, National Cancer Institute, Bethesda.

[10] B. W. BROWN, JR., "The use of controls in the clinical evaluation of cancer therapies," Symposium on the Statistical Aspects of Protocol Design, San Juan, Puerto Rico, December, 1970. Available through the Clinical Investigations Branch, National Cancer Institute, Bethesda.

[11] B. W. BROWN, JR., I. FRANTZ, H. C. McGILL, JR., G. W. McMILLAN, and J. P. STRONG, "The effect of accuracy of endpoint determination on the design of therapeutic trials with particular reference to coronary heart disease," Presented at Conference on Cardiovascular Disease Epidemiology, sponsored by the Council on Epidemiology, American Heart Association, San Diego, California, March 1 and 2, 1971.

[12] J. P. BUNKER, W. H. FORREST, JR., F. MOSTELLER, and L. D. VANDAM (editors), *The National Halothane Study*, Washington, D.C., U.S. Government Printing Office, 1969.

[13] P. L. CANNER, "Selecting one of two treatments when the responses are dichotomous," *J. Amer. Statist. Assoc.*, Vol. 65 (1970), pp. 293–306.

[14] T. C. CHALMERS, "A challenge to clinical investigators," *Gastroenterology*, Vol. 57 (1969), pp. 631–635.

[15] T. C. CHALMERS, "A clinician looks at the role of of statistics in clinical research," Symposium on the Statistical Aspects of Protocol Design, San Juan, Puerto Rico, December, 1970. Available through the Clinical Investigations Branch, National Cancer Institute, Bethesda.

[16] W. G. COCHRAN and G. M. COX, *Experimental Designs*, New York, Wiley, 1957 (2nd ed.).

[17] T. COLTON, "A model for selecting one of two medical treatments," *J. Amer. Statist. Assoc.*, Vol. 58 (1963), pp. 388–400.

[18] J. CORNFIELD, "A Bayesian test of some classical hypotheses—with applications to sequential clinical trials," *J. Amer. Statist. Assoc.*, Vol. 61 (1966), 577–594.

[19] ———, "The Bayesian outlook and its application," *Biometrics*, Vol. 25 (1969), pp. 617–58.

[20] J. CORNFIELD, M. HALPERIN, and S. W. GREENHOUSE, "An adaptive procedure for sequential clinical trials," *J. Amer. Statist. Assoc.*, Vol. 64 (1969), pp. 759–770.

[21] CORONARY DRUG PROJECT RESEARCH GROUP, "The Coronary Drug Project: initial findings leading to modifications of its research protocol," *J. Amer. Med. Assoc.*, Vol. 214 (1970), pp. 1303–1313.

[22] D. R. COX, *Planning of Experiments*, New York, Wiley, 1958.

[23] W. J. DIXON and F. J. MASSEY, JR., *Introduction to Statistical Analysis*, New York, McGraw-Hill, 1969 (3rd ed.).

[24] F. EDERER, "A parametric estimate of the standard error of the survival rate," *J. Amer. Statist. Assoc.*, Vol. 56 (1961), pp. 111–118.

[25] B. EFRON, "The two sample problem with censored data," *Proceedings Fifth Berkeley Symposium on Mathematical Statistics and Probability*, Berkeley and Los Angeles, University of California Press, Vol. 4, 1967, pp. 831–854.

[26] ———, "Forcing a sequential experiment to be balanced," Technical Report No. 14, Department of Statistics, Stanford University, 1970.

[27] A. R. FEINSTEIN, "Clinical biostatistics, III. The architecture of clinical research," *Clinical Pharmacology and Therapeutics*, Vol. 11 (1970), pp. 432–441 (and following notes in succeeding issues of this journal).

[28] ———, "What kind of basic science for clinical medicine?", *New England J. Med.*, Vol. 283 (1970), pp. 847–852.

[29] R. A. FISHER, *Statistical Methods and Scientific Inference*, New York, Hafner 1959 (2nd ed.).

[30] ———, *The Design of Experiments*, New York, Hafner, 1966 (8th ed.). (See pp. 17–21.)

[31] E. A. GEHAN, "Estimating survival functions from the life table," *J. Chronic Diseases*, Vol. 21 (1969), pp. 629–644.

[32] J. E. GRIZZLE, "The two-period change-over design and its use in clinical trials," *Biometrics*, Vol. 21 (1965), pp. 467–480.

[33] M. HALPERIN, E. ROGOT, J. GURIAN, and F. EDERER, "Sample sizes for medical trials with special reference to long-term therapy," *J. Chronic Diseases*, Vol. 21 (1968), pp. 13–24.

[34] J. L. HAYBITTLE, "A two-parameter model for the survival curve of treated cancer patients," *J. Amer. Statist. Assoc.*, Vol. 60 (1965), pp. 16–26.

[35] A. B. HILL (editor), *Controlled Clinical Trials*, Oxford, Blackwell Scientific Publications, 1960.

[36] ———, "The clinical trial," *Brit. Med. Bull.*, Vol. 7 (1951), pp. 278–282.

[37] ———, *Principles of Medical Statistics*, New York, Oxford University Press, 1971 (9th ed.).

[38] E. L. KAPLAN and P. MEIER, "Nonparametric estimation from incomplete observations," *J. Amer. Statist. Assoc.*, Vol. 53 (1958), pp. 457–481.

[39] T. J. KIRESUK, S. SALAZIN, and R. SHERMAN, "Goal attainment scaling: progress with implementation at a metropolitan community mental health center," pre-publication copy, 1971.

[40] C. R. KLIMT, G. L. KNATTERUD, C. L. MEINERT, and T. E. PROUT, "The University Group Diabetes Program: A study of the effects of hypoglycemic agents on vascular complications in patients with adult-onset diabetes," *Diabetes*, Vol. 19, Supp. 2 (1970).

[41] L. LASAGNA, "The controlled clinical trial: theory and practice," *J. Chronic Diseases*, Vol. 1 (1955), pp. 353–367.

[42] A. S. LITTELL, "Estimation of the T-year survival rate from follow-up studies over a limited period of time," *Hum. Biol.*, Vol. 24 (1952), pp. 87–116.

[43] D. MAINLAND, *Elementary Medical Statistics*, Philadelphia and London, W. B. Saunders, 1963.

[44] R. J. MAURICE, "A different loss function for the choice between two populations," *J. Roy. Statist. Soc. Series B*, Vol. 21 (1959), pp. 203–213.

[45] R. G. MILLER, JR., "A sequential signed-rank test," *J. Amer. Statist. Assoc.*, Vol. 65 (1970), pp. 1554–1561.

[46] L. E. MOSES and F. MOSTELLER, "Institutional differences in postoperative death rates," *J. Amer. Med. Assoc.*, Vol. 203 (1968), pp. 492–494.

[47] M. R. NOVICK and J. E. GRIZZLE, "A Bayesian approach to the analysis of data from clinical trials," *J. Amer. Statist. Assoc.*, Vol. 60 (1965), pp. 81–96.

[48] D. B. OWEN, *Handbook of Statistical Tables*, Reading, Addison-Wesley, 1962.

[49] B. S. PASTERNACK and H. S. GILBERT, "Planning the duration of long-term survival time studies designed for accrual by cohorts," *J. Chronic Diseases*, Vol. 24 (1971), pp. 681–700.

[50] M. A. SCHNEIDERMAN, "The proper size of a clinical trial: 'Grandma's Strudel' method," *J. New Drugs*, Vol. 4 (1964), pp. 3–11.

[51] G. W. SNEDECOR, *Statistical Methods*, Ames, Iowa State University Press, 1937 (1st ed.).

[52] G. W. SNEDECOR and G. W. COCHRAN, *Statistical Methods*, Ames, Iowa State University Press, 1967 (6th ed.).

[53] M. SOBEL and G. H. WEISS, "Play-the-winner sampling for selecting the better of two binomial populations," *Biometrika*, Vol. 57 (1970), pp. 357–65.

[54] S. M. STIGLER, "The use of random allocation for the control of selection bias," *Biometrika*, Vol. 56 (1969), pp. 553–560.

[55] VETERANS ADMINISTRATION COOPERATIVE UROLOGICAL RESEARCH GROUP, "Carcinoma of prostate: treatment comparisons," *J. Urology*, Vol. 98 (1967), pp. 516–22.

[56] L. J. WITTS (editor), *Medical Surveys and Clinical Trials*, London, Oxford University Press, 1964 (2nd ed.).

[57] WORLD HEALTH ORGANIZATION, "International drug monitoring (the role of the hospital)," Report of a WHO Meeting, World Health Organization Technical Report Series, No. 425, 1969.

[58] ———, "Principles for pre-clinical testing of drug safety," Report of a WHO Scientific Group, World Health Organization Technical Report Series, No. 341, 1966.

[59] ———, "Principles for the clinical evaluation of drugs," Report of a WHO Scientific Group, World Health Organization Technical Report Series, No. 403, 1968.

[60] M. ZELEN, "Play the winner rule and the controlled clinical trial," *J. Amer. Statist. Assoc.*, Vol. 64 (1969), pp. 131–46.

[61] M. ZELEN and P. FEIGL, "Estimation of exponential survival probabilities with concomitant information," *Biometrics*, Vol. 21, No. 4 (1965), pp. 826–38.

[62] C. ZIPPIN and P. ARMITAGE, "Use of concomitant variables and incomplete survival information in the estimation of an exponential survival parameter," *Biometrics*, Vol. 22 (1966), pp. 665–72.

[63] E. GEHAN, "A generalized Wilcoxon test for comparing arbitrarily single censored samples," *Biometrika*, Vol. 52 (1965), pp. 203–223.

[64] J. BERKSON and R. P. GAGE, "Survival curve for cancer patients following treatment," *J. Amer. Statist. Assoc.*, Vol. 47, No. 259 (1952), pp. 501–515.

AUTOMATED DIAGNOSIS IN MULTIPHASIC SCREENING

DANKWARD KODLIN and MORRIS F. COLLEN
PERMANENTE MEDICAL GROUP
OAKLAND, CALIFORNIA

1. Introduction

While efforts at mathematizing the medical diagnostic process continue [10] the current state of the art appears to be characterized by two observations:

(1) in applications where the "correct" diagnosis can be established (for example, by surgery or autopsy) the accuracy of diagnostic algorithms is comparable but not superior to the performance of experts [14], [16];

(2) different analytical techniques give similar results [6], [7], [9].

One is thus tempted to argue that if experts can effectively compete with Bayes' theorem (at least, with that version which assumes the independence of symptom variables [16]) or if experts can weigh the evidence as effectively as a discriminant function, a good case for the exploration of relatively simple decision schemes can be made. This would seem to apply, in particular, to medical areas in which no confirmation of physicians' diagnoses is routinely available and where the major purpose of "automated" diagnosis is to maximize agreement with "routine clinical diagnosis" rather than agreement with "ultimate authority." The so-called multiphasic screening [3] as practiced in the Kaiser Foundation Medical Care Program, provides a typical example; here responses to a battery of several hundred medical questions are recorded in addition to measurements from a standard series of laboratory tests. At the conclusion of such an examination, the patient sees a clinician who reviews the findings and records diagnostic impressions on a check list containing some two hundred diagnoses. This setting is thus quite different from the typical application area of "computer diagnosis" mentioned above where a relatively small set of variables are considered for a small set of mutually exclusive diagnoses as they can be defined in narrow specialty fields. The magnitude of the task inherent in multiphasic screening would seem to make computational simplicity a feature of extreme virtue.

For these reasons, we continue to be interested in diagnostic schemes involving a limited number of dichotomized variables (YES-NO Questions and/or Tests) such as the likelihood ratio method of Neyman [5], [12], [13] and the simple

Partial support came from the National Center for Health Services Research and Development (Grant HS00288) and the Kaiser Foundation Research Institute.

15

scoring procedure developed in conjunction with the Cornell Medical Index questionnaire by van Woerkom and Brodman [1], [2], [15]. We shall compare the performance of these two methods on an example of considerable medical interest, the diagnosis of coronary heart disease in multiphasic screening, and discuss the utility aspects of various decision alternatives in this context.

2. Material and methods

For some 26,000 persons who took the multiphasic screening examination within one year, we have records on "variables" (about 700 questions and some 50 "objective" tests ranging from X-ray films to chemical body fluid determinations) and "diagnoses," the latter recorded by the "followup" physician. The average number of diagnoses per person is close to two, about half the value recorded in medical settings that deal with the typical "office patient" [2] rather than with persons seeking a health checkup. We envision a computerized diagnostic system that will, for the ith diagnosis or at least for the ith set (if related diagnoses have to be combined) examine a predetermined "relevant variable set" V_i and on the basis of a critical region R_i make a decision concerning that diagnosis. Consequently, a "healthy" person will be one whose response pattern is such that he falls within all negative regions.

Selection of the relevant variable sets is accomplished on a "learning sample," consisting of half the number of cases with diagnosis D_i and a group of 1000 noncases. The remaining cases and another group of 1000 noncases are retained as a "validation sample." With the aid of the learning sample, we select the "best" relevant variable set V_i from an "initial variable list" L_i prepared by clinical judgment. The choice is made on the basis of the likelihood ratio (cases/noncases) for each item on the list L_i, by taking, for practical reasons, the eight "best" variables only. Since tests (T) are much more expensive than questions (Q) a limited number of combinations of "best" Q and T are also made up, such as "best $6Q$ + best $2T$," and so forth.

In the following, we shall concentrate on a particular D_i, the condition coronary heart disease (chd). For this group (made up of the three diagnoses angina pectoris, ischemic heart disease, and myocardial infarction) the initial variable list contained some fifty questions and six tests. On the basis of the learning sample (336 cases and 1000 noncases) the eight best questions are those on chest pain and shortness of breath with likelihood ratios between 5 and 3 and the best two tests appear to be EKG (most abnormalities) and serum cholesterol (upper five percentile) with likelihood ratios of 3.4 and 3. Two analytical methods, the likelihood ratio method θ and the scoring method β are now applied to the learning sample.

2.1. *Likelihood ratio method θ.* Briefly, the method [5], [13] orders the observed response patterns of the eight dichotomized variables by the pattern likelihood ratio θ and investigates the two types of classification errors at various cutting levels of this array. Following medical custom, we plot sensitivity $1 - \alpha$ and specificity $1 - \beta$ for each level to obtain a performance curve such as Figure 1. Amongst the 256 possible patterns only some 90 occur in our learning sample. When the validation sample (316 cases and 1000 noncases) is classified according to a given positive region derived from the learning sample, some of the remaining patterns appear; these "unknown" patterns are allocated, under current practice, to the positive region. With sample sizes of the magnitude indicated, the performance curve from the validation sample is noticeably, but not excessively, worse than the curve derived from the learning sample.

2.2. *Scoring method β.* The method uses the same learning and validation samples and considers the same variables. While, with β, there is no need, for practical reasons, to be restrictive on the number of variables, we have found that no improvement results from inclusion of seven variables in addition to the eight used with the θ method and for this reason we present results that are identical as to type and number of variables considered.

Each positive response is scored by the relative likelihood deviation

$$(2.1) \qquad s_i = \frac{p_i - P_i}{\sqrt{P_i}},$$

where p_i is the observed frequency of positive response to the ith variable amongst cases and P_i is the observed frequency in the general patient population. The quantity is summed over all positive responses giving the total score

$$(2.2) \qquad \beta = \sum_{\substack{i=1 \\ \text{YES}}}^{\kappa} \frac{p_i - P_i}{\sqrt{P_i}}$$

for a person having κ positive (YES) responses. From an empirical distribution of β amongst cases of the learning sample a number of critical β values are taken and a person in the validation sample is diagnosed as CHD if his β value is larger than the critical value under consideration.

The scoring procedure is similar to, but not identical with, that of van Woerkom and Brodman [15], who sum over all positive responses within the whole set of variables (150 questions), while we restrict ourselves to the relevant set V_i.

Since, approximately,

$$(2.3) \qquad s_i = \sqrt{p_i}(\sqrt{\theta_i} - \sqrt{1/\theta_i}),$$

where θ_i is the likelihood ratio (cases/noncases) for the ith variable and furthermore since the term in brackets is roughly equal to $\log \theta$ (in the θ range from one to ten), one would expect that a score

$$(2.4) \qquad s_i' = \sqrt{p_i} \log \theta_i, \qquad \lambda = \sum s_i',$$

would give results similar to those obtained with β. It also remains to be seen if inclusion of negative responses in β or λ would improve the performance.

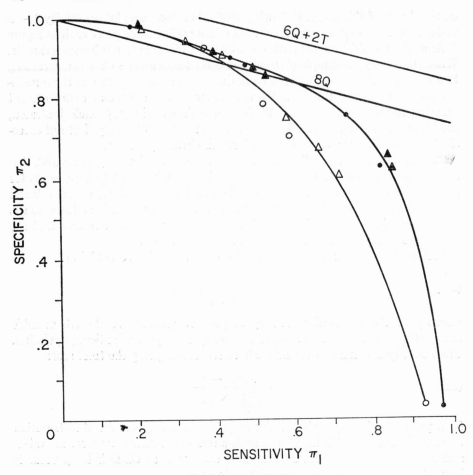

FIGURE 1

Performance of automated diagnosis of coronary heart disease on a
validation sample (316 cases and 1000 noncases).
Comparison of two analytical techniques: likelihood ratio method (o, ●)
versus scoring method (△, ▲).
Comparison of two variable sets: "8 Questions" (o, △) *versus* "6 Questions plus
2 Tests" [EKG and cholesterol] (●, ▲).
Upper straight line is the cost indifference line for "6 Questions plus 2 Tests";
lower straight line is the cost indifference line for "8 Questions."
Note that the methods have essentially the same performance and that, for the
cost matrix assumed, only the "8 Questions" procedure would be cost advantageous (against "no screening") and only at a sensitivity of less than 0.5 where
the corresponding curve crosses its indifference line.

3. Results

From Figure 1, it appears that θ and β have similar performance and corresponding plots for a number of different disease categories give no indication of consistent differences. Furthermore, the two techniques are comparable as to speed.

Differences between "questions alone" and "questions plus tests" are clearcut, the tests helping to improve specificity at sensitivity levels between 0.5 and 0.9. Even so, the performance is modest in comparison with other diagnostic achievements; for instance, for X-ray diagnosis of tuberculosis [10], a 94 per cent specificity can be achieved at a sensitivity level of 80 per cent. This may merely be an indication that diagnosis of tuberculosis is a relatively easy task. However, we believe that the performance curve for chd can be improved by reviewing the total medical record. The physician's diagnosis, as currently used, comes from a check list employed by him at the time of the followup examination and sometimes is at variance with the medical record. Such a review by an independent observer is time consuming. At least for the case of diabetes, where it has been carried out on a sampling basis, improvement of the automated diagnostic scheme was clearcut.

4. Decision theory

That the screening problem must be cast into the mold of decision theory has been clearly recognized for some time. Flagle [8] has reviewed this aspect of screening in a preceding Symposium and articles on utility and diagnosis are beginning to appear in the medical literature [11]. As Flagle [8] has pointed out, the utilities to be estimated for use in the decision process are *ad hoc*. That is to say, they do not only depend on the obvious factors such as the severity of the disease in question, but on the particular setting in which the subsequent *therapeutic* effort takes place. For this reason, we have decided to consider a cost matrix slightly more elaborate than that underlying the "regret" analysis of Flagle; the matrix in Table I contains the cost for each cell with its three components, the screening cost s, the "workup" or "referral" costs w (that is, costs of additional tests and physician time devoted to a patient declared positive by the screen), and the therapeutic costs T_{tp} for the true positive and T_{fn} for the false negative, both of which have to be carried, at least in part, by a "prepaid" medical care system such as ours.

For the three strategies:

S_1: "do nothing,"
S_2: "refer all,"
S_3: "refer those screened positive,"

we then have the respective costs

(4.1) $$C_1 = P(c_{21} - c_{22}),$$

(4.2) $$C_2 = P(c_{11} - c_{21}) + (1 - P)w,$$

(4.3) $$C_3 = P(c_{21} - \pi_1 e) + (1 - P)(c_{12} - \pi_2 w),$$

where P is the prevalence of the condition, π_1 the sensitivity, and π_2 the specificity, the remaining symbols being cost items defined in Table I.

TABLE I

ASSUMED COST MATRIX FOR CORONARY HEART DISEASE

T: treatment costs for true positive (tp), false positive (fp), false negative (fn), and true negative (tn); w: "workup" or referral cost; s: screening cost.

Note that $e = c_{21} - c_{11} = T_{fn} - T_{tp}$, "pure treatment differential" and $w = c_{12} - c_{22}$; T values of $100 and 200 are conjectural as is $w = 10$; $s = 1$ applies to the cost of EKG, Collen, Kidd, Feldman, and Cutler [4].

| | | Physician's diagnosis | |
		+	−
	+	$T_{tp} = 100$ $w = 10$ $s = 1$	$T_{fp} = 0$ $w = 10$ $s = 1$
		$c_{11} = 111$	$c_{12} = 11$
Screen	−	$T_{fn} = 200$ $w = 10$ $s = 1$	$T_{tn} = 0$ $w = 0$ $s = 1$
		$c_{21} = 211$	$c_{22} = 1$

Equating (4.1) and (4.3) and solving for π_2, we obtain

(4.4) $$\pi_2^* = 1 + \frac{s}{w}\frac{1}{1-P} - \frac{e}{w}\frac{P}{1-P}\pi_1,$$

the line of indifference between S_1 and S_3.

Equating (4.2) and (4.3) and solving for π_2, we obtain

(4.5) $$\pi_2^* = \frac{e}{w}\frac{P}{1-P} + \frac{s}{w}\frac{1}{1-P} - \frac{e}{w}\frac{P}{1-P}\pi_1,$$

the line of indifference between S_2 and S_3. Equations (4.4) and (4.5) are thus parallel lines, the slope of which is determined by the prevalence P and the ratio e/w. The two intercepts differ by the first term only and a plot of (4.5) quickly eliminates S_2 as a competitive strategy.

In Figure 1, two lines of cost indifference (S_1 versus S_3, equation (4.4) have been drawn, the upper one for a screening strategy involving only the cost of EKG with $s = 1$ (see Table I) and the lower one for $s = 0$, assuming that cost of questions is negligible. Since the performance curve rises only above the question line, but not above the EKG line, one would conclude that screening by questions is cost advantageous while screening by questions and EKG is not. The weak link in this argument is, of course, the uncertainty as to the magnitude of the value of e, the excess treatment cost due to delayed disease recognition.

5. Optimum screening level

Setting the derivative of (4.3) with respect to π_1 equal to zero, one obtains the relation

$$(5.1) \qquad f_0' = -\frac{e}{w}\frac{P}{1-P},$$

where f_0' is the derivative of the performance curve, the empirical function $\pi_2 = f(\pi_1)$, at the minimal cost.

Since (5.1) is identical to the slope of (4.4), one may locate the optimum screening level as the point at which the tangent of the performance curve is parallel to the indifference line. For Figure 1, this optimum is sensitivity π_1 between 0.2 and 0.3.

The expression (5.1) can be used to bring out the value system implied in the choice of particular screening levels [11]. For instance, for the case of X-ray screening for tuberculosis, Lusted [11] shows a preference for the point $\pi_1 = 0.8$ and $\pi_2 = 0.94$. At this point, his performance curve has a slope of -0.2. With a prevalence $P = 5 \times 10^{-4}$ from (5.1) we have $e/w = 400$.

It is interesting to note how much divergence can be produced on casual approach to this question. Rubin, Collen, and Goldman [13], discussing the optimal choice of a screening level, consider the function $U = a\pi_1 + b\pi_2$, and locate the pair π_1, π_2 which maximizes this function. The coefficients a and b are not defined, but from (4.3) it is clear that $a = Pe$ and $b = (1 - P)w$. Thus, maximization of U indeed minimizes the cost of the screening strategy. The writers remark that for "conditions such as tuberculosis a would probably be set several magnitudes higher than b." However, P values of the order of 5×10^{-4} still apply with population estimates of annual incidence rates of newly reported cases standing at 3×10^{-4}. Therefore, if we would take $w = 10$, and thus, $e = 4000$, then $a = 2$ and $b = 10$, indicating that divergence of opinion can be of the order of several magnitudes.

6. Discussion

The cost matrix postulated in Table I can be criticized for understating the benefits of screening. For instance, one may postulate that in the absence of screening facilities, a certain fraction ϕ of healthy persons would come for a "conventional" checkup, perhaps involving the cost w. Under these conditions, S_1, the "do nothing" strategy, would imply the cost

$$(6.1) \qquad C_1 = P(c_{21} - c_{22}) + \phi(1 - P)w,$$

giving the indifference line (S_1 versus S_3)

(6.2)
$$\pi_2^* = 1 + \frac{s}{w}\frac{1}{1-P} - \phi - \frac{e}{w}\frac{P}{1-P}\pi_1.$$

With ϕ values of the order of 0.1, the two indifference lines of Figure 1 would have to be displaced downwards by 0.1. As a consequence of this, screening with $6Q + 2T$ could now be justified on a cost basis for sensitivity levels below 0.5 and screening with $8Q$ for sensitivity levels below 0.65. The optimal screening level would remain at $\pi_1 \doteq 0.3$ at which π_2 is the same for these two alternatives (see Figure 1). In this case, as can be seen from equation (4.3), the "cheap" screen ($8Q$) is still saving the amount s in relation to the "expensive" screen ($6Q + 2T$). Once again, we wish to stress the speculative nature of these impressions, in the face of uncertainty about e/w and current reliance on diagnostic entries, as mentioned in Section 3. In general, we feel, however, that decision theoretical formalisms such as those presented, are useful in the way they point towards crucial items of information that are extremely difficult to acquire.

7. Summary

Multiphasic screening, the application of a large battery of questions and laboratory tests to large numbers of persons, has reached an advanced stage of automation, and rapid classification techniques that provide diagnostic categorization are of considerable interest in this field. With the example of automated diagnosis of coronary heart disease, we find the performance of two methods (likelihood ratio and scoring technique) in terms of characteristic curves to be comparable. Notions of test selection strategy are discussed in relation to the same disease although the precise nature of the cost matrix is speculative.

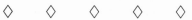

The authors wish to acknowledge contributions from Dr. Robert Feldman and programming work by Mrs. L. Lo and Mr. J. Standish.

REFERENCES

[1] K. BRODMAN and L. S. GOLDSTEIN, "The medical data screen. An adjunct for the diagnosis of 100 common diseases," Arch. Environ. Health, Vol. 14 (1967), pp. 821–826.
[2] K. BRODMAN and A. J. VAN WOERKOM, "Computer-aided diagnostic screening for 100 common diseases," J. Amer. Med. Assoc., Vol. 197 (1966), pp. 901–905.
[3] M. F. COLLEN, "Periodic health examinations using an automated multitest laboratory," J. Amer. Med. Assoc., Vol. 195 (1966), pp. 830–833.
[4] M. F. COLLEN, P. H. KIDD, R. FELDMAN, and J. L. CUTLER, "Cost analysis of a multiphasic screening program," New England J. Med., Vol. 280 (1969), pp. 1043–1045.
[5] M. F. COLLEN, L. RUBIN, J. NEYMAN, G. B. DANTZIG, R. M. BAER, and A. B. SIEGELAUB, "Automated multiphasic screening and diagnosis," Amer. J. Pub. Health, Vol. 54 (1964), pp. 741–750.

[6] J. M. DICKEY, "Estimation of disease probabilities conditioned on symptom variables," *Math. Biosciences*, Vol. 3 (1968), pp. 249–265.

[7] S. FELDMAN, D. F. KLEIN, and G. HONIGFELD, "A comparison of successive screening and discriminant function techniques in medical taxonomy," *Biometrics*, Vol. 25 (1969), pp. 725–734.

[8] C. D. FLAGLE, "A decision theoretical comparison of three procedures of screening for a single disease," *Proceedings of the Fifth Berkeley Symposium on Mathematical Statistics and Probability*, Berkeley and Los Angeles, University of California Press, 1967, Vol. 4, pp. 887–901.

[9] G. A. GORY and G. O. BARNETT, "Experience with a model of sequential diagnosis," *Comp. Biomed. Res.*, Vol. 1 (1968), pp. 490–507.

[10] J. A. JACQUEZ (editor), *Proceedings of the Second Conference on the Diagnostic Process*, held at the University of Michigan, 1971, Fort Lauderdale, Charles C Thomas, in press.

[11] L. B. LUSTED, "Decision-making studies in patient management," *New England J. Med.*, Vol. 284 (1971), pp. 416–424.

[12] J. NEYMAN, *First Course in Probability and Statistics*, New York, Holt, 1950, Chapter 5.

[13] L. RUBIN, M. F. COLLEN, and G. E. GOLDMAN, "Frequency decision theoretical approach to automated medical diagnosis," *Proceedings of the Fifth Berkeley Symposium on Mathematical Statistics and Probability*, Berkeley and Los Angeles, University of California Press, 1967, Vol. 4, pp. 867–886.

[14] A. W. TEMPLETON, K. BRYAN, R. WAIRD, J. TOWNES, M. HUQUE, and S. J. DWYER, "Computer diagnosis and discriminate analysis decision schemes," *Radiology*, Vol. 95 (1970), pp. 47–55.

[15] A. J. VAN WOERKOM and K. BRODMAN, "Statistics for a diagnostic model," *Biometrics*, Vol. 17 (1961), pp. 299–318.

[16] H. R. WARNER, A. F. TORONTO, and L. G. VEASY, "Experience with Bayes' theorem for computer diagnosis of congenital heart disease," *Ann. N.Y. Acad. Sci.*, Vol. 115 (1964), pp. 558–567.

SOME PRACTICAL PROBLEMS
IN CLINICAL TRIALS

WILLIAM F. TAYLOR and PETER C. O'BRIEN
MAYO CLINIC, MINNESOTA

1. Introduction

In 1971, the Mayo Clinic received a large grant to carry out clinical research on cancer. Twenty new projects were approved for support. Ordinarily these would be considered to be twenty independent projects and they would each have been provided with statistical services separately by our Medical Statistics Section. Something has been added, however, which provides a new set of problems. There exists now a new organization called a Clinical Cancer Center. It has been our problem (those of us in Medical Statistics) to try to define what a clinical cancer center is and to provide its statistical heart. At this writing we are still trying to develop a workable, unified record system tied in with appropriate computerization. So far the Center helps prepare protocols, designs the research records, handles randomization, edits data promptly, and prepares the data for analysis. Our intent is to examine results frequently, to provide summary reports frequently and, in general, to keep an aggressive watch over the course of the research. (There are a number of our statistical acquaintances around the country who have been through the same thing that we are going through now. They have our respect and admiration. Incidentally, we used to scoff at this sort of work as being pedestrian and dull. We scoff no more.)

In preparation for this grant, a massive effort was made at the Mayo Clinic to come up with suggestions of research projects that could be done with our large clinical practice. (It should be remembered that the Mayo Clinic has an enormous cancer patient load. About 6,000 new ones appear there each year.) As a result of this effort some 100 projects were proposed for support by a grant. These were whittled down by a committee to around 40 projects which were written up in formal NIH style and submitted to the National Cancer Institute. Site visits are never pleasant things if you are the one being visited. In this instance we were confronted by a distinguished panel of cancer experts. The visitors were both highly competent and highly critical. They examined our requests thoroughly. About half of our projects were turned down by the site visitors for one reason or another. Their report said, in part, the following.

"With respect to the scientific merit and design of the proposed studies, practically all suffered from primarily one weakness, namely, an improper experimental design from a biostatistical standpoint. Because of this, protocols were

25

left open ended and with too many options so that even with all the patient resources each year some of the studies would take years to accumulate enough data for analysis and by this time, of course, the time element would make comparisons impossible. The reviewers judged that those protocols illustrating this weakness were prepared without proper consultation with the biostatistical staff of the Mayo Clinic."

This statement is partly true. We had carefully worked over many of the projects using appropriate sample size considerations and revised protocols. But many were submitted without or in spite of our statistical criticism and some were difficult to love. Even so, a few projects we liked were turned down. On the other hand, some of the projects which were approved by the highly critical group of site visitors were ones that we had disapproved because we could not see that there would be enough patients in a reasonable length of time to come to any conclusions. There is an explanation of sorts. Some of the research topics involving only a few patients were exceedingly interesting to the reviewers and to the world of cancer research. While even the Mayo Clinic's case load might not be very large for some rare diseases, still it was one of the largest case loads in the country and some problems were considered interesting enough to look at in spite of small numbers of patients. We now feel in sympathy with the idea that a reasonable (inexpensive) randomized trial even on very infrequent cases may be better than the alternative we use now. If we had only started this ten years ago on myeloma, we would have some answers now which we need very much.

When we examined the officially accepted research proposals (and the several new ones which are now being prepared), we found, typically, that the research is clinical in nature requiring that each suitable patient be assigned at random to one of several treatment groups. The problem is to make a comparative evaluation of the treatments. How does one determine if a treatment is any good? It is not easy. For example, in the evaluation of patients with cancer of the prostate a "remission" is defined as (i) decrease in the size of the prostatic or paraprostatic mass or the size of the radiographic lesion as measured independently by two urologists, (ii) a decrease in the total acid phosphatase of 50 per cent or the tartrate inhibition fraction by 20 per cent, (iii) improvement in activity or resumption of normal activities since therapy. The first and third of these things are quite subjective and are difficult to measure with assurance. However, once remission occurs, then the usual problem is to determine how long it lasts. We are involved with survival time problems.

In clinical trials, survival time in some form or another is a very common object of study. The simple survival to death or survival to failure or survival to some sort of change of state is a fairly routine analysis. A first order complication is the case where survival alone is insufficient. Suppose a treatment is tried out in the hope of inducing remission of disease. However, remission may or may not be observed to occur. If a remission occurs, it may last for quite some time and a conditional "duration of remission" study can be carried out. But we really have the problem of total evaluation, determining both the proportion of patients in whom remission occurs and the duration of such remission. Similarly, when we resort to studying only total survival time, ignoring "quality of survival," we may lose the entire benefit of treatment. Our gynecologists were dismayed, for example, at finding no increase in survival of women with cancer of the ovaries in spite of new treatments which were felt to be helpful. Possibly the quality of life was all that could be improved in this dreadful disease, but as yet we do not know.

In the very large effort expended now in the evaluation of chemotherapy, there is a class of clinical trials called Phase II Research. This is research in which drugs which have been found to have interesting possibilities on the basis of animal research and on very tentative human research are submitted to various investigators to try out on suitable patients. The object is to find those drugs which seem to show some kind of beneficial activity. In spite of years of work, there are still gaps in the common sense of these experiments. One complicating problem is the fact that in most institutions patients are used repeatedly; those failing one drug are tried out on another, and upon failing a second time they are tried out on a third. One wonders how much is missed in a promising drug by testing it out predominantly on patients who have failed one or more previous trials. This occurs frequently in survival analyses.

Suppose a patient starts out with a certain treatment and is followed until he gets either a recurrence of the disease or a new disease. He then is removed from the study and re-entered into a new study to see how he survives under his new condition. The problem is what do you compare him with in his new condition? What kind of comparison survival curves can be constructed? For example, patients with chronic ulcerative colitis are treated without surgery for a certain disease. After a time certain patients are subjected to surgery. Did surgery do any good? Even if selection for surgery were random, the time of such selection in this progressive disease makes for difficulties. We have used a simple variation of a standard survival analysis [2], but we have also seen serious errors made in this situation. Surely our own methods are in need of improvement.

Another problem in the comparison of survival of two or more groups has to do with the differences in the groups due, perhaps, to lack of randomization, or due to "good" randomization which just turned out to be grossly unbalanced. In clinical trials, we think we should attempt to stratify where we think it is important and to randomize within each stratum. There are problems, then, of evaluating overall effects of treatment on the basis of observations from several strata, none of which has sufficient cases to stand alone.

Turn back now to the earlier part of this paper in which we discussed research protocols which we must help develop for the Mayo Clinic Cancer Center. We sometimes have to deal with small samples. The problems are interesting but the patients are slow in appearing at the Clinic. Lengthy observations must be made; research discipline must be maintained for years. It seems obvious that in these projects the investigators will be pushed for decisions as early as possible. Sequential analysis appears to be a reasonable approach to take in such cases. In addition, as part of the surveillance of the data collection system, the data must be examined. Waiting three or four years without analyzing the data, even though we edit it and query it and file it carefully away, simply leads to poor data and boredom. We cannot afford to let our data pile up unanalyzed. We must look at them frequently (much more frequently, in fact, than we used to think was necessary). Therefore, there is a natural incentive to evaluate research in progress and to see how we are doing. When our clinicians learn (as they will) of the results of our intermediate statistical analyses, they will say, "Don't we have enough now so we can stop?" It is an inevitable and a natural question. Therefore, it seems to us that in a carefully run data collection protocol, sequential analysis is thrust upon us by the nature of the needs for quality control. Early curiosity is not a scientific sin.

For example, in studying three treatments for chronic hepatitis, a double blind experiment was done. Patients as they came in were assigned at random to one of three groups. Every time a death occurred the investigators "broke the code" and looked at the treatment that the dead person had received. After all too short a time they began seeing deaths occur as follows: placebo, placebo, placebo, treatment 1, placebo, treatment 1, treatment 1. Treatment 2 had no deaths for a long time compared with the other two treatments. The investigators came in and they said, "Look, we think we are killing people with this experiment," but they also said, "We do not want to stop this experiment if we stop it so prematurely that somebody else is going to have to do it again." So faced with this compassionate, yet mature, outlook we made a sequential stopping decision.

2. Sequential methods

We have recently been studying the work of Robbins and others on sequential experimentation and have been attempting to apply some of these results to our survival time problems. So far our work is only a preliminary effort. We have also worked with Armitage's sequential pairing method [1], but wish to supplement this with sequential interval estimation methods such as those in Robbins' recent article in the *Annals* [3]. Robbins' work makes use of a theorem due to J. Ville [4]; also see A. Wald [5]. The probability that the likelihood ratio based on a sample of size n should exceed a quantity ε, for some n greater than 1, is $\leq 1/\varepsilon$, $\varepsilon > 1$. This theorem leads to many things; for example, to certain types of confidence interval estimates and to tests of hypotheses with power 1. One problem, discounted by Robbins, has to do with the fact that the sequential plans are open ended and the tests will rarely end under the null hypothesis. We give some examples of approaches that we have been examining.

The first approach is a sequential confidence interval estimate for an assumed constant risk of death. Consider a group of individuals who come under observation at intervals, one at a time. A treatment is applied and each individual is observed for the rest of his life. At the time of the nth death we observe the number of patients seen so far A_n, the time survived by each patient t_i and the state of each patient ($x_i = 0$ if alive, $x_i = 1$ if dead). We wish to estimate the value λ_0 of λ, the assumed constant risk of death. We carry out a paraphrase of Robbins' sequential confidence intervals. Let hypothesis H_0 specify $\lambda = \lambda_0$ and let alternative H_1 merely state that λ has been obtained at random from a distribution $F(\lambda)$. Let $g_n(\{t, x\})$ be the joint density function of the observations under H_0 and $g_n'(\{t, x\})$ that under H_1 at the time of the nth death. We use Ville's theorem

(1)
$$P\left\{\frac{g_n'}{g_n} \geq \varepsilon \text{ for some } n \geq 1\right\} \leq \frac{1}{\varepsilon}, \qquad \varepsilon > 1.$$

In this case,

(2)
$$\frac{g_n'}{g_n} = \frac{\int_0^\infty \exp\{-\lambda \sum t_i\} \lambda^n \, dF(\lambda)}{\exp\{-\lambda_0 \sum t_i\} \lambda_0^n},$$

where summation is over the number of patients A_n. If we choose $F(\lambda)$ as an exponential distribution with mean λ_0, this reduces to

(3)
$$P\left\{\frac{g_n'}{g_n} = \frac{e^{-1}/(n+1)}{[\exp\{-(\lambda_0 T_n + 1)\}(\lambda_0 T_n + 1)^{n+1}]/(n+1)!} \geq \varepsilon \text{ for some } n \geq 1\right\} \leq \frac{1}{\varepsilon},$$

where $T_n = \sum_{i=1}^{A_n} t_i$. Hence, the sequential confidence interval for λ_0 of size $1 - 1/\varepsilon$ can be defined as the interval $I(n)$ such that $\lambda_0 \in I(n)$, whenever an appropriate Poisson probability satisfies the inequality inside the braces below. Thus,

(4)
$$P\left\{\frac{\exp\{-(\lambda_0 T_n + 1)\}(\lambda_0 T_n + 1)^{n+1}}{(n+1)!} \geq \frac{e^{-1}}{(n+1)\varepsilon} \text{ for every } n \geq 1\right\} \geq 1 - \frac{1}{\varepsilon}.$$

A possible sequential test for two treatments might be to compute these sequential confidence intervals for the λ of each of the treatments and stop as soon as the two confidence intervals failed to overlap. This is quite crude and yet should provide a test of power 1. The expense might be great, for the expected sample size would doubtless be larger than for some other methods.

A second example is really an attempt to utilize more information than Armitage uses in his paired method of sequential experimentation analysis. Suppose the patients are coming in fairly rapidly compared with the rate of death, so that after a while we are pretty sure of having some extra patients alive whenever we observe a death. Consider two groups of patients. Suppose that at the time just before the jth death there are N_{1j} patients in one treatment group still alive and N_{2j} patients in the other. Suppose that the risk in treatment 1 is λ_1 and the risk in treatment 2 is λ_2. Then, given a death occurs, the probability that the death occurs in the first group can be expressed as $N_{1j}\lambda_1/(N_{1j}\lambda_1 + N_{2j}\lambda_2)$. Under the null hypothesis, $\lambda_1 = \lambda_2 = \lambda$. Under the alternative hypothesis $\lambda_1 =$

$c\lambda_2$. We then set up a sequential probability ratio test and arrive at a test of the hypothesis that $c = 1$. This is again sequential over the occurrence of successive deaths in the combined groups. Suppose we stop at the time of the nth death and look at the data. After cancelling λ_2 and λ, we obtain

$$(5) \quad P\left(\frac{g_n'}{g_n} = \prod_{j=1}^{n} \frac{[N_{1j}cx_j + N_{2j}(1 - x_j)]/(N_{1j}c + N_{2j})}{[N_{1j}x_j + N_{2j}(1 - x_j)]/(N_{1j} + N_{2j})} \geq \varepsilon \text{ for some } n \geq 1\right) - \frac{1}{\varepsilon},$$

where $x_j = 1$ if jth death occurs in first treatment group, $x_j = 0$ otherwise. Letting $\sum_j^n x_j = n_1$ and $\sum_{j=1}^{n}(1 - x_j) = n - n_1 = n_2$,

$$(6) \quad P\left(\log\frac{g_n'}{g_n} = n_1 \log c - \sum_{j=1}^{n} \log(N_{1j} + N_{2j}) + \sum_{j=1}^{n} \log(N_{1j}c + N_{2j}) \geq \log \varepsilon \right.$$
$$\left. \text{for some } n \geq 1\right)$$

$$= P\left(n_1 \geq \frac{1}{\log c}\{\log \varepsilon - \sum^{n} \log(N_{1j} + N_{2j}) + \sum^{n} \log(N_{1j}c + N_{2j})\}\right.$$
$$\left. \text{for some } n \geq 1\right) \leq \frac{1}{\varepsilon}$$

if $c > 1$. The inequality reverses (inside) if $c < 1$. If n_1 satisfies this inequality, we stop taking new cases and reject the hypothesis that $\lambda_1 = \lambda_2$. We can also define a confidence interval for c from (6).

A third example is still in the prenatal stage. Suppose we have two treatment groups which, by the nth death, have resulted in: A_{1n} cases started on 1st treatment, n_1 dead, and A_{2n} cases started on 2nd treatment, n_2 dead, where $A_{1n} = A_{2n}$ and $n_1 + n_2 = n$. These two groups have survival times totalling T_{1n} and T_{2n}, respectively. We test the hypothesis $\lambda_1 = \lambda_2 = \lambda$ against the alternative that $\lambda_1 = c\lambda_2$.

The likelihood ratio is

$$(7) \qquad \frac{g_n'}{g_n} = \frac{\exp\{-c\lambda_2 T_{1n}(c\lambda_2)^{n_1}\} \exp\{-\lambda_2 T_{2n}\lambda_2^{n_2}\}}{\exp\{-\lambda(T_{1n} + T_{2n})\}\lambda^n}.$$

If we replace λ_2 and λ by their maximum likelihood estimates, we get an expression of unknown characteristics but with, we feel, reasons for further examination:

$$(8) \quad P\left(\frac{g_n'}{g_n} \geq \varepsilon \text{ for some } n \geq 1\right) \approx P\left(\frac{e^{-n}e^{n_1}[n/(cT_{1n} + T_{2n})]^n}{e^{-n}[n/(T_{1n} + T_{2n})]} \geq \varepsilon \right.$$
$$\left. \text{for some } n \geq 1\right)$$

$$= P\left(n_1 \geq \frac{1}{\log c}\{\log \varepsilon - n \log(T_{1n} + T_{2n}) + n \log(cT_{1n} + T_{2n})\}\right.$$
$$\left. \text{for some } n \geq 1\right) \leq \frac{1}{\varepsilon}.$$

If $c < 1$, the inequality for n_1 reverses. Note the similarity to the previous example, (6).

Finally, as a fourth approach, we put the pair preference method of Armitage into the same context. At the nth death let there be M pairs of patients who have arrived in the study and who have been randomized (by pairs) into the two treatment groups. For each such pair, we can establish a preference only if at least one member has died on or before the time of the nth death. We prefer the treatment associated with longer survival. Let the number of preferences be m and let the number of these for which treatment 1 is *not* preferred be m_1. If p is the probability of not preferring treatment 1, the hypothesis to test here is that $p = \frac{1}{2}$. As shown by Armitage $p = \lambda_1/(\lambda_1 + \lambda_2) = c/(1 + c)$, where c, as above, is λ_1/λ_2. The likelihood ratio is now

$$(9) \qquad \frac{g_n'}{g_n} = \frac{p^{m_1}(1 - p)^{m - m_1}}{(\frac{1}{2})^m} = \left(\frac{p}{1 - p}\right)^{m_1} [2(1 - p)]^m = c^{m_1}\left(\frac{2}{1 + c}\right)^m.$$

Hence, we write Ville's theorem as

$$(10) \qquad P\left(m_1 \geq \frac{1}{\log c}\left\{\log \varepsilon - m \log \frac{2}{1 + c}\right\} \text{ for some } m \geq 1\right) \leq \frac{1}{\varepsilon}.$$

If $c < 1$, the inequality for m_1 reverses. We note once more a similarity in form among this expression and the two previous examples, (6) and (8).

3. Monte Carlo simulation

We produced by Monte Carlo methods a simulated situation in which patients "arrive" at the Clinic in a Poisson process at rate 0.2 per day. The first arrival was randomly assigned treatment R_x1 or R_x2; the second received the other treatment. Each odd numbered arrival was thus assigned a treatment at random. Those receiving R_x1 died according to a Poisson process at risk λ_1, those with R_x2 at risk λ_2. Every time a death occurred, we applied the three stopping rules defined by the inequalities in (6), (8), and (10). For each rule, we recorded the sample number defined as the number of deaths required for terminating the experiment.

We obtained 100 sequential experiments. In each experiment, we arbitrarily limited the number of cases to 200 (100 pairs), following each until death. We let $\lambda_1 = 0.003$, $\lambda_2 = 0.009$, and $c = \frac{1}{3}$. For each of the three stopping rules, each of the 100 experiments stopped before the 200 cases had arrived. For the method of (6), the "number at risk" method, the average sample number (ASN) was 23.2 with a range from 6 to 78. The 90th percentile was 44 and the standard deviation 14.6. For method (8), the "time at risk" method, the ASN was 23.0, range 6 to 78, the 90th percentile 41, and the standard deviation 14.8. These are quite close. Out of the 100 experiments the number at risk method led to a smaller n than the time at risk method 20 times, to a larger n 27 times, and to the same n 53 times.

The stopping rule (10), the pair preference method, tended to require a sample number larger than the above two methods. We found the ASN to be 35.7 with range from 8 to 161, the 90th percentile 61, and the standard deviation 28.2. Out of the 100 experiments this pair preference method was worse (larger n) than both the others 77 times. It was better than both 9 times.

The Monte Carlo procedure was repeated 100 times under the null hypothesis in which both λ_1 and $\lambda_2 = 0.009$ and 100 pairs of patients were followed until all had died. The value of c in (6), (8), and (10), however, was kept at $\frac{1}{3}$. The number at risk method did not stop 97 times, the time at risk method 96 times, and the pair preference method 97 times. In two of the 100 experiments all three methods stopped fairly early (between the 18th and 39th death).

4. Remarks

We have found that two sequential stopping rules (6) and (8) appear to be more sensitive on the average than Armitage's pair preference method (10) in a situation featuring a rather strong difference in the risk of death in two treatment groups. We have also found no apparent difference in the proportion of times the null hypothesis was rejected when really true. The methods used were preliminary. The number of simulated cases might have been too few in the null hypothesis situation. Surely the difference between treatment groups should be varied and simulation retried with smaller differences. Confidence intervals for the value of c in (6), (8), and (10) would also have been valuable.

A word in defense of the pair preference method. Its assumptions are somewhat less restrictive than those in the two other methods given here; the assumption of constant risk can be relaxed somewhat.

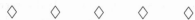

Our thanks go to Mr. Roger Oenning who programmed the Monte Carlo aspects of this study.

REFERENCES

[1] P. Armitage, *Sequential Medical Trials*, Oxford, Blackwell, 1960, Chapter 7.
[2] G. J. Devroede, W. F. Taylor, W. G. Sauer, R. J. Jackman, and G. B. Stickler, "Cancer risk and life expectancy of children with ulcerative colitis," *New England J. Med.*, Vol. 285 (1971), pp. 17–21.
[3] H. Robbins, "Statistical methods related to the law of the iterated logarithm," *Ann. Math. Statist.*, Vol. 41 (1970), pp. 1397–1409.
[4] J. Ville, *Étude Critique de la Notion de Collectif*, Paris, Gauthier-Villars, 1939.
[5] A. Wald, *Sequential Analysis*, New York, Wiley, 1947.

WHEN IS A FIXED NUMBER
OF OBSERVATIONS OPTIMAL?

D. A. DARLING

UNIVERSITY OF CALIFORNIA, IRVINE

1. Introduction

Many of the classical fixed sample size tests and estimates have sequential counterparts which are more economical, needing on the average fewer observations to ensure a given performance. It turns out, however, that under some circumstances, admittedly artificial, a sample of fixed, nonrandom size is optimal.

We determine here rather inclusive conditions ensuring that for a sequence of partial sums of independent, identically distributed random variables, a fixed sample size is optimal with respect to a given nonnegative payoff function.

2. Notations

Let $X_1, X_2, \cdots$ be independent and identically distributed replicates of a random variable X, and set $S_0 = 0$, $S_n = X_1 + X_2 + \cdots + X_n$, $n \geq 1$.

Let M be the set of all real numbers α for which $\varphi(\alpha)$, the moment generating function of X, is finite: $\varphi(\alpha) = E(\exp \{\alpha X\})$ and $M = \{\alpha | \varphi(\alpha) < \infty\}$. The set M is an interval containing $\alpha = 0$, and may consist of all the real numbers, a subinterval of them, or the sole value zero.

The nonnegative function $r_n(x)$, $n = 0, 1, \cdots$, x real, will be called the payoff function in the sense that if one stops observations after n trials his income is $r_n(S_n)$.

The optimal stopping problem is to determine a stopping time N, if possible, such that

$$(1) \qquad E(r_N(S_N)) = \sup_T E(r_T(S_T)),$$

where the sup on the right is taken over all stopping times T. When such a stopping time N exists, we denote its "value" by V; that is, V is the maximal expected payoff given by (1); $V = E(r_N(S_N))$.

The pair (n, x) is called *accessible* if S_n is contained in every neighborhood of x with positive probability. Clearly, the value of $r_n(x)$ at inaccessible points is irrelevant.

This investigation was supported by PHS Research Grant No. GM-10525-08, National Institutes of Health, Public Health Service.

3. The main result

THEOREM. *The fixed integer n_0 is an optimal stopping time for S_n if there exists a measure μ over the set M such that*

$$(2) \quad \int_M \exp\{\alpha x\} \, \varphi^{-n}(\alpha)\mu(d\alpha) \geq r_n(x), \qquad n = 0, 1, 2, \cdots, \qquad -\infty < x < \infty,$$

with equality holding in (2) at all x for which the pair (n_0, x) is accessible. The value is

$$(3) \qquad V = E(r_{n_0}(S_{n_0})) = \mu(M).$$

To prove this theorem, we introduce the space-time chain (n, S_n), $n = 0, 1,$ $\cdots$, and the harmonic functions $h_n(x)$ with respect to it. These are functions with the property that $h_n(x) = E(h_{n+1}(x + X))$, and it is known that any such function can be represented by the integral on the left side of (2), for an appropriate μ. This fact is proved for discrete valued random variables in [1] and [3], and is easily extended to the present case. The set M in the theorem is called the Martin boundary.

Suppose now that μ and n_0 are as stated in the theorem. Then for the corresponding harmonic function $h_n(x)$, the sequence $h_n(S_n)$ is a martingale, and if N is any bounded stopping rule, $h_0(S_0) = \mu(M) = E(h_N(S_N))$. Thus, denoting by $a \wedge b$ the minimum of a and b we have, by Fatou's lemma for any stopping time T,

$$(4) \qquad \mu(M) = E(h_{T \wedge n}(S_{T \wedge n})) = \lim_{n \to \infty} E(h_{T \wedge n}(S_{T \wedge n}))$$

$$\geq E(h_T(S_T)) \geq E(r_T(S_T)).$$

Consequently, for any T, $E(r_T(S_T)) \leq \mu(A)$, and by the definition of accessibility, equality holds everywhere in (4) for the stop rule given by $T = n_0$. Thus, $T = n_0$ is optimal and $V = E(r_{n_0}(S_{n_0})) = \mu(M)$.

There is a certain sense in which the conditions of the theorem are necessary in order that $T = n_0$ be optimal, but we do not discuss them here.

4. Some examples

Let the variables be normally distributed $N(\theta, 1)$ with unknown mean θ and variance 1. Suppose we always estimate θ by taking the sample mean $\overline{X}_n = (1/n)S_n$. Suppose the payoff for stopping after n trials with a sample mean $\overline{X}_n$ is

$$(5) \qquad r_n(S_n) = \exp\left\{\frac{n^2}{2(n+1)} \, (\overline{X}_n - \theta)^2\right\} d_n,$$

where d_n is some numerical sequence. Then if the sequence $d_n(n+1)^{\frac{1}{2}}$ attains its supremum at $n = n_0$, the fixed stopping time n_0 is optimal and the value is $V = d_{n_0}(n_0 + 1)^{\frac{1}{2}}$.

To prove this assertion let $W = d_{n_0}(n_0 + 1)^{\frac{1}{2}} = \sup d_n (n+1)^{\frac{1}{2}}$, and note that $\varphi(\alpha) = \exp\{\theta\alpha + \alpha^2/2\}$. If we take

$$(6) \qquad \mu(d\alpha) = \frac{W}{(2\pi)^{\frac{1}{2}}} \exp\left\{-\frac{\alpha^2}{2}\right\} d\alpha, \qquad -\infty < \alpha < \infty,$$

we obtain for the integral on the left side of equation (2)

$$(7) \qquad h_n(x) = \frac{W}{(2\pi)^{1/2}} \int_{-\infty}^{\infty} \exp\left\{ \alpha x - n\alpha\theta - \frac{n\alpha^2}{2} - \frac{\alpha^2}{2} \right\} d\alpha$$

$$= \frac{W}{(n+1)^{1/2}} \exp\left\{ \frac{(x - n\theta)^2}{2(n+1)} \right\}$$

$$= \frac{W}{(n+1)^{1/2}} \frac{r_n(x)}{d_n}.$$

Hence, $h_n(x) \geq r_n(x)$ if and only if $W \geq d_n (n+1)^{1/2}$. By the definition of W this is true, equality holds when $n = n_0$, and $V = W$.

As a second example, consider the case of the exponential payoff $r_n(S_n) = \exp\{aS_n\} d_n$, where $a \in M$ and d_n is a numerical sequence. Dynkin [2] has shown in this case that a fixed number of trials is optimal, using quite different methods.

This is a special case of the theorem when μ assigns a mass c to the point a, and μ assigns zero measure to any set not containing a.

Then

$$(8) \qquad h_n(x) = \int \exp\{\alpha x\} \varphi^{-n}(\alpha) \mu(d\alpha) = c \exp\{\alpha x\} \varphi^{-n}(a).$$

The condition $h_n(x) \geq r_n(x)$ becomes

$$(9) \qquad c \exp\{ax\} \varphi^{-n}(a) \geq \exp\{ax\} d_n,$$

or $c \geq \varphi^n(a) d_n$, $n = 0, 1, 2, \cdots$.

If we suppose that $\varphi^n(a) d_n$ assumes its supremum at $n = n_0$, and we set $c = \varphi^{n_0}(a) d_{n_0}$, the stopping rule $T = n_0$ is optimal by the theorem, and $V = c$.

REFERENCES

[1] J. L. DOOB, J. L. SNELL, and R. E. WILLIAMSON, "Applications of boundary theory to sums of independent random variables," *Contributions to Probability and Statistics*, Stanford University Press, 1960, pp. 182–197.

[2] E. B. DYNKIN, "Sufficient statistics for the optimal stopping problem," *Theor. Probability Appl.* (English translation), Vol. 13 (1968), pp. 152–153.

[3] J. NEVEU, "Chaînes de Markov et théorie du potentiel," *Ann. Fac. Sci. Clermont-Ferrand*, Vol. 24 (1964), pp. 37–89.

A CLASS OF STOPPING RULES FOR TESTING PARAMETRIC HYPOTHESES

HERBERT ROBBINS and DAVID SIEGMUND
COLUMBIA UNIVERSITY and HEBREW UNIVERSITY

Let $f_\theta(x)$, $\theta \in \Omega$, be a one parameter family of probability densities with respect to some σ-finite measure μ on the Borel sets of the line. Denote by P_θ the probability measure under which random variables $x_1, x_2, \cdots$ are independent with the common probability density $f_\theta(x)$. Let θ_0 be an arbitrary fixed element of Ω and ε any constant between 0 and 1. We are interested in finding stopping rules N for the sequence $x_1, x_2, \cdots$ such that

$$(1) \qquad P_\theta(N < \infty) \leqq \varepsilon \qquad \text{for every } \theta \leqq \theta_0,$$

and

$$(2) \qquad P_\theta(N < \infty) = 1 \qquad \text{for every } \theta > \theta_0.$$

Among such rules, we wish to find those which in some sense minimize $E_\theta(N)$ for all $\theta > \theta_0$.

A method of constructing rules which satisfy (1) and (2) by using mixtures of likelihood ratios was given in [3]. Here we sketch an alternative method.

Let $\theta_{n+1} = \theta_{n+1}(x_1, \cdots, x_n)$ for $n = 0, 1, 2, \cdots$, be any sequence of Borel measurable functions of the indicated variables such that

$$(3) \qquad \theta_{n+1} \geqq \theta_0.$$

In particular, θ_1 is some constant $\geqq \theta_0$. Define

$$(4) \qquad z_n = \prod_1^n \frac{f_{\theta_i}(x_i)}{f_{\theta_0}(x_i)}, \qquad\qquad n = 1, 2, \cdots,$$

and for any constant $b > 0$, let

$$(5) \qquad N = \begin{cases} \text{first } n \geqq 1 \text{ such that } z_n \geqq b, \\ \infty \text{ if no such } n \text{ occurs.} \end{cases}$$

We shall show that under a certain very general assumption on the structure of the family $f_\theta(x)$, the inequality (1) holds at least for all $b \geqq 1/\varepsilon$.

ASSUMPTION. *For every triple $\alpha \leqq \gamma \leqq \beta$ in Ω,*

$$(6) \qquad \int \frac{f_\alpha(x)f_\beta(x)}{f_\gamma(x)} \, d\mu(x) \leqq 1.$$

Research supported by Public Health Service Grant No. 1-R01-GM-16895-03.

We remark without proof that this holds for the general one parameter Koopman-Darmois-Pitman exponential family and many others.

Denote by $\mathfrak{F}_n$ the Borel field generated by $x_1, \cdots, x_n$. Then *for each fixed* $\theta \leqq \theta_0$, $\{z_n, \mathfrak{F}_n, P_\theta; n \geqq 1\}$ *is a nonnegative supermartingale sequence.* For, given any $n \geqq 1$,

$$
(7) \qquad E_\theta(z_{n+1}|\mathfrak{F}_n) = z_n E_\theta \left(\frac{f_{\theta_{n+1}}(x_{n+1})}{f_{\theta_0}(x_{n+1})} \,\middle|\, \mathfrak{F}_n \right)
$$

$$
= z_n \int \frac{f_\theta(x) f_{\theta_{n+1}}(x)}{f_{\theta_0}(x)} \, d\mu(x) \leqq z_n,
$$

since by hypothesis $\theta \leqq \theta_0 \leqq \theta_{n+1}$. We can therefore apply the following.

LEMMA. *Let* $\{z_n, \mathfrak{F}_n, P; n \geqq 1\}$ *be any nonnegative supermartingale. Then for any constant* $b > 0$,

$$
(8) \qquad P(z_n \geqq b \text{ for some } n \geqq 1) \leqq P(z_1 \geqq b) + \frac{1}{b} \int_{(z_1 < b)} z_2 \, dP \leqq \frac{E(z_1)}{b}.
$$

PROOF. Defining N by (5), we have

$$
(9) \qquad P(z_n \geqq b \text{ for some } n \geqq 1) = P(z_1 \geqq b) + P(1 < N < \infty).
$$

Since z_n is a nonnegative supermartingale,

$$
(10) \qquad \int_{(N>1)} z_1 \, dP \geqq \int_{(N>1)} z_2 \, dP = \int_{(N=2)} z_2 \, dP + \int_{(N>2)} z_2 \, dP \geqq \cdots
$$

$$
\geqq \sum_{i=2}^{n} \int_{(N=i)} z_i \, dP + \int_{(N>n)} z_n \, dP \geqq b P(1 < N \leqq n) + 0,
$$

because $z_i \geqq b$ on $(N = i)$ and $z_n \geqq 0$. Since n is arbitrary,

$$
(11) \qquad P(1 < N < \infty) \leqq \frac{1}{b} \int_{(z_1 < b)} z_2 \, dP,
$$

and hence from (9)

$$
(12) \quad P(z_n \geqq b \text{ for some } n \geqq 1) \leqq P(z_1 \geqq b) + \frac{1}{b} \int_{(z_1 < b)} z_2 \, dP
$$

$$
\leqq \frac{1}{b} \int_{(z_1 \geqq b)} z_1 \, dP + \frac{1}{b} \int_{(z_1 < b)} z_1 \, dP = \frac{E(z_1)}{b},
$$

which proves (8).

Applying this lemma to (4) and (5), we see that for each fixed $\theta \leqq \theta_0$,

$$
(13) \qquad P_\theta(N < \infty) \leqq P_\theta(z_1 \geqq b) + \frac{1}{b} \int_{(z_1 < b)} z_2 \, dP_\theta
$$

$$
\leqq \frac{E_\theta(z_1)}{b} = \frac{1}{b} \int \frac{f_\theta(x) f_{\theta_1}(x)}{f_{\theta_0}(x)} \, d\mu(x) \leqq \frac{1}{b},
$$

and hence, as claimed above, (1) holds at least for $b \geqq 1/\varepsilon$.

As an example, suppose that under P_θ the x are $N(\theta, 1)$, so that $f_\theta(x) = \varphi(x - \theta)$, where $\varphi(x)$ is the standard normal density, and that $\theta_0 = 0$. It is easily seen that if $\theta_1 > 0$ then

$$z_n = \prod_1^n \exp\left\{\theta_i x_i - \frac{\theta_i^2}{2}\right\}, \qquad E_\theta(z_1) = \exp\{\theta\theta_1\},$$

(14)

$$P_\theta(z_1 \geq b) = \Phi\left(\theta - \frac{\log b}{\theta_1} - \frac{\theta_1}{2}\right),$$

(15)
$$\int_{(z_1 < b)} z_2 \, dP_\theta = \int_{-\infty}^{\log b/\theta_1 + \theta_1/2} \int_{-\infty}^{\infty} z_2 \varphi(x_2 - \theta)\varphi(x_1 - \theta) \, dx_2 \, dx_1$$

$$\leq \exp\{\theta\theta_1\} \, \Phi\left(\frac{\log b}{\theta_1} - \frac{\theta_1}{2} - \theta\right),$$

where $\Phi(x) = \int_{-\infty}^{x} \varphi(t) \, dt$. Hence, (13) gives for any $\theta \leq 0$, the inequality

(16) $\quad P_\theta\left(\prod_1^n \exp\left\{\theta_i x_i - \frac{\theta_i^2}{2}\right\} \geq b \text{ for some } n \geq 1\right)$

$$\leq \Phi\left(\theta - \frac{\log b}{\theta_1} - \frac{\theta_1}{2}\right) + \frac{1}{b} \exp\{\theta\theta_1\} \, \Phi\left(\frac{\log b}{\theta_1} - \frac{\theta_1}{2} - \theta\right)$$

$$\leq \frac{1}{b} \exp\{\theta\theta_1\}.$$

The middle term of (16) is increasing in θ, so

(17) $\quad P_\theta\left(\prod_1^n \exp\left\{\theta_i x_i - \frac{\theta_i^2}{2}\right\} \geq b \text{ for some } n \geq 1\right)$

$$\leq \Phi\left(-\frac{\log b}{\theta_1} - \frac{\theta_1}{2}\right) + \frac{1}{b} \Phi\left(\frac{\log b}{\theta_1} - \frac{\theta_1}{2}\right) \leq \frac{1}{b}$$

for every $\theta \leq 0$.

We shall now suppose that in addition to the requirement that $\theta_{n+1} = \theta_{n+1}(x_1, \cdots, x_n) \geq 0$, *the sequence θ_n converges to θ with probability 1 under P_θ for each $\theta > 0$.* For example, both

(18)
$$\theta_{n+1} = \frac{\max(0, s_n)}{n}$$

and

(19)
$$\theta_{n+1} = \frac{s_n}{n} + \frac{\varphi(s_n/\sqrt{n})}{\sqrt{n}\Phi(s_n/\sqrt{n})},$$

where $s_n = x_1 + \cdots + x_n$, have this desired property (equation (19) is the posterior expected value of θ given $x_1, \cdots, x_n$ when the prior distribution of θ is flat for $\theta > 0$). Thus, for large n,

(20) $\quad z_n = \prod_1^n \exp\left\{\theta_i x_i - \frac{\theta_i^2}{2}\right\} \approx \prod_1^n \exp\left\{\theta x_i - \frac{\theta^2}{2}\right\} = \exp\left\{\theta s_n - \frac{n\theta^2}{2}\right\} = z_n(\theta),$

say. Now it has been remarked elsewhere [2], and a proof based on [1], pp. 107–108, is easily given, that for any fixed $\theta > 0$,

(21)
$$N_{\theta,b} = \begin{cases} \text{first } n \geq 1 \text{ such that } z_n(\theta) \geq b, \\ \infty \text{ if no such } n \text{ occurs,} \end{cases}$$

is optimal in the sense that if T is any stopping rule of $x_1, x_2, \cdots$ such that

$$(22) \qquad P_0(T < \infty) \leq P_0(N_{\theta,b} < \infty),$$

then $E_\theta(N_{\theta,b}) < \infty$ and $E_\theta(T) \geq E_\theta(N_{\theta,b})$. Thus, the N using (18) or (19) may be expected to be "almost optimal" simultaneously for all values $\theta > 0$. Monte Carlo methods will be needed to get accurate estimates of $P_0(N < \infty)$ and $E_\theta(N)$ for $\theta > 0$. We have, however, been able to find the asymptotic nature of $E_\theta(N)$ as $\theta \to 0$ or $b \to \infty$ in the normal and other cases for various choices of the θ_n sequence, and the results will be published elsewhere. For example, using (18), we can show that, for $\theta > 0$,

$$(23) \qquad E_\theta(N) \sim P_0(N = \infty) \left(\log \frac{1}{\theta} \Big/ \theta^2 \right) \qquad \text{as } \theta \to 0,$$

and

$$(24) \qquad E_\theta(N) = \frac{2 \log b + \log_2 b}{\theta^2} + o(\log_2 b) \qquad \text{as } b \to \infty.$$

By putting

$$(25) \qquad \theta_{n+1} = \begin{cases} \dfrac{s_n}{n} & \text{if } s_n \geq [n(2 \log_2^+ n + 3 \log_3^+ n)]^{1/2}, \\ 0 & \text{otherwise,} \end{cases}$$

where $\log_2 n = \log (\log n)$, and so on, equation (23) is replaced by

$$(26) \qquad E_\theta(N) \sim 2 P_0(N = \infty) \log_2 \frac{1}{\theta} \Big/ \theta^2 \qquad \text{as } \theta \to 0,$$

which is optimal for $\theta \to 0$.

In evaluating $P_\theta(N < \infty)$ for $\theta \leq 0$ with an arbitrary sequence $\theta_{n+1} = \theta_{n+1}(x_1, \cdots, x_n) \geq 0$, $n = 0, 1, 2, \cdots$, and $b > 1$, we see that this probability is equal to

$$(27)$$

$$P_\theta \left(\prod_1^n \exp \left\{ \theta_i x_i - \frac{\theta_i^2}{2} \right\} \geq b \text{ for some } n \geq 1 \right) = \sum_{n=1}^{\infty} \int_{(N=n)} \exp \left\{ \theta s_n - \frac{n\theta^2}{2} \right\} dP_0.$$

For any fixed x and n the function $f(\theta) = \exp \{\theta x - n\theta^2/2\}$ is increasing for $-\infty < \theta < x/n$. Hence if the condition

$$(28) \qquad s_n > 0 \quad \text{whenever} \quad N = n, \qquad n = 1, 2, \cdots,$$

is satisfied, then $P_\theta(N < \infty)$ will be an increasing function of $\theta \leq 0$ (as is the middle term of (16)). Recalling that

$$(29) \qquad N = \begin{cases} \text{first } n \geq 1 \text{ such that } \sum_1^n \left(\theta_i x_i - \dfrac{\theta_i^2}{2} \right) \geq \log b, \\ \infty \text{ if no such } n \text{ occurs,} \end{cases}$$

we see that if $N = 1$, then $\theta_1 x_1 \geq \log b + \theta_1^2/2$ so $s_1 = x_1 > 0$, while if $N = n > 1$, then

$$\sum_1^{n-1} \theta_i x_i < \log b + \frac{1}{2} \sum_1^{n-1} \theta_i^2,$$

(30)

$$\sum_1^n \theta_i x_i \geq \log b + \frac{1}{2} \sum_1^n \theta_i^2,$$

so $\theta_n x_n > 0$, and hence $\theta_n > 0$ and $x_n > 0$. In cases (18) and (25), it follows that $s_{n-1} \geq 0$, and hence $s_n = s_{n-1} + x_n > 0$. Thus, $P_\theta(N < \infty)$ is an increasing function of $\theta \leq 0$ in these cases. Whether this is true for the choice (19) we do not know. Likewise, we do not know whether $P_\theta(N \leq n)$ is an increasing function of θ for each fixed $n = 1, 2, \cdots$, even for (18) or (25). For $\theta > 0$, $P_\theta(N < \infty) = 1$ and $E_\theta(N) < \infty$ in all three cases.

In the case of a general parametric family $f_\theta(x)$, we can try to make $E_\theta(N)$ small for $\theta > \theta_0$ by choosing θ_n to converge properly to θ under P_θ for $\theta > \theta_0$, but a comparison with the methods of [3] remains to be made. The present method of sequentially estimating the true value of θ when it is $> \theta_0$ appears somewhat more natural in statistical problems.

If we do not wish to take advantage of the property (6), we can use, instead of (4),

(31)
$$z_n' = \prod_1^n \frac{f_{\theta_i}(x_i)}{h_n},$$

where $h_n = h_n(x_1, \cdots, x_n) = \sup_{\theta \leq \theta_0} \{\prod_1^n f_\theta(x_i)\}$. The use of (31) has been independently suggested by Edward Paulson. For $\theta \leq \theta_0$, we then have

(32) $\quad P_\theta(z_n' \geq b$ for some $n \geq 1) \leq P_\theta \left(\prod_1^n \frac{f_{\theta_i}(x_i)}{f_\theta(x_i)} \geq b$ for some $n \geq 1 \right) \leq \frac{1}{b}$,

by the lemma above. It would seem, however, that (31) should be less efficient than (4) when the assumption (6) holds.

REFERENCES

[1] Y. S. Chow, H. Robbins, and D. Siegmund, *Great Expectations: The Theory of Optimal Stopping*, Boston, Houghton-Mifflin, 1971.
[2] D. A. Darling and H. Robbins, "Some further remarks on inequalities for sample sums," *Proc. Nat. Acad. Sci.*, Vol. 60 (1968), pp. 1175–1182 (see p. 1181).
[3] H. Robbins, "Statistical methods related to the law of the iterated logarithm," *Ann. Math. Statist.*, Vol. 41 (1970), pp. 1397–1409.

SEQUENTIAL MEDICAL TRIALS WITH DATA DEPENDENT TREATMENT ALLOCATION

B. J. FLEHINGER*

IBM THOMAS J. WATSON RESEARCH CENTER

and

T. A. LOUIS**

COLUMBIA UNIVERSITY

1. Introduction

This paper is concerned with clinical trials intended to determine which, if either, of two treatments for a disease is the superior. The experimental situation is one in which patients arrive for treatment sequentially over some period of time. When a patient is admitted to the trial, he is immediately administered one of the two treatments. The effect of the treatment on the patient may be measured, either immediately, or after some delay. After a certain amount of data is collected, the trial is terminated with the conclusion that one of the two methods is superior or that there is no significant difference between them.

Emphasis in this study is on a search for protocols which assign fewer patients to the inferior treatment as compared to classical statistical methods, while retaining the error probabilities associated with these methods. In these protocols, the assignment of a patient to one of the two treatments being compared is determined by data about patients previously treated. The statistical properties (error probabilities, expected sample sizes, expected number to inferior treatment) of a variety of protocols have been explored by computer simulation, and it has been demonstrated that Wald type sequential procedures can be combined with data dependent assignment rules to reduce the expected number assigned to the inferior treatment. The Neyman-Pearson measures of significance and power remain unchanged.

2. Definition of a protocol

Treatments 1 and 2 are to be compared. The effect on the jth patient assigned to treatment i is assumed to be a random variable X_{ij} with density f_i which

* Also Visiting Associate Professor at Cornell University Graduate School of Medical Sciences and Visiting Investigator at Sloan-Kettering Institute, New York, N.Y.

** This work was done while the author was a consultant at the IBM Thomas J. Watson Research Center, Yorktown Heights, N.Y.

depends upon the treatment. The densities f_1 and f_2 may be characterized by parameters μ_1 and μ_2 with $\mu_1 - \mu_2 = \Delta$. The objective of the clinical trial is the acceptance of one of the following hypotheses:

(2.1)
$$H_0: \Delta = 0, \text{ the two treatments are equally effective,}$$
$$H_1: \Delta \geq \Delta^*, \text{ treatment 1 is better than treatment 2,}$$
$$H_2: \Delta \leq -\Delta^*, \text{ treatment 2 is better than treatment 1,}$$

where Δ^* is a positive constant.

A protocol consists of the following ingredients: (a) admission rule, (b) assignment rule, and (c) termination rule.

The admission rule effectively defines the population under study. It contains both the disease characteristics and the demographic properties that qualify a patient for admission to the trials. It cannot depend on knowledge of the particular treatment to be administered.

The assignment rule selects the particular treatment to be administered to a given patient. In order that bias not be introduced, it is important that the assignment be independent of the characteristics of the individual. Traditionally, this independence is achieved by randomization. In the following section, both deterministic and randomized assignment rules based on data about previous patients will be described.

The termination rule determines when the trials are ended and one of the hypotheses is accepted. This paper considers only Wald SPRT type tests which end when a generalized likelihood ratio crosses a specified boundary.

The performance of a protocol may be characterized by three surfaces, all of them functions of the two parameters μ_1 and μ_2: OC, the probability of rejecting H_0; ASN, the expected number of patients in the trial; ITN, the expected number of patients assigned to the inferior treatment.

3. Assignment rules

Both deterministic and randomized data dependent assignment rules have been thoroughly explored by simulation. All these rules require that at every patient arrival some estimate $\hat{\Delta}$ of Δ be constructed. This estimate can depend only on the effects of treatment on previous patients in the trial. Treatment 1 or 2 will be termed leading at any time according as $\hat{\Delta}$ is or is not greater than zero. The deterministic rules R_γ operate as follows.

Select $\gamma: 0 \leq \gamma \leq 1$, fixed throughout the trial. At the time of the Nth patient arrival, let M_i be the number of patients previously assigned to treatment i. If

(3.1)
$$|M_1 - M_2| < \gamma N, \text{ assign the patient to the leading treatment,}$$
$$|M_1 - M_2| \geq \gamma N, \text{ assign to the treatment with fewer patients}$$
$$\text{previously assigned.}$$

Note that $M_1 + M_2 = N - 1$.

A few observations shed light on the operation of these rules. By a simple calculation, it can be shown that an R_γ rule sets the following bounds on the fraction of patients assigned to either treatment at every stage of the trial:

$$(3.2) \qquad \frac{1-\gamma}{2} - \frac{1}{2N} \le \frac{M_i}{N} \le \frac{1+\gamma}{2} + \frac{1}{2N} \qquad \text{for } i = 1, 2, \text{ all } N.$$

From (3.1), R_0 is strict alternation, while R_1 always assigns to the leading treatment. This class of rules uses as input only data generated within the trial and does not reference data on the particular patient to be assigned.

A randomized rule $\bar{R}_\gamma$ which is approximately equivalent to R_γ with respect to OC, ASN, ITN, is the following. Assign the first patient to treatment 1 or 2 with equal probability and assign the second patient to the other treatment. Assign each succeeding patient to the currently leading treatment with probability $(1 + \gamma)/2$, and to the trailing one with probability $(1 - \gamma)/2$. Here, $\bar{R}_0$ assigns to either treatment with probability $\frac{1}{2}$ throughout the trials, while $\bar{R}_1$ always selects the leading treatment.

4. Termination rules

All the protocols considered in the paper are terminated when a generalized likelihood ratio crosses a specified boundary.

The assumptions in Section 2 on treatment responses can be restated:

$$(4.1) \qquad \begin{aligned} &X_{1j} \text{ has density } f(X_{1j}|\mu_1) = f(X_{1j}|\theta + \Delta/2), \\ &X_{2j} \text{ has density } f(X_{2j}|\mu_2) = f(X_{2j}|\theta - \Delta/2), \end{aligned}$$

where $\theta = (\mu_1 + \mu_2)/2$ is a nuisance parameter lying in some space Θ.

To form the generalized likelihood ratios (LR) used in termination, let

$$(4.2) \qquad \begin{aligned} L_1 = \text{LR } (H_1 \text{ versus } H_0) &= \frac{\sup_{\theta \in \Theta} \prod_{j=1}^{M_1} f(X_{1j}|\theta + \Delta^*/2) \prod_{j=1}^{M_2} f(X_{2j}|\theta - \Delta^*/2)}{\sup_{\theta \in \Theta} \prod_{j=1}^{M_1} f(X_{1j}|\theta) \prod_{j=1}^{M_2} f(X_{2j}|\theta)}, \\[2ex] L_2 = \text{LR } (H_2 \text{ versus } H_0) &= \frac{\sup_{\theta \in \Theta} \prod_{j=1}^{M_1} f(X_{1j}|\theta - \Delta^*/2) \prod_{j=1}^{M_2} f(X_{2j}|\theta + \Delta^*/2)}{\sup_{\theta \in \Theta} \prod_{j=1}^{M_1} f(X_{1j}|\theta) \prod_{j=1}^{M_2} f(X_{2j}|\theta)}. \end{aligned}$$

To terminate the clinical trial the following rule is used. Pick A, B, such that $0 < A < 1 < B < \infty$, and if ever

$$(4.3) \qquad \begin{aligned} &\max (L_1, L_2) < A, \text{ stop and accept } H_0, \\ &\max (L_1, L_2) > B, \text{ stop and accept the appropriate } H_1 \text{ or } H_2, \end{aligned}$$

otherwise continue the clinical trial.

The above procedure will be referred to as GSPRT(A, B). In any testing situation where $EX_{ij}^2 < \infty$, it is not difficult to show that ASN is finite for all R_γ, $\gamma < 1$.

5. Computational example

In general, the R_γ assignment rules coupled with GSPRT termination result in OC surfaces very close to those associated with conventional, data independent assignment rules. Appropriate choices of γ reduce the expected number of patients assigned to the inferior treatment (ITN) with only small increases in ASN.

As an example of the performance of the R_γ family of rules, we have studied, by simulation, the problem of testing for a difference in the means of two normal populations with known, equal variance. Specifically,

$$
\begin{aligned}
X_{11}, X_{12}, \cdots, &\text{ iid } N(\mu_1, 1), \\
X_{21}, X_{22}, \cdots, &\text{ iid } N(\mu_2, 1), \\
\Delta = \mu_1 &- \mu_2.
\end{aligned}
$$

(5.1)

After M_i patients have been administered treatment i, let

$$
(5.2) \qquad \bar{X}_i(M_i) = M_i^{-1} \sum_{j=1}^{M_i} X_{ij}, \qquad M_i > 0, \ i = 1, 2.
$$

The estimate $\hat{\Delta}$ of Δ which is used in the assignment rule (Section 3) is

$$
(5.3) \qquad \hat{\Delta} = \bar{X}_1(M_1) - \bar{X}_2(M_2).
$$

The two generalized likelihood ratios computed from (4.2) which are used in the termination rule are

$$
(5.4) \qquad
\begin{aligned}
L_1 &= \exp\left\{ \Delta^* \frac{M_1 M_2}{M_1 + M_2} (\hat{\Delta} - \Delta^*/2) \right\}, \\
L_2 &= \exp\left\{ \Delta^* \frac{M_1 M_2}{M_1 + M_2} (-\hat{\Delta} - \Delta^*/2) \right\}.
\end{aligned}
$$

Since the testing procedure is invariant under translations of θ, the three surfaces OC, ASN, and ITN are reduced to curves. For given values of Δ^*, γ, A, and B, these functions depend only on Δ, not on μ_1 and μ_2.

Simulation with 5,000 replications was carried out on an IBM 360/91 to investigate the effects of varying Δ^*, γ, A, and B on the three curves OC, ASN, and ITN. Although several pairs of stopping values were considered, $A = 0.1$ and $B = 30$ were used in the tables presented in this paper. The results for this pair are representative of the performance of the R_γ family with other stopping parameters. Simulations have been done for two values of Δ^*, three values of γ, and several values of Δ for each Δ^*, γ pair.

Table I summarizes the OC, ASN, and ITN data from these simulations and Figures 1, 2, and 3 display the curves for $\Delta^* = 0.5$ graphically. The first observation from these data concerns the remarkable constancy of the OC curve with variations of γ. Thus, within the accuracy of the simulation, the OC depends only on the termination parameters and Δ/Δ^*.

TABLE I

PERFORMANCE OF PROTOCOLS
Termination parameters: $A = 0.1$, $B = 30$.
ITN values are not applicable when $\Delta = 0$.

Δ	OC			ASN			ITN		
	$\gamma = 0$	$\gamma = .2$	$\gamma = .5$	$\gamma = 0$	$\gamma = .2$	$\gamma = .5$	$\gamma = 0$	$\gamma = .2$	$\gamma = .5$
$\Delta^* = .5$									
0	.06	.05	.05	125	127	160	—	—	—
.125	.14	.13	.14	139	141	181	70	63	66
.25	.45	.43	.43	160	164	211	80	68	62
.375	.77	.78	.77	141	146	186	71	59	50
.50	.94	.94	.94	102	107	136	51	43	36
.75	1.00	1.00	1.00	56	59	74	28	24	19
1.0	1.00	1.00	1.00	38	40	51	19	16	13
$\Delta^* = 1$									
0	.05	.05	.05	33	34	42	—	—	—
.25	.13	.13	.13	37	39	48	19	17	17
.5	.43	.45	.43	43	46	58	22	19	17
.75	.80	.78	.79	38	40	51	19	16	14
1.0	.96	.95	.96	27	28	36	14	11	10
1.5	1.00	1.00	1.00	15	16	19	8	6	5
2.0	1.00	1.00	1.00	10	10	13	5	4	4

Variations in the value of γ (for $0 \leq \gamma \leq 0.5$) affect only the ASN and ITN curves. In all cases simulated, ASN increases with γ. On the other hand, ITN always decreases initially as γ increases from zero. Changing γ from 0 to 0.2 causes only a small increase in ASN while markedly reducing ITN for all nonzero values of Δ considered. Thus, some of the rules in the R_γ class achieve the stated objective of reducing *ITN* without altering the error probabilities of the clinical trial, and, in fact, accomplish this end without sizable increases in ASN.

In [7] another model for comparing two treatments by data dependent assignment coupled with GSPRT termination was studied. In this model, it is assumed that the effect on a given patient can be measured by his survival time after treatment and that this time is exponentially distributed with a mean life which characterizes the treatment. Patients arrive at fixed intervals of time, so that the data about previous patients are truncated. A modification of the R_γ rule designed for this incomplete information case produced results very similar to those displayed in Table I.

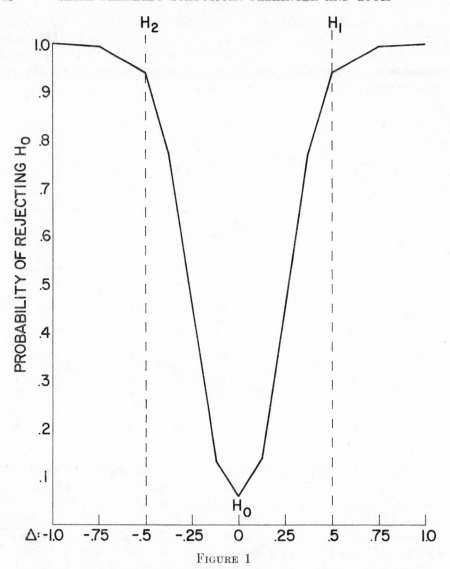

FIGURE 1

OC curves.
$A = 0.1, B = 30, \Delta^* = 0.5.$
Rules: $R_\gamma: \gamma = 0, 0.2, 0.5.$

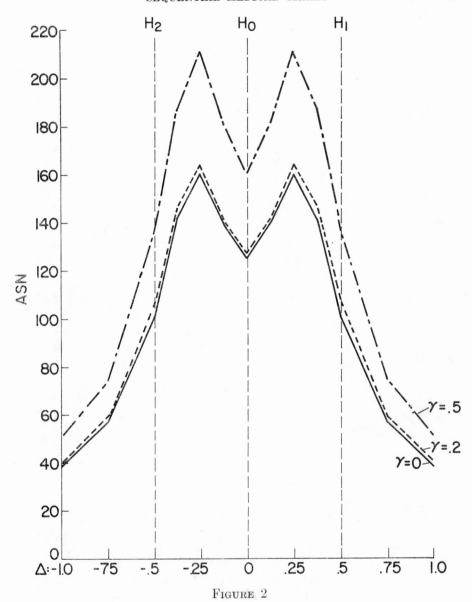

FIGURE 2

ASN curves.
$A = 0.1, B = 30, \Delta^* = 0.5.$
Rules: $R_\gamma: \gamma = 0, 0.2, 0.5.$

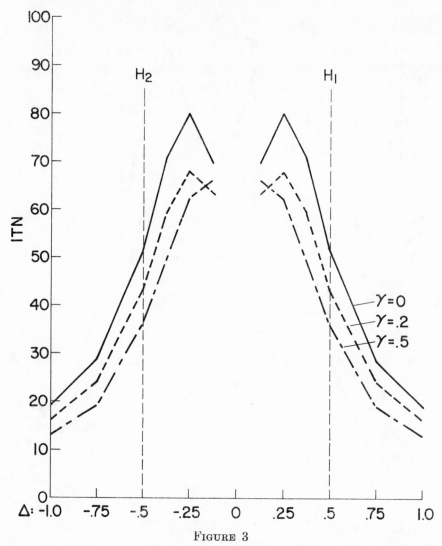

FIGURE 3

ITN curves.
$A = 0.1$, $B = 30$, $\Delta^* = 0.5$.
Rules: R_γ: $\gamma = 0, 0.2, 0.5$.

REFERENCES

[1] F. J. ANSCOMBE, "Sequential medical trials," *J. Amer. Statist. Assoc.*, Vol. 58 (1963), pp. 365–384.

[2] P. ARMITAGE, *Sequential Medical Trials*, Oxford, Blackwell, 1960.

[3] R. N. BRADT, S. M. JOHNSON, and S. KARLIN, "On sequential designs for maximizing the sum of n observations," *Ann. Math. Statist.*, Vol. 27 (1956), pp. 1060–1074.

[4] N. BRESLOW, "On large sample sequential analysis with applications to survivorship data," *J. Appl. Prob.*, Vol. 6 (1969), pp. 261–274.

[5] T. COLTON, "A model for selecting one of two medical treatments," *J. Amer. Statist. Assoc.*, Vol. 58 (1963), pp. 388–401.

[6] J. CORNFIELD, M. HALPERIN, and S. W. GREENHOUSE, "An adaptive procedure for sequential clinical trials," *J. Amer. Statist. Assoc.*, Vol. 64 (1969), pp. 759–770.

[7] B. J. FLEHINGER and T. A. LOUIS, "Sequential treatment allocation in clinical trials," *Biometrika*, Vol. 58 (1971), pp. 419–426.

[8] H. ROBBINS, "Some aspects of the sequential design of experiments," *Bull. Amer. Math. Soc.*, Vol. 58 (1952), pp. 527–535.

[9] ———, "A sequential decision problem with finite memory," *Proc. Nat. Acad. Sci.*, Vol. 42 (1956), pp. 920–923.

[10] M. SOBEL and G. H. WEISS, "Play-the-winner sampling for selecting the better of two binomial populations," *Biometrika*, Vol. 57 (1970), pp. 357–365.

[11] M. ZELEN, "Play-the-winner rule and the controlled clinical trial," *J. Amer. Statist. Assoc.*, Vol. 64 (1969), pp. 131–146.

COMPARISONS OF SEQUENTIAL PROCEDURES FOR SELECTING THE BEST BINOMIAL POPULATION

DAVID HOEL

NATIONAL INSTITUTE OF
ENVIRONMENTAL HEALTH SCIENCES
and
MILTON SOBEL

UNIVERSITY OF MINNESOTA

1. Introduction

Recently the problem of selecting the best one of several binomial populations has been studied from the point of view of different sampling rules. In this paper, we compare some sequential procedures with and without early elimination. The main breakdown is between those using the cyclic play the winner (PWC) sampling rule and those using the vector at a time (VT) sampling rule.

The PWC rule orders the k given populations at random at the outset and uses this ordering in a cyclic manner. After each success, we sample from the same population; after each failure, we switch to the next population in the ordering scheme. After the kth population, we complete the cycle by going back to the first population.

The VT rule consists of taking k tuple observations, one component from each population. In a variation of this, the cyclic (VTC) rule, we start as in the PWC rule by randomizing the order of the populations and then take one observation from each population using the fixed cyclic order; thus, we need not complete the last vector in the VTC rule.

Both of the above rules can be modified as follows. Let the order of the populations sampled be $\pi_1, \pi_2, \cdots, \pi_k$. From the beginning of sampling π_1 to the end of sampling π_k, we have gone through one complete sampling cycle. Our new modification is to reorder the k populations after each complete sampling cycle; this reordering *can* depend on the observed results. We denote such a modification of the PWC and VTC rules by PWO and VTO, respectively.

Several papers dealing with the PW and VT sampling rules [6], [9], [12], and [13] consider termination rules based on a fixed sample size or on inverse sampling, that is, we sample until at least one population reaches a fixed number of

The work of Milton Sobel was supported by NSF Grant GP-11021 at the University of Minnesota.

successes. In [10], $k = 2$ and the termination rule is based on the difference of the numbers of successes. The monograph [1] deals mainly with VT sampling and a stopping rule based on likelihood ratios. (A summary of the above work can be found in [11].) Paulson [7], [8] has brought in early elimination techniques, which (except for [1]) is not a feature of the above references; some discussion of elimination procedures does appear in Chapter 9 of [1].

In this paper, we introduce a new procedure that combines the likelihood approach to the stopping rule with the PWC sampling rule. In Section 4, we derive an extension of the rule in [10] to the case of k populations, which contains the feature of early elimination. Empirical results for the PWO sampling rules are obtained and analyzed for the inverse sampling rule in Section 6. Sections 3 and 4 deal with the PW sampling while Sections 5 and 7 are partly concerned with VT sampling. In Section 5 sequential techniques developed in [3] are applied to Wald's sequential double dichotomy formulation [14], producing a binomial selection procedure with VT sampling and early elimination features.

In Section 7, we briefly describe two other VT rules, originally given in [1] and [7]. Finally, we present empirical results for all of the above procedures in Sections 6 and 7 and make appropriate comparisons.

2. Notation, definition, and requirement

Let p_i denote the single trial success for population π_i and let $q_i = 1 - p_i$, $i = 1, 2, \cdots, k$. The ordered p values are denoted by $p_{[1]} \leq p_{[2]} \leq \cdots \leq p_{[k]}$. For $p_{[k]} > p_{[k-1]}$, a correct selection (CS) is defined as the selection of the population associated with $p_{[k]}$; for equality, either selection is correct. Let Δ denote the value of $p_{[k]} - p_{[k-1]}$. A procedure R is said to satisfy the (Δ^*, P^*) probability (of a correct selection) requirement if

$$(2.1) \qquad P\{CS|R\} \geq P^* \quad \text{whenever} \quad \Delta \geq \Delta^*;$$

here Δ^* (with $0 < \Delta^* < 1$) and P^* (with $1/k < P^* < 1$) are preassigned constants. All the procedures discussed in this paper satisfy this common requirement (2.1).

Let N_i denote the sample size taken from π_i, and let N denote the sum over i of these sample sizes, $i = 1, 2, \cdots, k$. Let $N_{(i)}$ denote the sample size from the population associated with $p_{[i]}$, $i = 1, 2, \cdots, k$. Then we define our loss function by

$$(2.2) \qquad L = \sum_{i=1}^{k} (p_{[k]} - p_{[i]}) N_{(i)}$$

and the corresponding risk function by

$$(2.3) \qquad \text{risk} = \sum_{i=1}^{k} (p_{[k]} - p_{[i]}) E\{N_{(i)}\}.$$

In the applications that we have in mind, the one dealing with clinical trials is uppermost, where p_i denotes the probability of a cure using treatment i. In this application, the primary concern is to reduce the use of poorer treatments. The risk function (2.3) represents the expected number of failures that could have been avoided if we had known beforehand which treatment (or population) is best.

In addition to the above risk function, we are also interested in reducing the expected total number of observations $E\{N|R\}$ for the procedure R.

3. Likelihood procedure for play the winner sampling

In this section, we consider the likelihood procedure that is appropriate for play the winner sampling. The case of general k is considered in Section 3.1 and this is specialized to $k = 2$ in Section 3.2.

3.1. *Likelihood rule for* PW *sampling with general k.*   A likelihood rule based on PW sampling and without early elimination can be developed in a manner similar to that given in [1]. We describe this procedure for $k = 3$ and specialize to $k = 2$ in Section 3.2; the generalization to arbitrary k is a straightforward extension of the case $k = 3$.

Let $S_1 \leq S_2 \leq S_3$ denote the current number of successes from the three populations and let F_i represent the current number of failures from the population associated with S_i, $i = 1, 2, 3$. If $S_3 = S_2 (> S_1)$, we associate S_3 with the smaller of the two corresponding F values; similarly for $S_1 = S_2 = S_3$, we assign S_3 to the one with the smallest F value. If it is still not determined, then we use randomization. However, it is shown below that for $P^* \geq \frac{1}{2}$ our rule never terminates sampling when randomization is used. Let $p_{[1]} \leq p_{[2]} \leq p_{[3]}$ be the ordered (unknown) probabilities of success on a single trial.

The method, based on the techniques in [1], is to write the most likely of the three possible assignments of the pair (S_3, F_3) with the ordered p values and to stop sampling when the minimum (over that part of the parameter space for which $p_{[3]} - p_{[2]} \geq \Delta^*$) of the corresponding likelihood ratio is at least P^*. More specifically, let the likelihood $L(\alpha, \beta, \gamma)$ be defined by

$$(3.1) \qquad L(\alpha, \beta, \gamma) = p_{[1]}^{S_\alpha}(1 - p_{[1]})^{F_\alpha} p_{[2]}^{S_\beta}(1 - p_{[2]})^{F_\beta} p_{[3]}^{S_\gamma}(1 - p_{[3]})^{F_\gamma},$$

where (α, β, γ) is a permutation of $(1, 2, 3)$. Let the likelihood ratio $\mathcal{L}(3)$ be defined by

$$(3.2) \qquad \mathcal{L}(3) = \frac{L(1, 2, 3) + L(2, 1, 3)}{\Sigma L(\alpha, \beta, \gamma)},$$

where the sum is over all $3! = 6$ possible permutations. This likelihood ratio $\mathcal{L}(3)$ associates S_3 with $p_{[3]}$ and $\mathcal{L}(j)$ is defined similarly to (3.2) and associates S_j with $p_{[3]}, j = 1, 2$. It is a basic result in [1] (pp. 17 and 18) that if any procedure R has the property at stopping time that

$$(3.3) \qquad \max_j \min \mathcal{L}(j) \geq P^*,$$

where the minimum is over all points in the parameter space for which $p_{[3]} - p_{[2]} \geq \Delta^*$, then R must satisfy the P^* condition (2.1). It is believed, also shown in [1] (part 1 of Theorem 6.1.1), that this minimum in (3.3) is generally attained at some generalized favorable configuration (GLF) in which

$$(3.4) \qquad p_{[1]} = p_{[2]} = p - \Delta^*,$$

where we now use p to designate $p_{[3]}$ (this has not been demonstrated). Assuming that $\mathcal{L}(3)$ yields the maximum in (3.3) at termination (which is also not yet shown), it follows by straightforward algebra that we can write (3.3) in the form

$$(3.5) \qquad \max_{\Delta^* \leq p \leq 1} \left\{ \frac{L(3, 2, 1) + L(2, 3, 1) + L(1, 3, 2) + L(3, 1, 2)}{L(1, 2, 3) + L(2, 1, 3)} \right\} \leq \frac{1 - P^*}{P^*}.$$

Using (3.1), we obtain for (3.5) the explicit form

$$(3.6) \qquad \max_{\Delta^* \leq p \leq 1} \left\{ \left(\frac{p - \Delta^*}{p}\right)^{T_1} \left(\frac{1 - p}{1 - p + \Delta^*}\right)^{U_1} + \left(\frac{p - \Delta^*}{p}\right)^{T_2} \left(\frac{1 - p}{1 - p + \Delta^*}\right)^{U_2} \right\}$$
$$\leq \frac{1 - P^*}{P^*},$$

where $T_i = S_3 - S_i$ and $U_i = F_i - F_3$, $i = 1, 2$. For the case of VT sampling, we note that $F_j - F_3 = S_3 - S_j$, $j = 1, 2$ and the stopping rule (3.6) reduces to that given in [1] and in Section 7 below. For PW sampling the above does not hold and we note that $F_j - F_3$ can only take the values -1, 0, and $+1$. If $F_j - F_3 = -1$ for either $j = 1$ or $j = 2$, then the left side of (3.6) clearly tends to ∞, and hence the inequality cannot be satisfied. Thus, we can state the following stopping rule.

Stopping rule for procedure R_{LPW}: stop sampling as soon as $F_3 \leq \min(F_1, F_2)$ and (3.6) holds.

The terminal decision rule is to select the population associated with S_3. If $S_3 = S_2$ and $F_3 = F_2$ at stopping time, then we randomize between these two populations with probability $\frac{1}{2}$ for each. Since $P^* > \frac{1}{3}$, we cannot terminate with both $S_3 = S_2 = S_1$ and $F_3 = F_2 = F_1$. Moreover, for $P^* \geq \frac{1}{2}$ the value of $(1 - P^*)/P^* \leq 1$ and the inequality (3.6) cannot hold if $S_3 = S_2$ and $F_3 = F_2$. Hence, we will never have to randomize in our termination rule when $P^* \geq \frac{1}{2}$.

It should be noted that the procedure R_{LPW} is carried out by computing the maximum in (3.6) after every single observation and this can be tedious. However, it is possible to use (3.6) to construct a set of stopping points for any given P^*. This set turns out to be fairly small and thus becomes a convenient method of describing the entire stopping rule. Illustrations of such stopping sets are given in Table I for $\Delta^* = 0.1, 0.2$ and $P^* = 0.75, 0.90, 0.95, 0.99$. For example, for the pair $(\Delta^* = 0.2, P^* = 0.90)$ there are 11 pairs of stopping points given in Table I. If $F_1 = F_2 = F_3$, then sampling terminates as soon as $T_2 = S_3 - S_2 \geq 10$ and $T_1 = S_3 - S_1 \geq 26$ *or* as soon as $T_2 \geq 11$ and $T_1 \geq 17$ *or*, and so forth.

A conservative variation of the above rule replaces $(1 - p)/(1 - p + \Delta^*)$ in (3.6) by its upper bound 1 when $F_3 \leq \min(F_1, F_2)$ and we obtain the following stopping rule.

TABLE I

STOPPING POINTS FOR THE SEQUENTIAL LIKELIHOOD PROCEDURE
R_{LPW} WITH $k = 3$ POPULATIONS
$T_1 = S_3 - S_1$, $T_2 = S_3 - S_2$ as defined in the text.
Note: some numerical results for these procedures are given in Tables V, VI, and VII.

$\Delta^* = 0.1$

P^*	$F_1 = F_2 = F_3$ T_1	T_2	$F_1 = F_2 = F_3 + 1$ T_1	T_2	$F_2 = F_3 = F_1 - 1$ T_1	T_2	$F_1 = F_3 = F_2 - 1$ T_1	T_2
0.75	18	17	11	10	13	13	13	13
	19	16	13	9	15	12	14	11
	20	15	14	8	20	11	15	10
	22	14	17	7			16	9
	25	13	23	6			18	8
	29	12					20	7
	38	11					26	6
0.90	28	27	20	19	23	23	23	21
	30	26	21	18	24	22	24	20
	31	25	22	17	30	21	25	19
	33	24	24	16			26	18
	37	23	28	15			27	17
	42	22	36	14			29	16
	61	21					32	15
							40	14
0.95	35	35	26	25	30	29	30	27
	36	34	27	24	37	28	31	26
	37	33	29	23			32	25
	38	32	31	22			33	24
	41	31	34	21			34	23
	44	30	42	20			36	22
	50	29					39	21
	78	28					47	20
0.99	51	50	40	39	45	44	45	42
	52	49	41	38			46	40
	54	48	42	37			47	39
	56	47	44	36			48	38
	58	46	47	35			49	37
	63	45	53	34			51	36
	75	44					54	35
							59	34

$\Delta^* = 0.2$

P^*	$F_1 = F_2 = F_3$ T_1	T_2	$F_1 = F_2 = F_3 + 1$ T_1	T_2	$F_2 = F_3 = F_1 - 1$ T_1	T_2	$F_1 = F_3 = F_2 - 1$ T_1	T_2
0.75	9	8	4	4	6	6	6	5
	10	7	6	3	9	5	7	4
	12	6	10	2			8	3
	24	5					11	2
0.90	13	13	8	8	11	10	11	8
	15	12	9	7			12	7
	17	11	11	6			14	6
	26	10						
0.95	17	16	11	10	14	14	14	11
	19	15	13	9			15	10
	22	14	20	8			17	9
							23	8
0.99	24	24	17	17	21	21	21	18
	25	23	18	16			22	17
	27	22	20	15			23	16
	32	21					24	15

Stopping rule for the conservative likelihood procedure R'_{LPW}: stop sampling as soon as $F_3 \leqq \min (F_1, F_2)$ and

$$(3.7) \qquad (1 - \Delta^*)^{T_1} + (1 - \Delta^*)^{T_2} \leqq \frac{1 - P^*}{P^*}.$$

It will be seen in Section 7 that when $P^* = 0.95$ and $\Delta^* = 0.2$, this conservative rule roughly causes a 20 per cent increase in the total expected number of observations, $E\{N\}$ above that for the procedure R_{LPW}.

3.2. *Likelihood rule for* PW *sampling with* $k = 2$. The special case $k = 2$ is of particular interest because we can make the procedure more explicit and because we can make comparisons with other procedures already studied, for example, the procedure R_{PW} in [10]. The derivation in Section 3.1 above gives for $k = 2$ the following stopping rule.

Stopping rule for $R_{\text{LPW}}(k = 2)$: stop as soon as $F_2 \leqq F_1$ (that is, $F_1 - F_2 = 0$ or 1) *and*

$$(3.8) \qquad \max_{\Delta^* \leqq p \leqq 1} \left\{ \left(\frac{p - \Delta^*}{p} \right)^{S_2 - S_1} \left(\frac{1 - p}{1 - p + \Delta^*} \right)^{F_1 - F_2} \right\} \leqq \frac{1 - P^*}{P^*}.$$

After randomization, let I denote the population that we sample from first and II the other population. Then $F_1 = F_2$ in (3.8) when we are sampling from I and $F_1 = F_2 + 1$ in (3.8) when we are sampling from II and II has more successes. Hence, we stop and select I as soon as $S_2 - S_1 = t$ (if this happens before another equality below), where $t > 0$ is the smallest integer equal to or greater than the solution of

$$(3.9) \qquad t = \frac{\log \left(\dfrac{1 - P^*}{P^*} \right)}{\log (1 - \Delta^*)}.$$

We stop and select II as soon as $S_2 - S_1 = s$ (if this happens first), where $s > 0$ is the smallest integer for which

$$(3.10) \qquad \max_{\Delta^* \leqq p \leqq 1} \left\{ \left(\frac{p - \Delta^*}{p} \right)^s \left(\frac{1 - p}{1 - p + \Delta^*} \right) \right\} \leqq \frac{1 - P^*}{P^*}.$$

It is easily seen that $t \geqq s$ and that we will only select a population after getting a success from that same population. This differs from the procedure R_{PW} in [10] only in that we allow $t \geqq s$ and in [10] only $t = s$ is considered (see Table II).

Using the recursion formula method given in [10], we can now derive an exact expression for the $P\{CS\}$, $E\{N\}$, and the expected number of observations $E\{N_B\}$ on the poorer treatment. This will be done for arbitrary positive s and t and, as a special case, we can then set s and t equal to the values obtained above by the likelihood approach. Let p (respectively, p') be associated with population I (respectively, II), let $NT = I$ mean that the next trial is on population I, let (s, t) denote the stopping points, and define

$$(3.11) \qquad \begin{aligned} P_n &= P_n(s, t) = P \{I \text{ is selected}|S_I - S_{II} = n, NT = I, (s, t)\}, \\ Q_n &= Q_n(s, t) = P \{I \text{ is selected}|S_I - S_{II} = n, NT = II, (s, t)\}. \end{aligned}$$

TABLE II

Stopping Points for the Sequential Likelihood Procedure
R_{LPW} with $k = 2$ Populations

P^*	$\Delta^* = 0.1$		$\Delta^* = 0.2$	
	$F_1 = F_2$ $S_2 - S_1$	$F_1 = F_2 + 1$ $S_2 - S_1$	$F_1 = F_2$ $S_2 - S_1$	$F_1 = F_2 + 1$ $S_2 - S_1$
0.75	11	6	5	2
0.90	21	14	10	6
0.95	28	20	14	8
0.99	44	34	21	15

The Common Values of r Required by the Procedure
R_{PW} of [10]
Use 7 and 8 with probability (weight) 0.679 and 0.321, respectively, in order to obtain a PCS of exactly $P^* = 0.75$
with $\Delta^* = 0.1$.

P^*	$\Delta^* = 0.1$	$\Delta^* = 0.2$
0.75	7.32	3.19
0.90	16.45	7.38
0.95	22.96	10.44
0.99	37.82	17.56

Then the PW sampling scheme, conditional on I being the better population leads to the recursion

$$(3.12) \qquad \begin{aligned} P_n &= pP_{n+1} + qQ_n, \\ Q_n &= p'Q_{n-1} + q'P_n, \end{aligned}$$

with boundary conditions $P_t = 1$ and $Q_{-s} = 0$.

From (3.12), we find that

$$(3.13) \qquad P_n(s, t) = \frac{q' - q\lambda^{s+n}}{q' - q\lambda^{s+t}}; \qquad Q_n(s, t) = \frac{q'(1 - \lambda^{s+n})}{q' - q\lambda^{s+t}},$$

where $\lambda = p'/p \leqq 1$. Setting $n = 0$, we obtain the conditional PCS $= P_0(s, t)$ given that I is the better population. For the same problem, we define the dual expressions

$$(3.14) \qquad \begin{aligned} P_n' &= P_n'(s, t) = P \{II \text{ is selected} | S_{II} - S_I = n, \ NT = II, \ (s, t)\}, \\ Q_n' &= Q_n'(s, t) = P \{II \text{ is selected} | S_{II} - S_I = n, \ NT = I, \ (s, t)\}, \end{aligned}$$

and let p (respectively, p') be associated with II (respectively, I). Then we find that the recursive scheme is exactly as in (3.12) with the new boundary conditions $P_s' = 1$ and $Q_{-t}' = 0$, which differ from the above only in that s and t are interchanged. It follows that the conditional PCS given that II is the better population is $Q_0'(s, t)$ and this is obtained from (3.13) by merely interchanging s and t, that is, $Q_0'(s, t) = Q_0(t, s)$. Hence, from these two conditional PCS results, we obtain

$$(3.15) \qquad P\{CS|R_{\text{LPW}}\} = \frac{P_0(s, t) + Q_0(t, s)}{2} = \frac{q' - \frac{1}{2}(q\lambda^s + q'\lambda^t)}{q' - q\lambda^{s+t}}.$$

It is easily seen that for the three extreme cases $p' \to 0$, $p' \to p > 0$, and $p \to 1$ we obtain from (3.15), $P(CS) = 1$, $\frac{1}{2}$, and $1 - (p')^t/2$, respectively.

Using an analogous method to obtain $E\{N_B\}$, the number of observations on the poorer population, we define

$$(3.16) \qquad \begin{aligned} U_n &= U_n(s, t) = E\{N_{II}|S_I - S_{II} = n, NT = I, (s, t)\}, \\ V_n &= V_n(s, t) = E\{N_{II}|S_I - S_{II} = n, NT = II, (s, t)\}, \end{aligned}$$

and associate p with population I. Then the PW sampling scheme leads to the recursion

$$(3.17) \qquad \begin{aligned} U_n &= pU_{n+1} + qV_n, \\ V_n &= p'V_{n-1} + q'U_n + 1, \end{aligned}$$

with boundary conditions $U_t = 0 = V_{-s}$. It can be shown (and it is sufficient to verify) that

$$(3.18) \qquad \begin{aligned} U_n(s, t) &= \frac{q(t - n)}{p(1 - \lambda)} - \frac{q[p + q(s + t)]\lambda^s(\lambda^n - \lambda^t)}{p(1 - \lambda)(q' - q\lambda^{s+t})}, \\ V_n(s, t) &= \frac{p + q(t - n)}{p(1 - \lambda)} - \frac{[p + q(s + t)]\lambda^s(q'\lambda^n - q\lambda^t)}{p(1 - \lambda)(q' - q\lambda^{s+t})}. \end{aligned}$$

The conditional $E\{N_B\}$ given that I is the better population is $V_0(s, t)$. We again define new quantities dual to (3.16) by writing

$$(3.19) \qquad \begin{aligned} U'_n &= U'_n(s, t) = E\{N_I|S_{II} - S_I = n, NT = II, (s, t)\}, \\ V'_n &= V'_n(s, t) = E\{N_I|S_{II} - S_I = n, NT = I, (s, t)\}, \end{aligned}$$

and letting p be associated with population II. Then we get the same recursion scheme as in (3.17) with the new boundary conditions $U'_s = 0 = V'_{-t}$, so that we need only interchange s and t in (3.18) to solve for (3.19). Hence, the conditional $E\{N_B\}$ given that II is the better population is $V'_0(s, t) = V_0(t, s)$. Hence, from (3.18),

$$(3.20) \quad E\{N_B|R_{\text{LPW}}\} = \frac{U_0(s, t) + V_0(t, s)}{2} = \frac{[p + q(s + t)](1 - \lambda^t)(q' - q\lambda^s)}{2p(1 - \lambda)(q' - q\lambda^{s+t})}.$$

Similarly, to find $E\{N_A\}$, we replace N_{II} by N_I in (3.16) and obtain, in place of (3.17),

$$(3.21) \qquad \begin{aligned} \tilde{U}_n &= p\tilde{U}_{n+1} + q\tilde{V}_n + 1, \\ \tilde{V}_n &= p'\tilde{V}_{n-1} + q'\tilde{U}_n, \end{aligned}$$

with boundary conditions $\tilde{U}_t = 0 = \tilde{V}_{-s}$. The solution of this set is

$$(3.22) \qquad \begin{aligned} \tilde{U}_n(s, t) &= \frac{q'(t - n)}{p(1 - \lambda)} - \frac{q[p' + q'(s + t)]\lambda^s(\lambda^n - \lambda^t)}{p(1 - \lambda)(q' - q\lambda^{s+t})}, \\ \tilde{V}_n(s, t) &= \frac{p' + q'(t - n)}{p(1 - \lambda)} - \frac{[p' + q'(s + t)]\lambda^s(q'\lambda^n - q\lambda^t)}{p(1 - \lambda)(q' - q\lambda^{s+t})}. \end{aligned}$$

Again, we set up the dual quantities

$$(3.23) \quad \begin{aligned} \tilde{U}'_n &= \tilde{U}'_n(s, t) = E\{N_{II}|S_{II} - S_I = n, NT = II, (s, t)\}, \\ \tilde{V}'_n &= \tilde{V}'_n(s, t) = E\{N_{II}|S_{II} - S_I = n, NT = I, (s, t)\}, \end{aligned}$$

and let p be associated with population II. Then the recursion is the same as in (3.21) with the boundary conditions $\tilde{U}'_s = 0 = \tilde{V}'_{-t}$, so that we need only interchange s and t in (3.22). Hence, the conditional $E\{N_A\}$ given that II is the better population is $\tilde{V}'_0(s, t) = \tilde{V}(t, s)$. It follows from (3.22) that

$$(3.24) \quad E\{N_A|R_{\text{LPW}}\} = \frac{U_0(s, t) + V_0(t, s)}{2} = \frac{[p' + q'(s + t)](q' - q\lambda^s)(1 - \lambda^t)}{2p(1 - \lambda)(q' - q\lambda^{s+t})}.$$

Adding $E\{N_A\}$ and $E\{N_B\}$, gives

$$(3.25) \quad E\{N|R_{\text{LPW}}\} = \left(\frac{\bar{p} + q(s + t)}{p}\right)\left(\frac{1 - \lambda^t}{1 - \lambda}\right)\left(\frac{q' - q\lambda^s}{q' - q\lambda^{s+t}}\right),$$

where $\bar{p} = (p + p')/2$ and $\bar{q} = 1 - \bar{p}$.

For the case $p = p'$, we take the limits in (3.20), (3.24), and (3.25) as $p' \to p$ and obtain

$$(3.26) \quad E\{N_B|R_{\text{LPW}}\} = E\{N_A|R_{\text{LPW}}\} = \tfrac{1}{2}E\{N|R_{\text{LPW}}\} = \frac{t(p + qs)}{2p},$$

which is comparable with $r(p + qr)/2p$ obtained in (2.11) in [11] for the procedure R_{PW} with $s = t \, (= r)$. If, as is usually the case, we have $t > r > s$ and $st < r^2$, then each of these three expectations is smaller under R_{PW} for q close to zero and each is smaller under R_{LPW} for p close to zero. Thus, neither of these procedures can be uniformly better than the other, that is, throughout the parameter space. Since t in (3.9) is asymptotically $(\Delta^* \to 0)$ like r in (2.13) of [11], it follows that the same lack of a uniform result holds in comparing R_{LPW} and the vector at a time procedure R_{VT}, that is, $E\{N|R_{\text{VT}}\}$ is smaller for $p \to 0$ and $E\{N|R_{\text{LPW}}\}$ is smaller for $p \to 1$.

To illustrate the results of procedure R_{LPW} and compare them with the procedure R_{PW} in [10], we consider the pair $(P^* = 0.95, \Delta^* = 0.2)$ and put the results in tabular form. For the procedure R_{PW}, we need to randomize between $r = 10$ (with probability 0.555) and $r = 11$ (with probability 0.445); this achieves the P^* value $0.555(0.945) + 0.445(0.956) = 0.950$ in the LF configuration. For the procedure R_{LPW}, we randomize between the pair $(s = 7, t = 11)$ with probability 0.434 and the pair $(s = 8, t = 12)$ with probability 0.566; this achieves the P^* value $0.434(0.943) + 0.566(0.955) = 0.950$ in the LF configuration. In randomizing between these two particular pairs $(7, 11)$ and $(8, 12)$, for procedure R_{LPW}, rather than other pairs, such as $(7, 12)$ and $(8, 12)$, our criterion was to minimize the maximum of $E\{N_B\}$, which generally occurs at $\bar{p} = \Delta^*/2$. This also seems to minimize the maximum for $E\{N\}$ and $E\{N_A\}$, which also generally occur at $\bar{p} = \Delta^*/2$.

The comparison of R_{PW} and R_{LPW} in Table III shows that the latter has a smaller $E\{N_B\}$ and $E\{N\}$ in 17 out of the 18 entries. Thus, we have effected a

TABLE III

A COMPARISON OF PROCEDURES R_{PW} AND R_{LPW} FOR $k = 2$, $P^* = 0.95$, AND
$\Delta^* = 0.2$ IN THE GLF CONFIGURATION $\Delta = 0.2$
Note that randomization was used to make $P^* = 0.95$ exactly in both cases;
see text for details.

$\bar{p} = \dfrac{p + p'}{2}$	$E\{N_B\}$		$E\{N_A\}$		$E\{N\}$	
	R_{PW}	R_{LPW}	R_{PW}	R_{LPW}	R_{PW}	R_{LPW}
0.1	42.28	38.76	52.22	47.83	94.50	86.59
0.2	37.31	34.22	47.25	43.29	84.55	77.51
0.3	32.29	29.56	42.22	38.59	74.51	68.15
0.4	27.13	24.71	36.99	33.61	64.12	58.33
0.5	21.85	19.80	31.55	28.51	53.40	48.31
0.6	16.60	15.04	26.08	23.50	42.68	38.54
0.7	11.55	10.54	20.77	18.80	32.32	29.33
0.8	6.77	6.33	15.79	14.50	22.56	20.83
0.9	2.26	2.31	11.23	10.69	13.49	13.00

fairly uniform improvement, with emphasis on the maximum value at $\bar{p} = \Delta^*/2$, although (as was expected) the improvement is not substantial anywhere. However, in the context of clinical trials even slight decreases in $E\{N_B\}$ are important.

4. An elimination procedure R_{EPW}

For $k > 2$, we define an elimination procedure which is an extension of the procedure R_{PW} defined for $k = 2$ and studied in [10]. Under R_{PW}, we stop sampling when $|s_i - s_j| = r$, where s_i is the number of successes from π_i, $i \neq j$, $i = 1, 2, j = 1, 2$. Assuming $s_i > s_j$, we then select π_i as the better population. The approximate value of r required to satisfy (2.1) is the smallest integer equal to or greater than r_2, where

$$(4.1) \qquad r_2 = \frac{\log 2(1 - P^*)}{\log (1 - \Delta^*)}.$$

We extend this procedure as follows. Population π_j is eliminated if for some π_i (not yet eliminated) $s_i - s_j = r$. Let π_k be the best population. Since

$$(4.2) \qquad 1 - P\{CS\} \leqq \Sigma P \{\pi_i \text{ eliminates } \pi_k\} \leqq (k - 1)(1 - P^*),$$

it follows that

$$(4.3) \qquad P\{CS\} \geqq 1 - (k - 1)(1 - P^*).$$

If we now set the right side of (4.3) equal to $\tilde{P}^*$, solve for P^*, and substitute the result in (4.1), then it is clear that the resulting procedure which uses throughout for r the smallest integer equal to or greater than

$$(4.4) \qquad r_k = \frac{\log\left\{ 2 \dfrac{(1 - \tilde{P}^*)}{k - 1} \right\}}{\log (1 - \Delta^*)}.$$

satisfies

(4.5) $$P\{CS|R_{\text{EPW}}\} \geq \tilde{P}^* \quad \text{whenever} \quad \Delta \geq \Delta^*.$$

Monte Carlo results for R_{EPW} and comparisons with other procedures can be found in Tables V, VI, and VII (below).

5. Elimination with Wald's double dichotomy

For $k \geq 2$, we investigate the numerical results of an elimination procedure which is derived in [5] and based on general methods from [3] applied to the double dichotomy problem as formulated by Wald [14].

This procedure R_{EVT} uses the VT sampling rule and eliminates population π_j if for some π_i (not yet eliminated),

(5.1) $$s_i - s_j \geq c + dn^*,$$

where $c > 0$ and $d \leq 0$ are predetermined constants and n^* is the number of unlike pairs from π_i and π_j (that is, observations in the same vector of the form S, F or F, S).

We now give the values of c and d that satisfy the requirement (2.1). Define τ_0 by

(5.2) $$\tau_0 = \left(\frac{1 - \Delta^*}{1 + \Delta^*}\right)^2 < 1,$$

and let τ_1 denote any value such that

(5.3) $$\tau_0 < \tau_1 \leq \frac{1}{\tau_0}.$$

It is shown in [5] that by taking

(5.4) $$c = \frac{2 \log \left(\frac{k - 1}{1 - P^*}\right)}{\log \frac{\tau_1}{\tau_0}}, \qquad d = \frac{2 \log \left(\frac{1 + \tau_1}{1 + \tau_0}\right)}{\log \frac{\tau_1}{\tau_0}} - 1,$$

the requirement (2.1) will be satisfied. We select $\tau_1 = 1/\tau_0$ for our Monte Carlo studies and this implies that $d = 0$, the reason being that asymptotically $(P^* \to 1)$ at the generalized least favorable configuration (that is, when $p_{[1]} = p_{[2]} = \cdots = p_{[k-1]} = p_{[k]} - \Delta^*$), the risk defined in (2.3) is minimized for this value of τ_1 (see [5]).

The use of $d = 0$ above also provides us with the analogous elimination procedure for extending the procedure R_{VT} in [10] to $k > 2$ in the same way that we extended R_{PW} in Section 4.

6. Comparisons of several play the winner procedures for $k = 2$

In this section, our aim is to make a comparison for $k = 2$ of the likelihood procedure developed in Section 3.2 with some other procedures that satisfy the

TABLE IV

EXPECTED SAMPLE SIZES FOR $k = 2$ UNDER FIVE PW PROCEDURES $(P^* = 0.95, \Delta^* = 0.2)$
The table gives $E\{N_B\}$, $E\{N\}$ for $\Delta = 0.2$ and $E_0\{N\}$ for $\Delta = 0$ in each cell.
For R_I and R_{IO}, use $r = 20$ and 21 with weights 0.958 and 0.042, respectively.
For R_H, use $r = 33$ and 34 with weights 0.6 and 0.4, respectively.
For R_{IT}, use $r = 20$ and 21 with weights 0.761 and 0.239, respectively.

$\bar{p} = \dfrac{p + p'}{2}$		R_{LPW}	R_I	R_{IO}	R_H	R_{IT}
0	$E_0\{N\}$	∞	∞	∞	65.8	40.5
	$E\{N_B\}$	38.8	80.7	80.2	26.8	20.2
0.1	$E\{N\}$	86.6	180.9	180.4	59.7	45.5
	$E_0\{N\}$	801.2	348.4	348.0	64.2	45.0
	$E\{N_B\}$	34.2	52.5	52.0	26.1	22.5
0.2	$E\{N\}$	77.5	119.3	118.8	59.0	51.4
	$E_0\{N\}$	362.6	173.0	172.5	63.2	50.6
	$E\{N_B\}$	29.6	38.2	37.5	25.2	24.9
0.3	$E\{N\}$	68.2	88.3	87.6	58.0	58.0
	$E_0\{N\}$	216.4	114.4	113.7	62.2	57.8
	$E\{N_B\}$	24.7	29.2	28.5	24.1	25.7
0.4	$E\{N\}$	58.3	69.1	68.4	56.9	61.1
	$E_0\{N\}$	143.2	84.8	84.2	61.4	65.3
	$E\{N_B\}$	19.8	22.9	22.1	22.6	22.7
0.5	$E\{N\}$	48.3	56.0	55.2	55.3	55.7
	$E_0\{N\}$	99.4	67.0	66.2	60.2	64.8
	$E\{N_B\}$	15.0	17.7	17.0	20.5	18.0
0.6	$E\{N\}$	38.5	46.0	45.2	53.2	46.6
	$E_0\{N\}$	70.0	54.8	53.9	59.0	55.3
	$E\{N_B\}$	10.5	13.5	12.5	17.5	13.6
0.7	$E\{N\}$	29.3	38.2	37.1	50.2	38.5
	$E_0\{N\}$	49.2	45.8	44.7	57.6	46.3
	$E\{N_B\}$	6.3	8.9	7.8	12.5	8.9
0.8	$E\{N\}$	20.8	30.8	29.7	45.3	31.1
	$E_0\{N\}$	33.6	38.4	37.1	55.2	38.9
	$E\{N_B\}$	2.3	2.5	2.5	2.5	2.5
0.9	$E\{N\}$	13.0	22.4	22.4	35.4	22.6
	$E_0\{N\}$	21.4	31.4	30.0	51.0	31.8
1.0	$E_0\{N\}$	11.6	20.0	20.0	33.4	20.2

same probability requirement (2.1) with $\Delta^* = 0.2$ and $P^* = 0.95$. All of our numerical entries for $k = 2$ (in Table IV) are based on exact formulas. In Table IV, we have included in each cell $E\{N_B\}$ for the LF configuration ($\Delta = 0.2$) and $E\{N\}$ for the LF ($\Delta = 0.2$) and equal parameter (EP) configuration ($\Delta = 0$). The procedures R_I and R_{IO} are inverse sampling procedures using PW sampling without and with reordering after each complete cycle, respectively.

The modified procedure R_H due to Hoel [3] uses PW sampling and scores, where the score W_A (for drug A, say) is defined by adding the successes of drug A and the failures of drug B and the termination rule is inverse sampling, that is, stop when max $(W_A, W_B) = r$. It has a bounded $E\{N\}$ value for $p = p' = 0$ and is therefore an improvement on R_I for small values of p.

Another procedure R_{IT}, due to Berry and Sobel [2], modifies the inverse sampling scheme by terminating the procedure either after a fixed number c of complete cycles or after one population reaches r successes, whichever occurs sooner. This procedure appears to have two preassigned constants (r, c) to specify, but both constants are used (with $r = c$) to satisfy (2.1).

Table IV (for $k = 2$) shows that for $\bar{p} = (p + p')/2 > \frac{1}{2}$ the likelihood procedure is preferable using either the risk criterion or $E\{N\}$. However, for $\bar{p} < \frac{1}{2}$ the value of $E\{N\}$ becomes infinite for all three of the procedures, R_{LPW}, R_I, and R_{IO} when $p = p'$. Procedures R_H and R_{IT}, on the other hand, have a bounded $E\{N\}$ function even for $p = p'$ and the numerical improvement for small $\bar{p}$ in Table IV, especially for $p = p'$, is very striking. It follows, as in the case of $k = 3$ in the next section, that if we had some *a priori* knowledge about the value of $\bar{p}$, we could more easily decide which of these procedures to use.

Procedure R_{IO} shows only a small improvement over procedure R_I, but it is uniform over the entire parameter space.

7. Monte Carlo simulation studies for $k = 3$

In this section, we bring together several procedures appropriate for $k = 3$ populations and make some Monte Carlo studies to compare them. The criteria for comparison are the risk function (2.3) and the expected total number of observations $E\{N\}$. The same formulation (2.1) applies to all these procedures with the common values $P^* = 0.95$ and $\Delta^* = 0.2$. Each entry in Table V corresponds to the average of the results of 1,000 experiments.

The main breakdown is between the procedures that use PW sampling and those that use VT sampling. We have included three previously published procedures. In the PW group, we include the inverse sampling procedure R_I studied in [13]. In the VT group, we include the procedure R_{BKS} which was developed in [1], by Bechhofer, Kiefer, and Sobel, for general k, but details of which are given in ([1], p. 270) only for $k = 2$. We also include in the VT group the procedure R_P due to Paulson [7]. A brief description of these procedures now follows.

Under procedure R_I, we sample cyclically from three populations with PW sampling until any one of them has r successes; it is then selected to be the best population. The Monte Carlo results for R_I given in Tables V, VI, and VII are very close to approximate values based on (3.35) and (3.37) in [13]. A table of these approximate values, not included here, gives values consistently smaller than the observed values in Table IV.

Under procedure R_{BKS}, we use vector sampling and stop as soon as

$$(7.1) \qquad \left(\frac{1 - \Delta^*}{1 + \Delta^*}\right)^{2T_1} + \left(\frac{1 - \Delta^*}{1 + \Delta^*}\right)^{2T_2} \leqq \frac{1 - P^*}{P^*}$$

and select the population associated with S_3. For $P^* > \frac{1}{2}$, we will not stop when $S_3 = S_2$, and hence, randomization will not be required at termination. It should be noted that the form of this procedure in (7.1) is similar to that of the conservative procedure in (3.7), but since the latter uses PW sampling there is no direct comparability.

Under procedure R_P, we take N_{ir} observations from population π_i, $i = 1, 2, 3$, where N_{ir} is a Poisson random variable with mean J. Let s_{ir} (respectively, f_{ir}) denote the total number of successes (respectively, failures) from π_i up to and including the rth stage. Then population π_j is eliminated at stage r if for some π_i (not yet eliminated), we have

$$(7.2) \qquad s_{jr} - f_{jr} \leqq s_{ir} - f_{ir} + \frac{\log \alpha}{\log \lambda} + rA(\lambda),$$

where $\alpha = (1 - P^*)/(k - 1)$,

$$(7.3) \qquad A(\lambda) = \frac{J[\Delta^*(\lambda^2 - 1) - (\lambda - 1)^2]}{\lambda \log \lambda},$$

and λ is any value between 1 and $(1 + \Delta^*)/(1 - \Delta^*)$. For our Monte Carlo studies, we use the same values for J and λ that were used in [7], namely, $J = 1$ and $\lambda = (1 + 0.75\Delta^*)/(1 - 0.75\Delta^*)$, which equals $23/17 = 1.353$ in our case. It should perhaps be remarked that the Poisson observations are not counted in computing $E\{N\}$ or the risk function.

Table V gives the empirical risk function, Table VI gives the empirical $E\{N\}$

TABLE V

RISK FOR VARIOUS PROCEDURES $k = 3$, $\Delta^* = 0.2$, AND $P^* = 0.95$
GLF configurations with 1,000 experiments per point.

	Play the winner sampling					Vector sampling	
	R_{EPW} Sobel-Weiss (elimination)	R_I Inverse sampling	R'_{LPW} Likelihood conservative	R_{LPW} Likelihood	R_{BKS} (see [1])	R_P Paulson (elimination)	R_{EVT} Wald's double dichotomy (elimination)
max p_i							
.20	22.82	45.47	27.57	22.83	9.95	10.14	9.95
.25	21.35	35.73	25.84	21.03	10.28	10.12	9.80
.30	19.67	29.08	23.99	20.05	10.29	10.01	9.61
.35	18.25	24.78	22.85	18.90	10.35	10.17	9.49
.40	17.25	21.34	21.58	17.60	10.25	9.95	9.44
.45	15.73	18.33	19.39	16.06	10.38	9.90	9.33
.50	14.72	16.26	18.18	14.95	10.40	10.14	9.21
.55	13.08	14.44	16.62	13.51	10.20	9.97	9.24
.60	12.02	12.63	14.61	11.89	10.23	10.01	9.32
.65	10.41	11.25	13.20	10.73	10.32	10.21	9.16
.70	8.71	9.85	11.40	9.22	10.44	10.07	9.18
.75	7.42	8.77	9.74	8.13	10.84	10.07	9.45
.80	6.13	7.41	7.85	6.36	10.70	9.95	9.52
.85	4.88	6.08	6.04	5.01	10.88	10.14	9.70
.90	3.62	4.71	4.36	3.48	10.79	10.19	9.72
.95	2.27	3.00	2.65	2.32	10.73	10.17	9.73
1.00	1.02	1.09	0.95	1.00	10.68	10.20	9.91

TABLE VI

EXPECTED TOTAL NUMBER OF OBSERVATIONS FOR VARIOUS PROCEDURES
$k = 3$, $\Delta^* = 0.2$, AND $P^* = 0.95$
GLF configurations with 1,000 experiments per point.

	Play the winner sampling					Vector sampling	
	R_{EPW}	R_I	R'_{LPW}	R_{LPW}	R_{BKS}	R_P	R_{EVT}
	Sobel-						Wald's
	Weiss		Likelihood			Paulson	double
	(elimi-	Inverse	conserva-	Likeli-		(elimi-	dichotomy
max p_i	nation)	sampling	tive	hood	(see [1])	nation)	(elimination)
.20	184.7	368.5	223.3	184.8	74.6	81.1	74.6
.25	177.9	291.1	210.3	171.2	77.1	81.0	76.0
.30	166.5	238.4	196.6	164.1	77.2	80.6	75.8
.35	156.4	204.1	188.2	155.5	77.6	81.7	75.8
.40	149.6	176.9	178.8	145.9	76.9	79.8	75.8
.45	138.8	153.6	162.5	134.5	77.9	79.4	75.4
.50	131.6	137.3	153.5	126.1	78.0	81.2	74.6
.55	118.3	123.1	141.8	115.1	76.5	80.0	74.8
.60	109.2	109.6	126.8	103.0	76.7	80.2	75.2
.65	97.2	99.2	116.3	94.5	77.4	82.0	74.6
.70	84.5	89.0	102.9	83.0	78.3	80.8	74.8
.75	73.4	80.9	90.3	74.7	81.3	80.6	76.9
.80	62.3	71.8	75.9	61.4	80.2	80.2	77.4
.85	52.1	63.1	62.4	51.0	81.6	81.0	79.1
.90	42.9	54.3	49.6	39.3	80.9	81.5	78.9
.95	31.4	44.3	36.5	30.2	80.4	81.7	78.8
1.00	21.2	33.4	23.7	20.2	80.1	81.3	79.7

function, and Table VII gives the estimated PCS function (or observed frequency of success).

As a group, the PW sampling procedures are different from the group of VT sampling procedures. The latter procedures have remarkably constant risk and $E\{N\}$ for varying values of max p_i, $i = 1, 2, 3$ while the former procedures appear to be monotonically decreasing with max p_i; the cross over point is about 0.65 in Table V and about 0.75 in Table VI. It follows that if we had some prior knowledge about max p_i (only), we might be better able to decide which type of sampling to use.

Among the PW sampling rules, the procedures R_{EPW} and R_{LPW} are quite similar and uniformly better than both the procedures R_I and the conservative likelihood procedure. However, from Table VI, it appears that the procedure R_{LPW} is slightly better than R_{EPW}.

For the VT sampling procedures, the procedure R_{EVT} is preferable to both R_{BKS} and R_P using either the risk or the $E\{N\}$ criterion; the differences between the latter two procedures appear to be small.

In Table VII we note, as expected, that all procedures satisfied the requirement (2.1) in all the experiments that were carried out. The PW procedures, except for conservative likelihood, came closer to the nominal value $P^* = 0.95$ than the VT procedures, and hence, were slightly more efficient in the sense that

TABLE VII

PROBABILITY OF CORRECT SELECTION FOR VARIOUS PROCEDURES
$k = 3$, $\Delta^* = 0.2$, AND $P^* = 0.95$
GLF configurations with 1,000 experiments per point.

	Play the winner sampling					Vector sampling	
	R_{EPW}	R_I	R'_{LPW}	R_{LPW}	R_{BKS}	R_P	R_{EVT}
	Sobel-Weiss (elimination)	Inverse sampling	Likelihood conservative	Likelihood	(see [1])	Paulson (elimination)	Wald's double dichotomy (elimination)
max p_i							
.20	1.000	1.000	1.000	1.000	1.000	.968	1.000
.25	1.000	1.000	1.000	1.000	1.000	.968	1.000
.30	1.000	1.000	1.000	1.000	.998	.966	.999
.35	1.000	1.000	1.000	1.000	.993	.973	.993
.40	1.000	.998	1.000	1.000	.984	.971	.993
.45	1.000	.991	1.000	.997	.984	.960	.989
.50	1.000	.984	1.000	.999	.980	.970	.982
.55	.996	.983	.997	.990	.957	.971	.974
.60	.991	.967	.997	.987	.961	.961	.970
.65	.994	.970	.997	.987	.964	.972	.977
.70	.991	.963	.995	.981	.973	.976	.969
.75	.972	.952	.990	.976	.983	.974	.981
.80	.970	.957	.985	.977	.983	.969	.989
.85	.967	.965	.987	.968	.994	.970	.997
.90	.968	.969	.981	.962	.999	.965	.997
.95	.952	.986	.978	.955	1.000	.966	1.000
1.00	.957	.996	.989	.969	1.000	.964	1.000

they have less "excess over the boundary". In addition, the columns of Table VII give some indication of where the least favorable configuration is for the pair ($\Delta^* = 0.2$, $P^* = 0.95$).

We wish to point out that we have not observed the expected number of stages required for termination since (1) it is not clearly defined for all procedures, and (2) it is not crucial for the application to clinical trials. It should also be pointed out that our Monte Carlo results are only for GLF configurations, where $p_{[1]} = p_{[2]} = p_{[3]} - 0.2$. In other configurations, the elimination procedures are even more preferable, because noncompeting populations can be eliminated early.

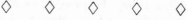

The authors wish to thank Professor R. E. Bechhofer of Cornell University for his helpful comments.

REFERENCES

[1] R. E. BECHHOFER, J. KIEFER, and M. SOBEL. *Sequential Identification and Ranking Problems*, Chicago, University of Chicago Press, 1968.
[2] D. BERRY and M. SOBEL, "A truncated inverse sampling procedure for selecting the best binomial population," Department of Statistics Technical Report No. 154, University of Minnesota, 1971.

[3] D. G. Hoel, "A method for the construction of sequential selection procedures," *Ann. Math. Statist.*, Vol. 42 (1971), pp. 630–642.

[4] ———, "An inverse stopping rule for play-the-winner sampling," *J. Amer. Statist. Assoc.*, Vol. 67 (1972), pp. 148–151.

[5] ———, "A selection procedure based upon Wald's double dichotomy test," Oak Ridge National Laboratory Technical Report No. TM-3237, Oak Ridge, Tennessee, 1971.

[6] E. Nebenzahl, "Play the winner sampling in selecting the better of two binomial populations," Department of Statistics Technical Report No. 147, University of Minnesota, 1970.

[7] E. Paulson, "Sequential procedures for selecting the best one of several binomial populations," *Ann. Math. Statist.*, Vol. 38 (1967), pp. 117–123.

[8] ———, "A new sequential procedure for selecting the best one of k binomial populations," Abstract, *Ann. Math. Statist.*, Vol. 38 (1969), p. 1865.

[9] M. Sobel and M. Huyett, "Selecting the best one of several binomial populations," *Bell System Tech. J.*, Vol. 36 (1957), pp. 537–576.

[10] M. Sobel and G. H. Weiss, "Play-the-winner for selecting the better of two binomial populations," *Biometrika*, Vol. 57 (1970), pp. 357–365.

[11] ———, "Recent results on using the play the winner sampling rule with binomial selection problems," *Proceedings of the Sixth Berkeley Symposium on Mathematical Statistics and Probability*, Berkeley and Los Angeles, University of California Press, 1972, Vol. 1, pp. 717–736.

[12] ———, "Play-the-winner rule and inverse sampling in selecting the better of two binomial populations," *J. Amer. Statist. Assoc.*, Vol. 66 (1971), pp. 545–551.

[13] ———, "Play-the-winner rule and inverse sampling for selecting the best of $k \geq 3$ binomial populations," *Ann. Math. Statist.*

[14] A. Wald, *Sequential Analysis*, New York, Wiley, 1947.

CRITICAL AGE DEPENDENT BRANCHING PROCESSES

HOWARD J. WEINER

UNIVERSITY OF CALIFORNIA, DAVIS

1. Introduction

This paper is a survey of some recent work which generalizes standard results in the Bellman-Harris single type critical age dependent branching process, especially the asymptotic probability of nonextinction of the process, and a limiting conditional exponential limit law. Also included are new results combining existing extensions and suggestions for further research and techniques in relaxing conditions on the processes.

2. Definition

The classical Bellman-Harris age dependent branching process ([8], Chapter 6) is defined as follows. At time 0, one new born cell starts the process with nonlattice lifetime distribution function $G(t)$, with $G(0) = 0$. At the end of its life, the cell disappears and is replaced by k daughter cells with probability p_k, $k = 0, 1, 2, 3, \cdots$. Each daughter cell behaves independent of all other cells, and has the lifetime distribution $G(t)$. Denote by $h(s)$ the generating function

$$(2.1) \qquad h(s) = \sum_{k=0}^{\infty} p_k s^k.$$

If $h'(1) \equiv m$, the mean number of daughter cells born to a parent cell, then the cases $m > 1$, $m = 1$, and $m < 1$ form a trichotomy for the behavior of the process in crucial respects, where $m = 1$ is the critical case (see [8]). We will consider now results for $Z(t)$, the number of cells alive at t.

3. Early results

When $m = 1$, $h^{(2)}(1) > 0$ and $h^{(3)}(1) < \infty$, and $G(t) = 1 - \exp\{-\lambda t\}$, Sevast'janov (see [8], Chapter 5) showed, by consideration of a differential equation satisfied by the generating function $F(s, t) \equiv \sum_{k=0}^{\infty} P[Z(t) = k]s^k$, that

$$(3.1) \qquad \lim_{t \to \infty} tP[Z(t) > 0] = 2[\lambda h^{(2)}(1)]^{-1}$$

and

$$(3.2) \qquad \lim_{t \to \infty} P[2(\lambda h^{(2)}(1)t)^{-1}Z(t) > u | Z(t) > 0] = \exp\{-u\},$$

for $u \geqq 0$.

The first generalization of the result (3.1) was a basic paper by Chover and Ney [1] which stated that for $m = 1$, $1 - G(t) = 0(t^{-3})$, and $h^{(3)}(1) < \infty$, that

$$(3.3) \qquad \lim_{t \to \infty} tP[Z(t) > 0] = \frac{2 \int_0^\infty u \, dG(u)}{h^{(2)}(1)} \equiv b.$$

Goldstein [7] has obtained this result by using the corresponding discrete time result first given by Kolmogorov and Yaglom (see [8], Chapter 5) to approximate the $P[Z(t) > 0]$ above and below.

By means of Abelian and Tauberian arguments satisfied by the integral equations for $E(Z^n(t))$, $n \geq 1$, Weiner [20] showed that

$$(3.4) \qquad \lim_{t \to \infty} t^{-(n-1)} E[Z^n(t)] = n! b^{-(n-1)}.$$

Since

$$(3.5) \qquad E[(bt^{-1}Z(t))^n | Z(t) > 0] \equiv \frac{E[bt^{-1}Z(t))^n]}{P[Z(t) > 0]} \to n!$$

by (3.4) and (3.5) above, and since $n!$ is the nth moment of an exponential law with parameter 1, Carleman's moment theorem yields that

$$(3.6) \qquad \lim_{t \to \infty} P[bt^{-1}Z(t) > u | Z(t) > 0] = \exp\{-u\}.$$

Sevast'janov [17] also claimed to prove (3.3) and (3.6) by different methods, but his proof contained a gap [20] which was acknowledged and presumably corrected.

4. One dimensional generalizations

Durham [3] has defined a generalization of the age dependent branching process in which each cell is allowed to give birth to daughter cells throughout its lifetime. This process is the same as the classical Bellman-Harris process except that we define $N(t)$ to be the number of daughter cells born to the initial parent cell by time t, if the parent cell lives longer than t. Assume $N(t) \uparrow N < \infty$, where N is a bona fide random variable. The case $EN = 1$ corresponds to the critical case.

Let $M(t) \equiv EN(t)$ and $A \equiv \frac{1}{2}E(N(N-1))$. If $a = A \int_0^\infty u \, dG(u) \Big/ \left(\int_0^\infty t \, dM(t) \right)^2$, and $m_1 = \int_0^\infty u \, dG(u) \Big/ \int_0^\infty t \, dM(t)$, then

$$(4.1) \qquad \lim_{t \to \infty} t^{-(n-1)} E[Z^n(t)] = n! m_1 a^{n-1}.$$

Suppose that $\infty > E[N(N-1)] - E[N(t)(N(t)-1)] = O(t^{-2})$ and that $1 - G(t) = O(t^{-2})$. Then, using an extension of the method of Chover and Ney [1],

$$(4.2) \qquad \lim_{t \to \infty} tP[Z(t) > 0] = \frac{b}{A}.$$

These two results (4.1) and (4.2) along with $EN^n < \infty$ for all $n \geq 1$ yield, by the argument in (3.5), that

(4.3) $$\lim_{t\to\infty} P[(at)^{-1}Z(t) > u | Z(t) > 0] = \exp\{-u\}.$$

Fildes [5] has considered an extension to the Bellman-Harris process, where the lifetime distributions of different generations may differ, with the lifetime distributions of each member of the nth generation denoted by $G_n(t)$. The basic results are that for $m = 1$, $1 - G_n(t) = o(t^{-2-\delta})$ uniformly in n, $\lim_{n\to\infty} G_n(t) \to G(t)$ with $\mu = \int_0^\infty t\, dG(t)$ and if X_n are independent with $P[X_n < t] = G_n(t)$, and $(1/n) \sum_{\ell=1}^\infty X_\ell \xrightarrow{p} \mu$ and if $h^{(n)}(1) < \infty$ for all n, then if $b = 2\mu(h^{(2)}(1))^{-1}$, and letting $Z_\ell(t)$ denote the number of cells alive at t starting with one cell newborn at $t = 0$ of generation ℓ, then

(4.4) $$\lim_{t\to\infty} tP[Z_\ell(t) > 0] = b$$

and

(4.5) $$\lim_{t\to\infty} P[bt^{-1}Z_\ell(t) > u | Z(t) > 0] = \exp\{-u\}.$$

The proofs of (4.4) and (4.5) are formally the same as for (3.4) and (3.6). We recall that Durham's proofs for (4.2) and (4.3) were along these lines.

Hence, one may state a theorem combining the extensions of Durham and Fildes as follows. We consider an age dependent branching process with generation dependent cell lifetime distributions and with each cell giving birth to offspring throughout its lifetime. Explicitly, the process starts at $t = 0$ with one new born cell of generation ℓ. Let $N_\ell(t)$ be the number of daughter cells born to a parent cell of generation ℓ, given that the parent cell is alive at t. Then we can state the following.

THEOREM 4.1. *Assume* $N_\ell(t) \uparrow N_\ell < \infty$ *as* $t \uparrow \infty$ *and that all* ℓ *and* $\{N_\ell\}$ *are independent random variables. Assume* $G_\ell(t) \to G(t)$ *as* $\ell \to \infty$, *with* $0 < \mu = \int_0^\infty t\, dG(t) < \infty$, *and that* $1 - G_\ell(t) = o(t^{-2-\delta})$ *uniformly in* ℓ *as* $t \to \infty$. *Assume that* $N_\ell(t) \to N(t)$ *for all* t *as* $\ell \to \infty$ *and that* $\lim_{t\to\infty} N(t) = \lim_{\ell\to\infty} N_\ell = N < \infty$ *a bona fide random variable. Assume further that if* $\{X_n\}$ *are independent random variables with* $P[X_n < t] = G_n(t)$, *that* $(1/n) \sum_{\ell=1}^\infty X_\ell \xrightarrow{p} \mu$. *Assume that* $\lim_{n\to\infty} (1/n) \sum_{\ell=1}^\infty N_\ell = EN = 1$, *the critical case.*

Define $M(t) \equiv EN(t)$; $b = \int_0^\infty t\, dM(t)$; $m_1 = \mu/b$; $A = E(\frac{1}{2}N(N-1))$; *and* $a = m_1 A/b$. *Let* $E(N_\ell(t)(N_\ell(t) - 1)(N_\ell(t) - 2) | cell\ lives\ longer\ than\ t) = B_\ell(t)$. *If* $B_\ell(t) \to B_\ell < \infty$ *as* $t \to \infty$ *and* $B_\ell \to B$ *as* $\ell \to \infty$, *and if* $EN^k < \infty$ *for all* $k \geq 1$, $B - B_\ell(t) = o(1/t^2)$ *uniformly in* ℓ *for* t *sufficiently large and* $1 - G_\ell(t) = o(1/t^2)$ *uniformly in* ℓ *for* t *sufficiently large, then*

(4.6) $$\lim_{t\to\infty} tP[Z_\ell(t) > 0] = \frac{b}{A}$$

and

(4.7) $\lim_{t \to \infty} P[(at)^{-1} Z_t(t) > u | Z_t(t) > 0] = \exp\{-u\}.$

Sevast'janov has considered an extension of the Bellman-Harris process to the case of variable offspring generating functions depending on the age at death of the parent.

Let a Bellman-Harris process start with one cell at time 0 with lifetime distribution $G(t)$. If the parent cell dies at time u, then n independent daughter cells, each proceeding as the parent cell with lifetime distribution $G(t)$, are born with probability $p_n(u)$, where $p_n(u) > 0$ and $\sum_{n=0}^{\infty} p_n(u) = 1$ for all $u > 0$.

Let $h(u, s) = \sum_{n=0}^{\infty} p_n(u) s^n$. Let

$$a(u) = \left. \frac{\partial h}{\partial s} \right|_{s=1},$$

(4.8) $$b(u) = \left. \frac{\partial^2 h}{\partial s^2} \right|_{s=1},$$

$$c(u) = \left. \frac{\partial^3 h}{\partial s^3} \right|_{s=1}.$$

Then Sevast'janov has shown by Taylor expansions and approximations in the basic integral equation for $F(s, t) = \sum_{k=0}^{\infty} P[Z(t) = k] s^k$ the following results.

THEOREM 4.2 [18]. *Assume* $\int_0^{\infty} a(u)\, dG(u) = 1$ *(critical case)*; $\infty > \int_0^{\infty} b(u)\, dG(u) > 0; \int_0^{\infty} u^3\, dG(u) < \infty; \int_0^{\infty} u^3 c(u)\, dG(u) < \infty;$ *and* $\int_0^{\infty} c(u)\, dG(u) < \infty.$
Then

(4.9) $$\lim_{t \to \infty} t P[Z(t) > 0] = \frac{2 \int_0^{\infty} u a(u)\, dG(u)}{\int_0^{\infty} b(u)\, dG(u)}.$$

THEOREM 4.3 [19]. *In addition to the assumptions of Theorem 4.2, assume further that*

$$EZ(t) = \frac{\int_0^{\infty} u\, dG(u) \cdot \int_0^{\infty} a(u)\, dG(u)}{\int_0^{\infty} u a(u)\, dG(u)} + o\left(\frac{1}{t}\right),$$

(4.10)

$$E[(Z(t))(Z(t) - 1)] = \frac{\int_0^{\infty} b(u)\, dG(u) \left(\int_0^{\infty} u\, dG(u)\right)^2 \left(\int_0^{\infty} a(u)\, dG(u)\right)^3}{\left(\int_0^{\infty} u a(u)\, dG(u)\right)^3} t$$
$$+ B_2 + o(1),$$

where B_2 is some constant, then

(4.11) $$\lim_{t \to \infty} P\left[\frac{Z(t)}{E(Z(t) | Z(t) > 0)} > u | Z(t) > 0\right] = \exp\{-u\}.$$

It is conjectured that adding the assumption that $(\partial^n / \partial s^n) h|_{s=1} < \infty$ for all n, and lumping together the extensions and assumptions of Fildes, Durham, and

Sevast'janov into a generalization of the Bellman-Harris critical age dependent branching process, to allow for generation dependent lifetimes, births of daughter cells throughout the life of a parent, and parent age at death dependent daughter cell generating functions, one could formulate a theorem giving that

$$(4.12) \qquad \lim_{t \to \infty} t P[Z(t) > 0] = c$$

and that

$$(4.13) \qquad \lim_{t \to \infty} P\left[\frac{Z(t)}{E(Z(t)|Z(t) > 0)} > u | Z(t) > 0\right] = \exp\{-u\},$$

but this will not be attempted here.

5. Multitype processes

We will consider a branching process with $m > 1$ distinguishable particle types as follows. At time 0, one newly born cell of type i is born, $i = 1, 2, \cdots, m$. Cell type i lives a random lifetime with continuous distribution function $G_i(t)$, $G_i(0+) = 0$. At the end of its life, cell i is replaced by j_1 new cells of type 1, j_2 new cells of type 2, $\cdots$, j_m new cells of type m with probability $p_{ij_1 \cdots j \cdots}$, and we define the generating functions

$$(5.1) \quad h_i(s_1, \cdots, s_m) \equiv h_i(s) = \sum_{j_1 \cdots j \cdots} p_{ij_1 \cdots j_m} s_1^{j_1} s_2^{j_2} \cdots s_m^{j_m} \equiv \sum_j p_{ij} s^j$$

for $i = 1, \cdots, m$, where $s = (s_1, \cdots, s_m)$, $j = (j_1, \cdots, j_m)$ and $s^j \equiv s_1^{j_1}, \cdots, s_m^{j_m}$. Each new daughter cell proceeds independently of the state of the system, with each cell type j governed by $G_j(t)$ and $h_j(s)$.

We will assume second moments of $h_i(s)$, $i = 1, \cdots, m$ to exist. Define $m_{ij} \equiv (\partial h_i(s)/\partial s_j)|_{s-1}$, where $1 = (1, \cdots, 1)$, an $m \times 1$ row vector, and let $M = (m_{ij})$ be the $m \times m$ matrix of first moments of the offspring distribution. Assume $m_{ij} > 0$ for all i, j.

DEFINITION 5.1. *Let $Z_{ij}(t) =$ number of cells of type j alive at t given that the process started at time 0 with one new cell type i, $1 \leq i, j \leq m$.*

DEFINITION 5.2. *Let $Z_i(t) = (Z_{i1}(t), Z_{i2}(t), \cdots, Z_{im}(t))$ denote the row vector of the numbers of cells alive at t given that the process started at time $t = 0$ with one cell of type i.*

DEFINITION 5.3. *Define*

$$(5.2) \qquad P_i(t) = P[Z_i(t) > 0].$$

We have from Frobenius' theory [12] that, assuming

$$(5.3) \qquad M = (m_{ij}) = \frac{\partial h_i(1)}{\partial s_j}, \qquad 0 < m_{ij} < \infty,$$

is a positive matrix (it suffices that $M^n > 0$ for some n), we can make the basic assumption of criticality.

DEFINITION 5.4. *Let ρ be that positive eigenvalue of M such that $\rho \geq |v|$, where v is any other eigenvalue of M.*

The basic assumption of criticality of the branching process throughout this paper is $\rho = 1$.

It follows that there are strictly positive eigenvectors $u > 0$, $v > 0$ such that

$$(5.4) \qquad Mu = u, \qquad vM = v, \qquad \sum_{i=1}^{m} u_i \equiv u \cdot 1 = 1$$

and

$$(5.5) \qquad u \cdot v \equiv \sum_{i=1}^{n} u_i v_i = 1.$$

ASSUMPTION 5.1. *The second moments of $h(s) \equiv (h_1(s), \cdots, h_m(s))$ exist at 1.*
DEFINITION 5.5. *The sum*

$$(5.6) \qquad Q(u) = \frac{1}{2} \sum_{i=1}^{m} \sum_{\ell=1}^{m} \sum_{r=1}^{m} \frac{\partial^2 h_i(1)}{\partial s_\ell \partial s_r} u_\ell u_r v_i < \infty$$

and is strictly positive.

ASSUMPTION 5.2. *The partial derivative*

$$(5.7) \qquad \frac{\partial^2 h_i(1)}{\partial s_j \partial s_k} \equiv a_{ijk} > 0 \qquad \qquad for\ all\ 1 \leqq i, j, k \leqq m.$$

ASSUMPTION 5.3. *All moments of $h_i(s)$ exist at $s = 1$.*
ASSUMPTION 5.4.

$$(5.8) \qquad \lim_{t \to \infty} t^2 (1 - G_i(t)) = 0, \qquad \qquad 1 \leqq i \leqq m.$$

DEFINITION 5.6. *Let $\mu_i \equiv \int_0^\infty t \, dG_i(t)$.*

Then we have the following.

THEOREM 5.1 [21]. *Under all assumptions except Assumption 5.3 we have,*

$$(5.9) \qquad \lim_{t \to \infty} t P_i(t) = \left(\sum_{\ell=1}^{m} \mu_\ell u_\ell v_\ell \right) \frac{u_i}{Q(u)}.$$

This behavior of the extinction rate contrasts with the cases $\rho > 1$, where the process becomes extinct with probability less than one [17], and with the case $\rho < 1$, where the process becomes extinct with probability one at an exponential rate [16].

Goldstein [7] has also obtained this result, but by using upper and lower bounds for $P_i(t)$ based on the corresponding multitype Galton-Watson result in discrete time [11].

Using (5.9), one can then, by moment methods similar to the one dimensiona case, and a Frobenius decomposition used by Mode [13], obtain Theorem 5.2.

THEOREM 5.2 [21]. *Let $Z_i(t)$ be the vector of the number of cells alive at time t, $i = 1, 2, \cdots, m$, starting with one new cell of type i in a critical multitype branching process satisfying all the assumptions stated. Then for all $r = (r_1, \cdots, r_m)$, $r_i \geqq 0$, $i = 1, \cdots, m$,*

$$(5.10) \quad \lim_{t \to \infty} P \left[\frac{Z_i(t)}{t} > r \,\Big|\, Z_i(t) > 0 \right] = \exp \left\{ \frac{- \left(\sum_{j=1}^{m} u_j v_j \mu_j \right)^2}{Q(u)} \max_{1 \leqq k \leqq m} \frac{r_k}{v_k \mu_k} \right\}.$$

A special case of these results has been obtained by Nair [15] (see also Mode [14]).

6. Related work

Goldstein's heavy use of imbedded Galton-Watson process results to obtain similar results for the corresponding age dependent cases suggests that this method perhaps can be used to obtain further results on other extensions of the Bellman-Harris process from corresponding discrete time results.

We briefly indicate some recent critical case Galton-Watson discrete time results which may be so used. Foster [6] has obtained limiting conditional distributions for a Galton-Watson process subject to immigration, as has Heathcote [9]. Fearn [4] has shown that a Galton-Watson process with generation dependent offspring distributions $h_n(s)$ = generating function of the number of offspring born to a cell in the nth generation has the following property. If $m_n \equiv h_n'(1) \to 1$ sufficiently fast, Z_n denotes the number of cells alive at time n starting with one cell in generation 0, then if Var $(Z_n/EZ_n) \to \infty$,

$$(6.1) \qquad P[Z_n > 0] \sim \frac{2}{\text{Var } (Z_n/EZ_n)},$$

generalizing the discrete time result of Kolmogorov and Yaglom (see [7], Chapter 5).

Another generalization concerns sequences of Bellman-Harris processes. Let $Z_n(t)$ denote the number of cells alive at t in an ordinary Bellman-Harris process starting with n new born cells alive at $t = 0$, and lifetime distribution $G(t)$. Assume also that the daughter cell generating function for each parent in this "nth process" is $h_n(s)$, where $h_n^{(1)}(1) \equiv m_n = 1 + \alpha/n + o(1/n)$, and $h_n^{(2)}(1) \to 2\beta$ as $n \to \infty$, and $h_n^{(3)}(1) < C$ all n.

Then Jagers [10] has shown that

$$(6.2) \qquad \frac{1}{n} Z_n(nt) \xrightarrow{L} X(t),$$

where $X(t)$ is a diffusion process of a simple kind. If tightness conditions [2] can be established under reasonable conditions, then perhaps study of $X(t)$ can lead to boundary crossing results about the underlying Bellman-Harris processes. Work is proceeding along these lines.

REFERENCES

[1] J. CHOVER and P. NEY, "The non-linear renewal equation," *J. Analyse Math.*, Vol. 21 (1968), pp. 381–413.
[2] P. BILLINGSLEY, *Convergence of Probability Measures*, New York, Wiley, 1968.
[3] S. DURHAM, "Limit theorems for a general critical branching process," *J. Appl. Probability*, Vol. 8 (1971), pp. 1–16.
[4] D. FEARN, "Branching processes with generation dependent birth distributions," Ph.D. Thesis, University of California, Davis, 1971.

[5] R. FILDES, "The age-dependent branching process with variable lifetime distribution," Ph.D. Thesis, University of California, Davis, 1971.

[6] J. FOSTER, "Branching processes involving immigration," Ph.D. Thesis, University of Wisconsin, 1970.

[7] M. I. GOLDSTEIN, "Critical age-dependent branching processes: single and multitype," *Z. Wahrscheinlichkeitstheorie und Verw. Gebiete*, Vol. 17 (1971), pp. 74–96.

[8] T. E. HARRIS, *The Theory of Branching Processes*, New York, Prentice-Hall, 1963.

[9] C. R. HEATHCOTE, "Corrections and comments on 'A branching process allowing immigration,'" *J. Roy. Statist. Soc. Ser. B*, Vol. 28 (1966), pp. 213–217.

[10] P. JAGERS, "Diffusion approximations of branching processes," Report of Stanford University Department of Statistics, October, 1970.

[11] A. JOFFE and F. SPITZER, "On multitype branching processes with $\rho \leq 1$," *J. Math. Anal. Appl.*, Vol. 19 (1967), pp. 409–430.

[12] S. KARLIN, *A First Course in Stochastic Processes*, New York, Academic Press, 1966.

[13] C. J. MODE, "A multidimensional age-dependent branching process with applications to natural selection I," *Math. Biosci.*, Vol. 3 (1968), pp. 1–18.

[14] ———, *Multitype Branching Processes-Theory and Applications*, New York, American-Elsevier, 1971.

[15] K. A. NAIR, "Multitype age-dependent branching processes," Ph.D. Thesis, State University of New York at Buffalo, 1970.

[16] T. A. RYAN, JR., "On age-dependent branching processes," Ph.D. Thesis, Cornell University, 1968.

[17] B. A. SEVAST'JANOV, "Age-dependent branching processes," *Theor. Probability Appl.*, Vol. 9 (1964), pp. 577–594.

[18] ———, "Asymptotic behavior of the probability of nonextinction of a critical branching process," *Theor. Probability Appl.*, Vol. 12 (1967), pp. 152–154.

[19] ———, "Limit theorems for age-dependent branching processes," *Theor. Probability Appl.*, Vol. 13 (1968), pp. 237–259.

[20] H. J. WEINER, "Asymptotic properties of an age-dependent branching process," *Ann. Math. Statist.*, Vol. 36 (1965), pp. 1565–1568.

[21] ———, "On a multitype critical age-dependent branching process," *J. Appl. Probability*, Vol. 7 (1970), pp. 523–543.

EQUILIBRIA FOR GENETIC SYSTEMS WITH WEAK INTERACTION

SAMUEL KARLIN
WEIZMANN INSTITUTE OF SCIENCE, ISRAEL
and
STANFORD UNIVERSITY
and
JAMES McGREGOR
STANFORD UNIVERSITY

1. Introduction

The following principle (stated here in rough form) bears many applications in the study of ecological and genetic systems.

PRINCIPLE I. *If a system of transformations acting on a certain set (in finite dimensional space) has a "stable" fixed point, then a slight perturbation of the system maintains a stable fixed point nearby.*

The theme of this principle is quite intuitive although care in its application and interpretation is vital. Its validity does not require the stability hypothesis to apply in a geometric sense. In fact, for numerous important nonrandom mating genetic models the stability of the relevant equilibrium is manifested only in an algebraic sense. The result is basic in the domain of global analysis and occurs in many other mathematical contexts as well. With the aid of this principle, we are able to establish the existence of equilibria for quite complicated genetic models and these have interesting interpretations for population phenomena.

A converse proposition to Principle I of considerable value in ascertaining *all* possible equilibria is also now stated in rough form. For a precise mathematical statement the reader should consult Karlin and McGregor [9].

PRINCIPLE II. *If $f(x)$ is a differentiable transformation acting on a certain set S (in finite dimensional space) having a finite number of fixed points, say y_1, y_2, $\cdots$, y_r, with the property that the linear approximation to $f(x)$ in the neighborhood of each fixed point has no eigenvalue of absolute value one, then a slight differentiable perturbation of $f(x)$ maintains* at most *a single fixed point $z_i \in S$ in the neighborhood of each y_i. Moreover, z_i is locally stable if and only if y_i is locally stable.*

It is worth noting that some fixed points of $f(x)$ (but none of the stable ones) may disappear under small perturbations.

We illustrate the scope of these principles by indicating the application to the investigation of three types of population models subject to a variety of genetic

Supported in part by National Institutes of Health Grant USPRS 10452-09.

79

factors. In Section 2, we treat the effect of small intermigration flow among several genetic subsystems or niches with different selection forces operating in the separate niches. Section 3 highlights the possibilities of mutation selection balance for two locus haploid and diploid populations. The small perturbation in this model arises due to the mutation pressure. The final section reviews results emanating from Principles I and II applied to the study of multilocus viability selection models with small recombination parameters. Some implications for evolutionary theory are also noted.

2. Stable equilibrium for multipopulation systems with migration coupling

In this section, we present a general framework for application of Principles I and II for population models involving slight intermigration flow among several separate subpopulations. More specifically, suppose there exists a number (say ρ) of ecological or genetic systems $\mathcal{P}_1, \mathcal{P}_2, \cdots, \mathcal{P}_\rho$, for example, separate communities, niches, with a finite number (say r) of possible types $A_1, A_2, \cdots, A_r$ that may be represented in each system. We generally denote the frequencies of types A_1, $A_2, \cdots, A_r$ in population (or system) $\mathcal{P}_\alpha$ by $\bar{p}_\alpha = (p_{\alpha 1}, \cdots, p_{\alpha r})$, and frequently subscript α is suppressed when no ambiguity of interpretation is possible. Suppose each system reproduces independently in some fashion such that the frequencies $\bar{p}' = (p'_{\alpha 1}, \cdots, p'_{\alpha r})$ in the next generation are determined by the relations

$$(2.1) \qquad p'_{\alpha j} = f_{\alpha j}(p_{\alpha 1}, \cdots, p_{\alpha r}), \qquad j = 1, 2, \cdots, r.$$

We sometimes write (2.1) in vector notation taking the form

$$(2.2) \qquad \bar{p}'_\alpha = \bar{f}_\alpha(\bar{p}_\alpha).$$

In most genetic models, the transformation (2.1) is displayed as a ratio of two algebraic polynomials in the frequency variables. These transformations naturally reflect mating and ecological behavior, segregation pattern, selection, migration and mutation pressures, temporal and spatial (cyclical or other) changes, the influence of recombination when more than one locus is involved, and other relevant factors of the process.

In each system $\mathcal{P}_\alpha$ there usually exist certain equilibria (invariant points under the transformation (2.1)) which are locally stable. The collection of equilibria include polymorphic (all types represented) and peripheral (that is, boundary equilibrium) points, where in the latter case some types are not represented. Local stability is to be understood in the following generalized sense. A frequency vector p^* is said to be locally stable if for any prescribed neighborhood U of p^* there exists another neighborhood V, $p^* \in V \subset U$ such that $f(\bar{V}) \subset V$ ($\bar{V}$ denotes the closure of V), and therefore the iterates of $\bar{f}_\alpha^{(n)}(\bar{p}) = \bar{f}_\alpha^{(n-1)}(\bar{f}_\alpha(\bar{p}))$ for any starting point $p \in \bar{V}$ never depart from V. In most cases, local stability of an equilibrium p^* actually entails that if the initial frequency vector $\bar{p}$ is sufficiently close to p^*, the iterates $\bar{f}_\alpha^n(\bar{p})$ indeed converge to p^*.

The notion of stability prescribed above makes no stipulations on the rate of convergence to the equilibrium. However, in most genetic and ecological systems when the equilibrium expresses a stable polymorphic balance, then convergence takes place at a geometric rate. But on the other hand when the equilibrium is of the boundary kind (mostly a population of a single type), then convergence not uncommonly occurs at an algebraic rate.

Suppose now that the system $(\mathcal{P}_1, \cdots, \mathcal{P}_\rho)$ is coupled by some form of interaction. To fix the ideas, we consider here the example when there are migration coefficients $m_{\alpha\beta}$ with the interpretation that after reproduction a proportion $m_{\alpha\beta}$ of individuals from $\mathcal{P}_\beta$ migrate to $\mathcal{P}_\alpha$. The recursion relations describing the evolution of type frequencies in the migration coupled system are then

$$(2.3) \qquad p'_{\alpha i} = \sum_{\beta=1}^{\rho} m_{\alpha\beta} f_{\beta i}(p_{\beta 1}, \cdots, p_{\beta r}), \qquad \alpha = 1, \cdots, \rho; i = 1, \cdots, r.$$

It is naturally assumed that $m_{\alpha\beta} \geq 0$ and $\sum_{\beta=1}^{\rho} m_{\alpha\beta} = 1$.

The migration specified by the ρ square matrix $M = ||m_{\alpha\beta}||$ would be called weak if M is sufficiently close to the identity matrix, that is, the $m_{\alpha\beta}$ with $\alpha \neq \beta$ are all sufficiently small. In this event, the flow between systems is slight. (All subsystems are presumed in the present theory to be of large size.) *If the uncoupled system has a locally stable equilibrium point p^* (that is, set of equilibrium vectors $\bar{p}_\alpha^*$), then we expect the coupled system to have a locally stable equilibrium point q^* near p^* provided the migration coupling is sufficiently weak.*

The above statement is a special case of the general Principle I.

We say a *full* polymorphism is attainable in the uncoupled system $(\mathcal{P}_1, \mathcal{P}_2, \cdots, \mathcal{P}_\rho)$ if there is a set of equilibrium frequency vectors p_α^*, $\alpha = 1, 2, \cdots, \rho$, where p_α^* is a *locally stable* solution of

$$(2.4) \qquad p_\alpha^* = f_\alpha(p_\alpha^*), \qquad \alpha = 1, 2, \cdots, \rho,$$

such that for each i, $1 \leq i \leq r$, $p_{\alpha i}^*$ is positive for at least one α (α may depend on i). The set of equilibrium frequency vectors p^* comprise a fixed point p_α^* of the uncoupled system in which every possible type is represented in at least one subsystem. Now if q^* is the nearby equilibrium point of the system under weak coupling, then every type will still be represented in at least one subsystem provided the coupling is sufficiently weak. In the migration coupling example, there is a simple condition which will guarantee that at the equilibrium state q^* each possible type is actually represented in every subsystem. The matrix $M = ||m_{\alpha\beta}||$ is called irreducible if there is a power M^k whose elements are all strictly positive. This means that a kth generation descendent of an individual from any subsystem has a positive probability to be in any other subsystem.

Our first application of Principle I is the following. *If a full polymorphism (defined in paragraph above) is attainable in the uncoupled system and if the migration matrix is irreducible and sufficiently weak (that is, M close to I = identity matrix), then the coupled system has a locally stable equilibrium state in which actually every possible type is represented in every subsystem.*

As a simple application of the assertion stated above, consider the case of a simple genetic system involving two alleles A_1 and A_2 at a single locus with two niches with selection coefficients $1, 1 - \sigma, 1$ for the genotypes $A_1 A_1$, $A_1 A_2$, and

A_2A_2, respectively, or more generally, we can suppose that the fitness coefficients of the genotypes are s_1, s_2, s_3 in niche 1; σ_1, σ_2, σ_3 in niche 2, where $s_2 < \min(s_1, s_3)$ and $\sigma_2 < \min(\sigma_1, \sigma_3)$. Thus, in each separate niche disruptive selection operates and ordinarily the population would be fixed. However, invoking the above result, we find that if a small fraction m (necessarily small) of the population of each niche migrates to the other niche then there are possible sets of stable polymorphisms with both alleles represented in each population. Of course, the possibility of stable global fixations also exists.

The polymorphic equilibria of this example have the property that a preponderance of one homozygote occurs in one niche while a preponderance of the alternative homozygote is maintained in the second niche. It is reasonable to speculate that some forms of habitat selection confer an advantage, say on A_2A_2 in niche 2, on A_1A_1 in niche 1, while the heterozygote (or hybrid type) bears marked disadvantage to both homozygotes in each of the niches, yet a global balance is preserved.

What evolves depends crucially on the initial composition of all the subpopulations. Thus, whether fixation transpires or polymorphism is attained could be a function of founders and random fluctuation effects determining the initial conditions. Small colonies of different homozygotes could inhabit neighboring localities with selection favoring both homozygotes over the heterozygotes in each locality. Subsequently, population size grows and presumably some slight gene flow binds the two localities. A suitable application of the principle then points to a polymorphism with most existing types being homozygotes (see Karlin and McGregor [10] for a more detailed quantitative analysis of this two niche model).

The extension to the case of three alleles is as follows. Consider a three allele model involving alleles A_1, A_2, A_3 with viabilities of A_iA_j specified by the matrix with the obvious interpretation

$$(2.5) \qquad \begin{pmatrix} 1 + \alpha_1 & 1 - \varepsilon_1 & 1 - \varepsilon_2 \\ 1 - \varepsilon_1 & 1 + \alpha_2 & 1 - \varepsilon_3 \\ 1 - \varepsilon_2 & 1 - \varepsilon_3 & 1 + \alpha_3 \end{pmatrix}, \qquad \varepsilon_i, \alpha_i > 0; \ i = 1, 2, 3,$$

so that each homozygote is favored. Consider two replicate systems of the above structure with slight migration between them. It can be proved that there exists no stable polymorphism with all genotypes represented. (The proof involves the converse version of Principle I, that is, Principle II.) However, if the above three allele genetic population is replicated in *three* systems with slight gene flow between them, then a stable polymorphism is possible involving all types. (The proof is accomplished by application of Principle I.)

3. On mutation selection balance for two locus models with small mutation rate

The haploid model considered is the traditional one. The parameters are listed in Table I. The recombination fraction is denoted by r. The mutation rate of

TABLE I

Gamete	AB	Ab	aB	ab
Fitness coefficient	σ_1	σ_2	σ_3	1
Frequencies in a given generation of haploid individuals	x_1	x_2	x_3	x_4

$a \to A$ or $b \to B$ is μ in both cases with mutations occurring independently at each locus. (All our results carry over as well for different mutation rates at each locus; specifically, rate μ_1 for $a \to A$ and μ_2 for $b \to B$.) Thus, we are assuming unidirectional mutation to the AB gamete.

For definiteness, we postulate as in most of the literature cited (although irrelevant to the qualitative conclusions deduced in this paper) that the effects occur in the order mutation $\to$ random union of gametes $\to$ segregation $\to$ selection. Thus, the population can be envisioned as consisting of mature haploids who produce gametes to be fertilized at which stage mutations occur. After segregation, selection operates.

The recursion relations connecting the gamete frequencies in two successive generations $(x_1, x_2, x_3, x_4) \to (x_1', x_2', x_3', x_4')$ are derived in the standard way yielding

$$(3.1) \quad \begin{aligned} W x_1' &= \sigma_1 \{ x_1 + \mu(x_2 + x_3) + \mu^2 x_4 - r(1 - \mu)^2 D \}, \\ W x_2' &= \sigma_2 \{ (1 - \mu)x_2 + \mu(1 - \mu)x_4 + r(1 - \mu)^2 D \}, \\ W x_3' &= \sigma_3 \{ (1 - \mu)x_3 + \mu(1 - \mu)x_4 + r(1 - \mu)^2 D \}, \\ W x_4' &= (1 - \mu)^2 x_4 - r(1 - \mu)^2 D, \end{aligned}$$

where $D = x_1 x_4 - x_2 x_3$ (the disequilibrium expression) and W, as usual, stands for the sum of the right members of the four equations and is a quadratic function of the variables x_1, x_2, x_3, x_4.

We shall deal mostly with the situation

$$(3.2) \qquad\qquad 1 > \sigma_2, \qquad 1 > \sigma_3, \qquad 1 < \sigma_1,$$

that is, a single mutation has a deleterious effect while a double mutant AB is endowed with a selective advantage relative to the wild type ab. The assumption (3.2) is a major case of interest in Crow and Kimura [2], Eshel and Feldman [3], especially relevant to their discussions concerning the advantages of recombination in evolution.

Let the conditions (3.2) prevail; that is, $\sigma_2 < 1$, $\sigma_3 < 1$, $\sigma_1 > 1$. If $(1 - r)\sigma_1 < 1$, then there exists a positive μ_0 such that for μ satisfying $0 < \mu < \mu_0$ there exists a stable polymorphism $\bar{x}^* = (x_1^*, x_2^*, x_3^*, x_4^*)$ of the system (that is, $x_i^* > 0$, $i = 1, \cdots, 4$) satisfying $x_1^* + x_2^* + x_3^* \le \varepsilon_0$, where $\varepsilon_0(\mu_0)$ tends to zero as μ_0 tends to zero. When $(1 - r)\sigma_1 > 1$ holds, fixation of the AB gamete occurs independent of the rate of mutation.

We can write the transformations (3.1) in the form

$$(3.3) \qquad x_i' = f_i(x_1, x_2, x_3) + \mu g_i(x_1, x_2, x_3, \mu), \qquad i = 1, 2, 3,$$

where $0 \leqq g_i(x_1, x_2, x_3, \mu) \leqq C$ and C is independent of μ and x_i.

The proof then involves an appropriate application of Principles I and II. We refer to Karlin and McGregor [8] for details and further discussion of the implications of the results. There are versions of the above result valid also in the corresponding diploid model.

The result of our Theorem 1 also has relevance to the finding of Feldman [4] that in a haploid two locus population, selection pressures alone cannot maintain a stable polymorphism. Thus, to achieve polymorphism some other influences apart from selection pressures should be operating.

Along these lines, it is implicit in the work of Raper and others that random mating is not applicable to a number of haploid models of fungi populations. In these cases, certain incompatibility mechanisms are in force. For such two locus haploid populations, a stable polymorphism can be maintained by the balance of the force of selection in conjunction with the incompatibility mating behavior.

We can also prove that selection coupled with certain assortative (and not only disassortative or incompatability) patterns of mating can produce stable polymorphisms for a two locus haploid population. Also, *multiniche* two locus haploid populations subject only to selection forces can exhibit stable polymorphism (see Karlin and McGregor [9]).

4. Applications of the basic principle to the study of multilocus models with small recombination parameters

We record some results on multilocus genetic models deduced by appropriate application of Principle I. The rigorous proofs and further developments on multilocus phenomena will be set forth in a separate publication.

Consider first a two locus diploid population. The notation adopted is the traditional one (Bodmer and Felsenstein [1]). The selection parameters of the ten genotypes are listed below

$$(4.1) \qquad \begin{array}{c} \\ AA \\ Aa \\ \\ aa \end{array} \begin{array}{ccc} BB & Bb & bb \\ \left(\begin{matrix} w_{11} & w_{12} & w_{22} \\ w_{13} & w_{14} & w_{24} \\ & w_{23} & \\ w_{33} & w_{34} & w_{44} \end{matrix} \right), \end{array} \qquad w_{14} = w_{23},$$

such that the subscripts 1, 2, 3, 4 refer to the gametes AB, Ab, aB, and ab, respectively, and w_{ij} is the fitness parameter of the genotype composed from gametes i and j. It is convenient to write the parameters in the form

$$(4.2) \qquad \begin{pmatrix} 1 - \alpha_1 & 1 - \beta_1 & 1 - \alpha_2 \\ 1 - \beta_2 & 1 & 1 - \beta_3 \\ 1 - \alpha_3 & 1 - \beta_4 & 1 - \alpha_4 \end{pmatrix}.$$

We will concentrate on the situation where $0 < \alpha_i < 1, 0 < \beta_i < 1, i = 1, 2,$ 3, 4, so that the two double heterozygotes have equal viability and are most fit. The unperturbed system is that where recombination is zero (complete linkage). The model then reduces to a standard four allele viability set up. Principle I can be applied where the small mixing parameter is the recombination fraction r. The following result can be achieved.

THEOREM 1. *If the viability matrix* (4.2) *satisfies one of the following:*

(i) *symmetric viability pattern* (that is, $\alpha_1 = \alpha_4$, $\alpha_2 = \alpha_3$, $\beta_1 = \beta_4$, $\beta_2 = \beta_3$, so that the viabilities are symmetric with respect to the two loci and the labeling of the alleles);

(ii) *multiplicative viabilities* (that is, the selection coefficients are determined as multiplicative effects of the viabilities at each locus);

(iii) *additive viabilities* (that is, the selection coefficients result as the additive effects of the viabilities at each locus), *then for r sufficiently small there exists at least one and at most two locally stable polymorphic equilibria; and*

(iv) *more generally, for r small enough and any viability pattern there exists at most two stable polymorphic equilibria.*

It is conjectured that the bound 2 on the number of stable polymorphic equilibria persists for all r.

Some additional special information applies in the situations of (i) and (ii).

(a) In the additive viability model with overdominance (meaning here that the double heterozygotes are most fit), there exists a unique interior stable polymorphism exhibiting linkage equilibrium with global convergence to this equilibrium occurring from any initial composition involving all gametes. This occurs for all recombination values $r > 0$ (see Karlin and Feldman [7]).

(b) By appropriate choices of the selection parameters for the case of multiplicative viabilities, we always have two stable internal equilibria provided r is near 0. On the other hand, when r is near $\frac{1}{2}$ Moran [12] established global convergence to an internal equilibrium which is in linkage equilibrium.

Extensions to multilocus model. Consider the corresponding model of k loci and assume all complete multiple heterozygotes have equal viability and are of superior fitness to all other genotypes. The following general result prevails. *There exists a prescription of viability parameters leading to 2^{k-1} distinct locally stable polymorphic equilibria. Moreover, for the multiplicative viability model if all the pairwise recombination parameters are sufficiently small then there exists at most 2^{k-1} distinct stable polymorphic equilibria. Any even number $\leqq 2^{k-1}$ can occur.*

These results suggest that there are generally more cases of stable polymorphism for multilocus selection models involving tight linkage than for weak linkage. The relevant polymorphisms for small recombination parameters are usually in substantial linkage disequilibrium, where a preponderance of a few special chromosome types are abundantly present. These facts argue for the conclusion that if variability (latent or actual) is desired for a population to cope with a multitude of environments, then recombination reducing mechanism may be favored in order to produce increased possibilities of polymorphism. Actually, tight linkage is a vehicle for maintaining diverse forms of polymorphism and, of course, also serve for easy transcription of a series of actions (biochemical or otherwise) controlled by a sequence of closley linked loci. On the other hand, loose linkage or large recombinations parallel more the effects of mutation and sexuality. Moderate recombination appears to serve less well both the objectives of maintaining polymorphism and/or simple regular gene transcription.

The analysis of multilocus models provides an important application of the general principle of Section 2. Principle I can be interpreted as a perturbation or continuity theorem. Starting with a given genetic system for which the nature of the equilibria can be fully delineated (for example, the classical multiallelic viability model), it is desired to investigate a perturbed version of the model. The perturbing factors can be in the form of small mutation and/or migration pressures, weak selection effects, slight seed load or some other genetic carry over from previous generations or small recombination effects superimposed on a multiallelic selection model corresponding to a multilocus situation with no recombination. In this last case, we have established the remarkable fact that in a k locus genetic model with multiplicative viability selection coefficients, provided all pairwise recombination parameters are sufficiently small, there exist at most 2^{k-1} stable polymorphic equilibria and for certain specifications of the selection coefficients this upper bound is achieved. This result underscores the increased potentialities for polymorphism corresponding to large cistrons or supergene complexes with slight intragenic recombination present.

The validation of these assertions for multilocus selection genetic model is not accomplished by determining explicitly the actual equilibria in the perturbed system and testing their stability properties (undoubtedly a prohibitive task), but rather the procedure exploits continuity methods coupled with the implicit function theorem and certain fixed point theorems.

The assertions of this section, their proofs, and implications for evolutionary theory will be elaborated elsewhere.

REFERENCES

[1] W. F. Bodmer and J. Felsenstein, "Linkage and selection: theoretical analysis of the deterministic two locus random mating model," *Genetics*, Vol. 57 (1967), pp. 237–265.
[2] J. F. Crow and M. Kimura, "Evolution in sexual and asexual populations," *Amer. Natur.*, Vol. 99 (1965), pp. 439–450.
[3] I. Eshel and M. W. Feldman, "On the evolutionary effect of recombination," *Theor. Pop. Biol.*, Vol. 1 (1970), pp. 88–101.
[4] M. W. Feldman, "Equilibrium studies of two locus haploid populations with recombination," *Theor. Pop. Biol.*, Vol. 2 (1971), pp. 299–318.
[5] I. Franklin and R. C. Lewontin, "Is the gene the unit of selection?," *Genetics*, Vol. 65 (1970), pp. 707–734.
[6] S. Karlin and M. W. Feldman, "Linkage and selection: the two locus symmetric viability model," *Theor. Pop. Biol.*, Vol. 1 (1970), pp. 39–72.
[7] ———, "Convergence to equilibrium of the two locus additive viability model," *J. Appl. Probability*, Vol. 7 (1970), pp. 262–271.

[8] S. KARLIN and J. McGREGOR, "On mutation selection balance for two-locus haploid and diploid populations," *Theor. Pop. Biol.*, Vol. 2 (1971), pp. 60–70.

[9] ———, "Polymorphisms for genetic and ecological systems with weak coupling," *Theor. Pop. Biol.*, Vol. 3 (1972), pp. 210–238.

[10] ———, "Application of methods of small parameters to multi-niche population genetic models," *Theor. Pop. Biol.*, Vol. 3 (1972), pp. 186–209.

[11] ———, "Polymorphisms for multi-locus selection system with tight linkage," to appear, 1973.

[12] P. A. P. MORAN, "On the theory of selection dependent on two loci," *Ann. Hum. Genet.*, Vol. 32 (1968), pp. 183–190.

THE MATHEMATICS OF SEX
AND MARRIAGE

NATHAN KEYFITZ

UNIVERSITY OF CALIFORNIA, BERKELEY

1. Introduction

The models of this paper attempt to account for the age, sex, and marital status distributions of human populations. A marriage market develops around preferences for mates of different ages, and we study this market as changes in age distributions change the availability of mates. Unless we know how to relate marriages to the exposed population, we cannot even calculate rates that will tell us whether marriage is increasing or decreasing. Sections 11 to 16 below attempt an empirically based solution of the two-sex problem.

2. Separate treatment of the sexes

To suggest what constitutes a "solution" from a demographic viewpoint, think of the sense in which the one-sex problem is solved. A given and fixed set of birth and death rates, specific by age, say for females, determines the entire trajectory of a closed population. Theory permits a calculation of exactly how many individuals would be present at each future time if those rates applied; the ultimate stable age distribution, the ultimate stable rates of birth, death, and natural increase, are similarly calculable. For the shorter term, a spectral analysis specifies the waves through which the population at each age would move on its way to the stable exponentially increasing condition; we can in particular trace the echo effect by which an initial hollow in the age distribution tends to be reflected in later generations with gradually diminishing relative amplitude until it disappears.

Aside from this, the one-sex theory enables us to say just what a given degree of emigration will do to the level of the ultimate population; how birth control applied by women aged 40 will affect the rate of increase of the population, as compared with birth control applied by women aged 20; when we find that the United States has a much higher mean age than Mexico, the theory enables us to trace this to our low birth rates rather than to any advantage that we may have in lower mortality. Within its own assumptions, often a close approximation to reality, the model gives complete and consistent results.

Acknowledgment is made of NSF grant GZ995 and NIH Research Contract 69-2200. The text was prepared while I was Visiting Professor at the University of Wisconsin in September 1971.

This is not true of the two sexes considered simultaneously, where models typically produce selfcontradictions. Consider two separate, uncoupled equations, one for the trajectory of each sex. Between the number F_t of females at time t and its derivative F'_t we might have the relation

$$(2.1) \qquad\qquad F'_t = r_F F_t,$$

where r_F is the observed rate of increase, to which the solution is $F_t = F_0 \exp \{r_F t\}$. For males M_t at time t, we would correspondingly have

$$(2.2) \qquad\qquad M'_t = r_M M_t,$$

with solution $M_t = M_0 \exp \{r_M t\}$.

If the parameters r_F and r_M are taken from a given period of observation of a real population, the two equations will provide solutions in which the male and female populations increase unequally, so that the sex ratio ultimately becomes zero or infinity. We know that in real populations the male and female populations do adjust in numbers so as to maintain equality, and the mechanism by which they do this eludes the representation (2.1) and (2.2).

3. Female dominance without recognition of age

The simplest way of coupling the equations is by supposing male or female *dominance* in the generation of births. In female dominance, both boy and girl babies are generated in fixed proportion to the number of females at time t. The pair of equations for the population trajectory becomes, if the birth rate is λ and the death rate μ,

$$(3.1) \qquad\qquad \begin{aligned} M'_t &= -\mu_M M_t + \lambda_M F_t, \\ F'_t &= -\mu_F F_t + \lambda_F F_t. \end{aligned}$$

The form of these equations, with $\mu_M = \mu_F$ and $\lambda_M = \lambda_F$, is due to Kendall [15]; Goodman [7] permitted the male and female parameters to differ from one another. The ratio λ_M/λ_F is not arbitrary, but holds close to 1.05 for human populations.

The equations (3.1) are coupled in one direction only—the first depends on the second, but the second does not depend on the first. The second member of (3.1) is in fact the same as (2.1) if we identify $\lambda_F - \mu_F$ with r_F, and hence must be satisfied by $F_t = F_0 \exp \{(\lambda_F - \mu_F)t\}$. From the solution for females in the second member of (3.1), that for males follows by substitution in the first member, and it turns out that the male population ultimately increases according to the same exponential as the female.

To find the asymptotic ratio of males to females is to find the value at which M_t/F_t has a zero derivative. Where the derivative of M_t/F_t is zero, M_t/F_t will be equal to the ratio of derivatives M'_t/F'_t, and hence from (3.1),

$$(3.2) \qquad\qquad \frac{M_\infty}{F_\infty} = \frac{M'_\infty}{F'_\infty} = \frac{-\mu_M M_\infty + \lambda_M F_\infty}{(\lambda_F - \mu_F) F_\infty},$$

or if R_∞ is the ratio M_∞/F_∞,

$$(3.3) \qquad R_\infty = \frac{-\mu_M R_\infty + \lambda_M}{\lambda_F - \mu_F}.$$

Solving this for R_∞, gives easily

$$(3.4) \qquad R_\infty = \frac{\lambda_M}{\lambda_F - \mu_F + \mu_M}.$$

The one sided coupling of the equations (3.1) is a decided improvement on the one sex model. It leads to (3.4) which accords with common sense in telling us that insofar as male mortality is heavier than female the ultimate sex ratio of the population of all ages will be less than the sex ratio at birth (Goodman [7], Keyfitz [16], p. 297). But it has the drawback of supposing that births continue unchanged in the total absence of males.

A similar argument applies to male dominance and to an average of male and female dominance taken with fixed weights. A degree of male dominance D would mean that each male produces at the rate of $D\lambda_M$ male births, and each female produces at the rate of $(1 - D)\lambda_M$ male births, per unit time, so that male births would be $\lambda_M(DM_t + (1 - D)F_t)$. Similarly, female births would be $\lambda_F(DM_t + (1 - D)F_t)$. If D is unity, then the rate of increase of the system is $\lambda_M - \mu_M$. If D is zero, the rate of increase is $\lambda_F - \mu_F$. If D is fixed at some intermediate value, then the ultimate rate of increase of the system is a weighted average of the male rate of increase $\lambda_M - \mu_M$ and of the female rate $\lambda_F - \mu_F$. This is better than female dominance, where births depend not at all on males. Nonetheless, births would still continue, though at a lower rate, in the mixed dominance case if either sex was entirely absent, as long as D is fixed.

4. The harmonic mean birth function

The defect may be rectified by making dominance vary with time, say letting the degree of male dominance be given by

$$(4.1) \qquad D_t = \frac{F_t}{M_t + F_t}.$$

In support of such a value of D_t we note that when there are few females D_t would be low, which is to say that the model would make births depend largely on the number of females, and on males when males are few. The equations are now

$$(4.2) \qquad \begin{aligned} M'_t &= -\mu_M M_t + \lambda_M(D_t M_t + (1 - D_t)F_t), \\ F'_t &= -\mu_F F_t + \lambda_F(D_t M_t + (1 - D_t)F_t), \\ D_t &= \frac{F_t}{M_t + F_t}, \end{aligned}$$

where as usual λ_M/λ_F equals the sex ratio at birth. By entering $D_t = F_t/(M_t + F_t)$ in the first two equations, we obtain

$$(4.3) \qquad \begin{aligned} M'_t &= -\mu_M M_t + 2\lambda_M \frac{M_t F_t}{M_t + F_t}, \\[2mm] F'_t &= -\mu_F F_t + 2\lambda_F \frac{M_t F_t}{M_t + F_t}. \end{aligned}$$

These equations are homogeneous and of the first degree in M_t and F_t, though not linear.

We can study the asymptotic properties of the system (4.3) by entering me^{rt} for M_t and fe^{rt} for F_t. Making this substitution and eliminating m and f, we obtain the condition for consistency, and it may be arranged to provide the intrinsic rate of natural increase as

$$(4.4) \qquad r = \frac{2}{\dfrac{1}{\lambda_M} + \dfrac{1}{\lambda_F}} - \frac{\dfrac{\mu_M}{\lambda_M} + \dfrac{\mu_F}{\lambda_F}}{\dfrac{1}{\lambda_M} + \dfrac{1}{\lambda_F}}.$$

Of the two terms the first is the harmonic mean of the given birth rates λ_M and λ_F, and the second a weighted arithmetic mean of the given death rates μ_M and μ_F, the weights being the reciprocals of the birth rates.

The corresponding ultimate sex ratio is m/f or

$$(4.5) \qquad \frac{m}{f} = \frac{\lambda_M - \frac{1}{2}(\mu_M - \mu_F)}{\lambda_F + \frac{1}{2}(\mu_M - \mu_F)},$$

whose numerator and denominator, respectively, are the averages of the numerator and denominator of the male and female dominant models.

Robert Traxler has gone on to solve (4.3) more completely. He divides the first equation by M_t and the second by F_t, subtracts the first equation from the second, substitutes $\log z$ for M_t/F_t, and so reduces the problem to a standard quadrature in z.

Our set (4.3) was reached by making dominance a function D_t of time. Fredrickson ([6], p. 121) and Pollard [26] reach the same equations by a different and instructive argument. They suggest the conditions that: (1) if linear equations are not possible, then let us at worst have equations that are homogeneous of degree one; (2) when either males or females are lacking, the births must be zero; and (3) when males are relatively plentiful the number of births must be proportional to the number of females, and *vice versa*. The quantity $M_t F_t/(M_t + F_t)$ tends simply to F_t when M_t is large:

$$(4.6) \qquad \lim_{M_t \to \infty} \frac{M_t F_t}{M_t + F_t} = \lim_{M_t \to \infty} \frac{F_t}{1 + \dfrac{F_t}{M_t}} = F_t.$$

A similar result holds when F_t becomes large and M_t remains finite.

The theoretical argument in favor of the harmonic mean birth function $2M_t F_t/(M_t + F_t)$ applies to marriage as well as to birth. But, as we will see in an empirical test below, the fluctuations in available males and females existing in real populations are not great enough to enable the harmonic mean to stand out over the arithmetic and geometric means.

5. An asymmetric birth function

A desirable degree of asymmetry is introduced by replacing $M_t F_t/(M_t + F_t)$ in (4.3) by $M_t^{1-\varepsilon} F_t^{1+\varepsilon}/(M_t + F_t)$. The homogeneity is retained, and setting ε greater than zero would make births depend more on fluctuations in the number of females than of males.

The pair of equations corresponding to (4.3), but with $M_t F_t$ on the right replaced by $M_t^{1-\varepsilon} F_t^{1+\varepsilon}$, may again be studied by entering $M_t = me^{rt}$ and $F_t = fe^{rt}$. We have two homogeneous equations in m and f:

(5.1)
$$mr = -\mu_M m + 2\lambda_M \frac{m^{1-\varepsilon} f^{1+\varepsilon}}{m + f},$$

$$fr = -\mu_F f + 2\lambda_F \frac{m^{1-\varepsilon} f^{1+\varepsilon}}{m + f},$$

equivalent to two nonhomogeneous equations in r and the ultimate sex ratio $m/f = x$:

(5.2)
$$r = -\mu_M + 2\lambda_M \frac{x^{-\varepsilon}}{1 + x},$$

$$r = -\mu_F + 2\lambda_F \frac{x^{1-\varepsilon}}{1 + x}.$$

First seeking x by equating the two right sides, we have

(5.3)
$$x \equiv \frac{m}{f} = \frac{\lambda_M - \frac{1}{2}(\mu_M - \mu_F)x^\varepsilon}{\lambda_F + \frac{1}{2}(\mu_M - \mu_F)x^\varepsilon},$$

which expresses x in terms of the other quantities including x^ε. This can be used for iteration, starting with an arbitrary x, say 1, entered on the right side to start the process. With ε zero, this is the same as (4.5), and with ε small, convergence will be rapid.

Once x is known, r may be obtained from either member of the pair (5.2):

(5.4)
$$r = 2\lambda_M \left(\frac{x^{-\varepsilon}}{1 + x} \right) - \mu_M.$$

If x were unity, then r would be $\lambda_M - \mu_M$. Having x greater than unity and ε positive lowers the value of r. In words, if there are fewer women than men, then making births depend more on women than on men reduces the birth rate. This is hardly surprising, but it shows that the model makes sense in one important respect.

6. A simple marriage model

Permanent monogamous marriage modifies the two-sex problem by fixing the difference between ages of father and mother through any sequence of births to a particular couple. We can here, in preliminary fashion because age is omitted, follow Kendall ([15], p. 248) and Goodman ([7], p. 216) in setting down the conditions for marriage and reproduction with the two sexes. This section is confined to female marriage dominance, meaning that the number of marriages is proportional to the number of females. The equations for single females F_t and for married couples N_t are

$$
(6.1) \qquad
\begin{aligned}
F'_t &= -(\mu_F + \nu)F_t + (\lambda_F + \mu_M)N_t, \\
N'_t &= \nu F_t - (\mu_F + \mu_M)N_t,
\end{aligned}
$$

where ν is the fraction of females marrying per unit time, applied continuously to F_t. We suppose that all births occur to married couples, at rate λ_F for girl babies, and that death rates are the same for the married and single population, conditions that could be relaxed at the cost of a slight complication in the equations. The first of the equations (6.1) says that the number of single females (a) declines with female mortality and with marriage, and (b) increases with births and with the death of married males. (We are counting the widows as "single.") The equation for single males can be easily written down, but is omitted here because it cannot affect the trajectory of females in our female dominant model.

Unlike equations that we will meet later, the pair (6.1) is easily solved. The trajectory from any starting point F_0 and N_0 and any set of the Greek letter fixed parameters is a sum of two exponentials each multiplied by a constant. But to try to answer our questions without explicit solution will be more suggestive for the unsolvable models that follow. We may be interested in the ratio of married to single females N_t/F_t and especially its rate of change. This is given by

$$
(6.2) \qquad \frac{d\left(\dfrac{N_t}{F_t}\right)}{dt} = \frac{N'_t}{F_t} - \frac{N_t}{F_t}\frac{F'_t}{F_t},
$$

in which we may enter the derivatives from (6.1):

$$
(6.3) \qquad \frac{d\left(\dfrac{N_t}{F_t}\right)}{dt} = \nu + \frac{N_t}{F_t}(\nu - \mu_M) - \left(\frac{N_t}{F_t}\right)^2 (\lambda_F + \mu_M).
$$

Equation (6.3) tells us that the ratio of married to single women goes up with ν, the marriage rate, and it goes down with increased births of females or deaths of males. These entirely reasonable results are evidence that we have not put into our equations (6.1) conditions that contradict common sense. It also follows from (6.3) that the proportion married is not affected by the female death rate, provided, as in this model, mortality is the same for single and married females.

7. Introduction of age in a continuous model

However, we cannot be satisfied with any model that fails to take account of age, since we are hoping to answer questions concerning the marriage market, which is clearly sorted out by age as well as sex. Sets of equations such as (3.1) or (6.1) can distinguish ages if we interpret F_t and other variables as column vectors of age distributions—say in five year age intervals, with the first item the number of persons aged zero to four at last birthday, the second element the numbers five to nine, and so forth. The Greek letter constants in (3.1) or (6.1) would now be interpreted as square matrices, with as many rows and columns as the number of ages recognized.

In fact there is good reason to object to matrix differential equations in this application. To take the same interval of time as of age offers a real advantage in population analysis, because then the whole group of one age moves into the next age interval in the time interval. If the time interval is shorter than the age interval only a part of the group moves on, and we face the complication of calculating what part. Thus, staying with discrete ages while making the time interval infinitesimal is to be avoided. We could easily write an analogue to any of our equations in discrete time; that for the first member of (6.1) would be given by replacing F'_t on the left by $F_{t+1} - F_t$. The Leslie [17] theory then applies in full detail.

Here we will proceed to infinitesimal intervals for both age and time, a device developed by von Foerster [5] in his work on cellular proliferation. In application to equations (2.1) and (2.2), F_t becomes a function of age and time, say $F_{a,t}$, and the female population of age $a + \Delta a$ at time $t + \Delta t$ is $F_{a+\Delta a, t+\Delta t}$. These latter include the same individuals as were counted in $F_{a,t}$, only a little older and subject to deductions for mortality (as well as for emigration if one wishes, but we shall confine ourselves here to populations closed to migration). The equation corresponding to (2.1) and (2.2) becomes

$$(7.1) \qquad F_{a+\Delta a, t+\Delta t} = F_{a,t} - \mu_a F_{a,t} \Delta t.$$

Expanding on the left by Taylor's theorem for two independent variables and cancelling $F_{a,t}$ from both sides, we have

$$(7.2) \qquad \frac{\partial F_{a,t}}{\partial t} \Delta t + \frac{\partial F_{a,t}}{\partial a} \Delta a = -\mu_a F_{a,t} \Delta t.$$

Dividing by Δa, which is supposed to be the same as Δt, and allowing $\Delta a = \Delta t$ to tend to zero, we have

$$(7.3) \qquad \frac{\partial F_{a,t}}{\partial t} + \frac{\partial F_{a,t}}{\partial a} = -\mu_a F_{a,t}.$$

This is von Foerster's equation for one sex, for all values of $0 < a < \omega$, where ω is the oldest age to which anyone lives. The corresponding equation for males at age a' is

$$(7.4) \qquad \frac{\partial M_{a',t}}{\partial t} + \frac{\partial M_{a',t}}{\partial a'} = -\mu_{a'} M_{a',t}$$

(Fredrickson [6]). Note that (7.3) and (7.4) are concerned with mortality only; $\mu_{a'}$ is our way of writing the male force of mortality. Deaths are uncoupled as usual; the numbers of males and their deaths are not taken as having any effect on the deaths of females.

Births enter as a boundary condition at age zero:

$$(7.5) \qquad F_{0,t} = \int_\alpha^\beta F_{a,t}\lambda_{a,t}\, da,$$

where α is the youngest age of childbearing and β the oldest, and $\lambda_{a,t}$ is the age specific birth rate at time t. We will consider birth rates fixed in time and accordingly write $\lambda_{a,t}$ as λ_a. But this is unsatisfactory once again, because births really depend on males as well as on females, and our model must somehow take account of this.

To improve on the female model with fixed (female, male, or mixed) dominance we need a simultaneous birth function of the females aged a to $a + da$ *and* males aged a' to $a' + da'$. By an extension of the varying D_t incorporated in (4.3), we could use here an analogue to the harmonic mean for births

$$(7.6) \qquad F_{0,t} = \frac{1}{F_t + M_t} \int_\alpha^\beta \int_\alpha^\beta \lambda_{a,a'} F_{a,t} M_{a',t}\, da\, da',$$

where $F_t + M_t$ is the total population of both sexes and all ages. This substantially meets the requirements mentioned earlier; for example, if the male population of all ages becomes very large then the birth rate $\lambda_{a,a'}$ is multiplied by a number proportional to $F_{a,t}$. Only if some ages and not others became very large would (7.6) be unsatisfactory.

Since in any large population the ratio of boy to girl babies is nearly constant, we can take for the boundary condition on males,

$$(7.7) \qquad M_{0,t} = sF_{0,t},$$

s being the sex ratio at birth.

Finally, to start the system on its way we need initial age distributions for males and females:

$$(7.8) \qquad \begin{array}{ll} F_{a,0} = F_a, & 0 < a < \omega \\ M_{a',0} = M_{a'}, & 0 < a' < \omega. \end{array}$$

To convert (7.3) to a homogeneous form, apply the substitution

$$(7.9) \qquad F_{a,t} = \exp\left\{-\int_0^a \mu_b\, db\right\} G_{a,t},$$

which results in

$$(7.10) \qquad \frac{\partial G_{a,t}}{\partial a} + \frac{\partial G_{a,t}}{\partial t} = 0.$$

But any function of $t - a$, say $G_{a,t} = f(t - a)$, obviously satisfies this homogeneous equation. Hence, a general solution of (7.3) is

$$(7.11) \qquad F_{a,t} = f_0 \exp\left\{-\int_0^a \mu_b\, db\right\} f(t - a),$$

where f_0 is an arbitrary constant, and $f(t - a)$ an arbitrary function.

To deal more easily with the boundary conditions, we will specialize $f(t - a)$ to an exponential, writing $f(t - a) = \exp\{(t - a)r\}$. Entering in (7.6) the value

(7.12)
$$F_{a,t} = f_0 \exp\{(t - a)r\} \exp\left\{-\int_0^a \mu_b \, db\right\}$$

and the corresponding function for $M_{a',t}$, we can solve for the asymptotic sex ratio and rate of increase as t becomes large.

We will make the usual assumption that the sex ratio at birth is the same for all ages of mothers and fathers, that is, in the present notation that $s = \lambda'_{a,a'}/\lambda_{a,a'}$, where $\lambda'_{a,a'}$ is defined as the rate of birth of boy babies to couples of which the mother is aged a and the father a'. For ease in writing let $\exp\left\{-\int_0^a \mu_b \, db\right\}$ be called ℓ_a as is usual in demographic work.

Then we have from (7.6) and the corresponding equation for $M_{0,t}$

(7.13)
$$\frac{M_{0,t}}{F_{0,t}} = \frac{\int_\alpha^\beta \int_\alpha^\beta \lambda'_{a,a'} \exp\{-r(a + a')\} \ell_a \ell_{a'} \, da \, da'}{\int_\alpha^\beta \int_\alpha^\beta \lambda_{a,a'} \exp\{-r(a + a')\} \ell_a \ell_{a'} \, da \, da'},$$

and with the supposition $\lambda'_{a,a'} = s\lambda_{a,a'}$, the ratio of integrals reduces to s. The assumption of a fixed ratio of boy to girl babies at each age of parents evidently leads to a fixed sex ratio for total births at all times. The sex ratio in the population as a whole is obtained from (7.12) and the corresponding equation for males as

(7.14)
$$\frac{M_t}{F_t} = \frac{\int_0^\omega M_{a,t} \, da}{\int_0^\omega F_{a,t} \, da} = \frac{s \int_0^\omega e^{-ra} \ell'_a \, da}{\int_0^\omega e^{-ra} \ell_a \, da}.$$

The boundary condition (7.6) provides the intrinsic rate of increase of the system r. Entering the general solution for $F_{a,t}$ of (7.12) and the corresponding solution for $M_{a,t}$, (7.6) becomes

(7.15)
$$1 = \frac{\int_\alpha^\beta \int_\alpha^\beta \lambda_{a,a'} e^{-ra} \ell_a e^{-ra'} \ell'_{a'} \, da \, da'}{\int_0^\omega (e^{-ra} \ell_a + s e^{-ra} \ell'_a) \, da},$$

on cancelling e^{rt} from both sides. (See Fredrickson [6], Equation (38).) This equation for r in the two sex model corresponds to Lotka's characteristic equation for one sex. It is solvable by iterative methods—for example, multiplying both sides by $e^{27.5r}$ and taking $1/27.5$ of the logarithms gives an improved r on the left when an arbitrary r is inserted on the right. (The method is exhibited in detail for the characteristic equation of the one-sex model in Keyfitz [16], p. 108.) P. Das Gupta [2] has developed and applied in some detail a two-sex model similar to that of the present section.

The model consisting of equations (7.3), (7.4), (7.6), (7.7), and (7.8) can be shown to reduce to the Lotka integral equation, where one sex only, say females, is under consideration and the analysis is concentrated on female births $F_{0,t}$.

The discrete approach using matrices (Leslie [17]) and that of Goodman [7] reduce to the above partial differential equations when the intervals of time and age, always remaining equal to one another, tend to zero. The partial differential equations may be extended to an explicit incorporation of marriage, and to this we proceed.

8. Age and marriage in a continuous model

If husbands and wives were always of exactly the same age, the contradictions between the male and female uncoupled models could be easily overcome, and much of the problem with which we are here concerned would disappear. In fact husbands are of different ages from their wives, but not independently for the several children: for any given marriage the difference of ages remains always the same. We take advantage of this fact by distinguishing the married population from the single, and suppose that all births are to married couples (Fredrickson, [6]).

Now let $M_{a',t} \, da'$ be the number of single males of age a' to $a' + da'$, let $F_{a,t} \, da$ be single females of age a to $a + da$, and let $N_{a,a',t} \, da \, da'$ be the number of couples in which the age of the wife is a to $a + da$ and of the husband a' to $a' + da'$. The partial differential equation for unmarried females that corresponds to (7.3) is

$$(8.1) \quad \frac{\partial F_{a,t}}{\partial t} + \frac{\partial F_{a,t}}{\partial a} = -\mu_a F_{a,t} - \int_0^\omega \nu_{a,a'} f(M_{a',t}, F_{a,t}) \, da'$$

$$+ \int_0^\omega \mu_{a'} N_{a,a',t} \, da' + \frac{1}{1+s} \int_0^\omega \lambda_{a,a'} N_{a,a',t} \, da',$$

where μ_a is the death rate of females of age a; $\nu_{a,a'}$ is the marriage rate between girls aged a and men aged a'; $\mu_{a'}$ is the death rate of males of age a'; $\lambda_{a,a'}$ is the rate of childbearing at time t of couples of which the wife is aged a and the husband aged a'; and f is a function whose nature will be discussed below. Of the four terms shown on the right side of (8.1) the first allows for the deaths of unmarried females, the second for marriages of women to men of all ages, the third for the deaths of married males, each of which releases one female into the unmarried group, and the fourth for childbearing among married couples.

The last term of (8.1) makes births perfectly straightforward in the two sex model. Admittedly its $\lambda_{a,a'}$ demands a kind of data that is not commonly produced, namely births by age of father and of mother, along with the number of married couples in the population by age of husband and of wife. These could easily be tabulated from existing censuses and vital statistics, and such tabulations are available for a few countries. The two items of data, on births and population, provide a discrete version of $\lambda_{a,a'}$; birth rates specific for age of father and of mother, say in five year age intervals, would be obtained by dividing births by population in each class. If seven age intervals are recognized for women, and nine for males, this means 63 rates altogether, not an impossible number to handle.

9. Varying marriage dominance

The second term on the right of (8.1), to allow for the women who leave the single state for marriage, now inherits the difficulties that appeared for births in models not recognizing marriage. All the possibilities in the function $f(M_{a',t}F_{a,t})$ that were previously open for births are now possibilities for marriage, and each brings with it the earlier disadvantages. To use female dominance would cause marriages to take place in the model even in the absence of males, and with male dominance in the absence of females. Mixed dominance in any fixed ratio would entail at least part of the same drawback.

The only escape is to allow the degree of dominance to vary according to the availabilities of individuals of the two sexes at the ages in question. The analogue for marriage and age to (4.3) would give for the second term on the right side of (8.1)

$$(9.1) \qquad - \int_0^\omega \nu_{a,a'} \frac{2M_{a',t}F_{a,t}}{M_{a',t} + F_{a,t}} \, da'.$$

Yet (9.1) does not embrace the full complexity of the problem. For marriages between women of age a and men of age a' evidently depend on much more than $F_{a,t}$ and $M_{a',t}$. They depend also on the numbers of individuals at other ages. If for example the number of women at ages $a - 1$ and $a + 1$ is increased, all other circumstances remaining the same, then the number of marriages between women aged a and men aged a' will be reduced. To take this into account we would have to make the second term on the right of (8.1) depend on other ages of women, say represented by x, so it would become

$$(9.2) \qquad - \int_0^\omega \int_0^\omega \nu_{a,x,a'} f(M_{a',t}, F_{a,t}, F_{x,t}) \, dx \, da',$$

where the function f would have to be specified. Equally, it could be argued that other ages of men should be taken into account.

10. Measuring the marriage rate

Until we know the form of the marriage function, we have no denominator constituting exposures that will permit calculation of a marriage rate. With a suitable marriage function, we can calculate marriage rates just as we calculate death rates. An example will suffice to present the problem and the proposed solution.

Let us try to decide whether marriage among single persons 20 to 24 years of age went up or down between 1963 and 1967 in the registration area of the United States. The facts are that 207,211 first marriages at those ages were reported for 1963, and 315,650 first marriages for 1967, in official vital statistics. In 1963, the estimated number of single males 20 to 24 was 2,355,000, and in 1967 it was 3,379,000, so in relation to single males the marriage rate was 0.0880 in 1963 and 0.0934 in 1967, a six per cent increase. But relating the marriages to the number of single women in the two years (1,339,000 and 2,183,000, respectively) produces the ratios 0.1547 for 1963 and 0.1446 for 1967, a seven per cent decline. Did the marriage rate go up or down?

Clearly, the best denominator for the rate is some kind of average of the single men and women. If we take the geometric mean the rate declines from 0.1167 to 0.1162 or 0.4 per cent. We will see, however, that such a symmetric treatment of the men and women exposed is not quite appropriate.

11. The marriage coefficients—response of preferences to availabilities

Running through all work on this subject is an implicit juxtaposition between the ages of mates preferred by young people and the demographic availabilities of persons of those ages. (Griffith Feeney [3], Henry [10], Hirschman and Matras [12], Hoem [13], and others have elaborated this point.) It is this juxtaposition that must somehow be incorporated in the marriage function. We want a function that will apply in the face of considerable departures from the availabilities that are "normal," that is, from those pertaining to a population of fixed marriage, birth and death rates and no migration.

A substantial departure from normal availabilities occurs in the wake of the postwar baby boom. United States births in 1947 numbered 3,817,000 (*Historical Statistics*, p. 22). About twenty years later the girls of this cohort reach marrying age, and they would ordinarily marry men about two years older than themselves, which is to say men born about 1945. But the births of 1945 numbered only 2,858,000, about one quarter fewer than those of 1947. This is what Paul Glick [24] has termed the marriage squeeze, and it is occurring in most western countries. When the births decline, on the other side of the baby boom, the squeeze will be in the opposite direction—the shortage will be of girls. This has already come about in Japan, and will gradually appear in the United States towards the end of the 1970's. Insofar as the fall of births from 1957 to 1968 was more gradual than the rise from 1945 to 1947 the squeeze of the mid-1980's will be less spectacular than that of the early 1970's.

Having now brought the presentation of the problem to its maximum of difficulty, I shall show how it can be simplified again, and how data may be made to bear on at least some aspects. What is needed is a way of using the observation of marriages in successive years, along with the known availabilities by age, to tell what function of the ages of available men and women determines the unions that take place. If the availabilities were always the same, we could not make the inference I propose, and under this condition of stability the problem would not arise. It is the changing availabilities that both give rise to the problem of this paper and provide the data for its solution.

12. Forcing the data to decide among marriage functions

The first confrontation with data in effect asks the observed marriages to discriminate among the five marriage functions:

$$(12.1) \qquad N_{i,j,t} = \nu_{i,j} F_{i,t} \qquad \text{(female dominance),}$$

$$(12.2) \qquad N_{i,j,t} = \nu_{i,j} M_{j,t} \qquad \text{(male dominance),}$$

$$(12.3) \qquad N_{i,j,t} = \nu_{i,j}(0.5 F_{i,t} + 0.5 M_{j,t}) \qquad \text{(arithmetic mean),}$$

$$(12.4) \qquad N_{i,j,t} = \nu_{i,j}(F_{i,t}^{0.5} M_{j,t}^{0.5}) \qquad \text{(geometric mean),}$$

$$(12.5) \qquad N_{i,j,t} = 2\nu_{i,j} \frac{F_{i,t} M_{j,t}}{F_{i,t} + M_{j,t}} \qquad \text{(harmonic mean),}$$

and to tell us which fits the observed marriages best.

We should be able to decide which of the functions (12.1) to (12.5) above is appropriate once we know marriages by age of bride and groom for two dates t and t', and the numbers of males and females exposed to the risk of marriage at the two dates. If the marriage function to be used is $f(F_{i,t}, M_{j,t})$, where f stands for any of (12.1) to (12.5) or some other function altogether, and if f contains one constant $\nu_{i,j}$ for each combination of ages as do (12.1) to (12.5), then the constant can be evaluated for time t and the f so completely specified can be applied to time t'. Suppose that the resulting estimate of marriages between brides aged i and grooms aged j at time t' is

$$(12.6) \qquad \hat{N}_{i,j,t'} = f(F_{i,t'}, M_{j,t'}).$$

Then the difference $d_{i,j,t'}$ between this estimate $\hat{N}_{i,j,t'}$ and the observation $N_{i,j,t'}$,

$$(12.7) \qquad d_{i,j,t'} = N_{i,j,t'} - \hat{N}_{i,j,t'},$$

averaged somehow over the ages of women i and of men j, is a measure of the appropriateness of the marriage function f.

Three kinds of average of (12.7) will be used—its root mean square, mean $\frac{3}{2}$ power, and mean absolute value, shown as the columns of Table I. The mean square gives relatively more weight to the large deviations, and the mean absolute value more weight to the smaller ones. We will see that the three measures do not always report in quite the same way on a given set of data.

The work will be confined to first marriages, partly because the exposure to risk is more clearcut for these. If divorce is easy the whole of the married population is at risk of further marriage, but the degree of risk varies greatly among individuals and we have no way of establishing a cutoff. For first marriages the single population is the obvious measure of exposure, even though some members may be immune and others highly susceptible.

TABLE I

MEASURE OF DEPARTURE FROM OBSERVATIONS OF ESTIMATES OF MARRIAGES BASED ON
FIVE MARRIAGE FUNCTIONS, DATA FOR UNITED STATES 1963 AND 1967, AND SWEDEN 1959
AND 1963
n is 9 for the U.S. and 36 for Sweden.

	$[\sum (d^2/n)]^{1/2}$	$[\sum |d|^{3/2}/n]^{2/3}$	$\sum |d|/n$
United States 1963 and 1967			
(12.1) Female dominance	16,256	14,465	12,079
(12.2) Male dominance	18,860	16,498	13,642
(12.3) Arithmetic mean	14,316	11,896	9,069
(12.4) Geometric mean	14,678	11,874	8,608
(12.5) Harmonic mean	15,320	12,421	9,195
Sweden 1959 and 1963			
(12.1) Female dominance	309.0	227.9	149.1
(12.2) Male dominance	375.9	266.4	160.9
(12.3) Arithmetic mean	291.2	201.0	120.7
(12.4) Geometric mean	297.6	202.6	115.1
(12.5) Harmonic mean	309.8	214.4	125.9

13. Measuring departures of observed from expected marriages

The first set of data on which the several marriage functions are to be tested is for the registration area of the United States, 1963 and 1967, using age groups 15–19, 20–24, and 25–44 at last birthday. (The official publication does not show any finer breakdown of ages of the single under 45.) The second set of data for Sweden in 1959 and 1963, in which six age groups (15–19, 20–24, 25–29, 30–34, 35–39, and 40–44) are recognized, was provided to me by David McFarland [23].

The measures of departure of Table I correspond to the two sets of data and three criteria of fit ranging from mean square to mean absolute value. They show the one-sex models (12.1) and (12.2) to be generally inferior to the various averages of the two sexes (12.3), (12.4), and (12.5). The sequence is essentially the same for the three measures of departure, and for the United States and Sweden, with the arithmetic and geometric means tied for first place.

A surprising feature of the outcome is that the theoretical merits of the harmonic mean over the arithmetic and geometric do not assert themselves. Our theoretical argument revolved around ensuring that when one sex was altogether lacking there would be no marriages, and when one sex was plentiful marriages would be proportional to the other. The data apparently vary too little from the stable case to discriminate on the basis of what happens when the number of one sex goes towards zero or infinity.

14. Asymmetry

The second question we will put to the data concerns the degree of dominance: whether males or females are more important for marriage. Merely to illustrate the logic that will be employed in this argument, suppose that we have statistics for available men and women, along with the year's marriages, in three situations that are in all other respects identical, as in Table II.

TABLE II

HYPOTHETICAL MARRIAGES WITH DIFFERING NUMBERS OF
SINGLE MEN AND SINGLE WOMEN

	Single men	Single women	Year's marriages
(a)	100,000	100,000	10,000
(b)	120,000	100,000	11,000
(c)	100,000	120,000	11,500

Apparently the extra 20,000 males in (b) increase marriages by 1000, while the extra 20,000 females in (c) increase them by 1500. Various mechanisms are imaginable; we will not attempt to discriminate among them.

Instead, we empirically investigate whether fluctuations in the number of females affect marriages more or less than do equal fluctuations in the number of males. To test for such asymmetry requires some kind of weighting of the numbers of males and females, and the easiest way to weight is by modifying the arithmetic or geometric mean. Weighting the females with $0.5 + \varepsilon$ and the males with $0.5 - \varepsilon$ alters the arithmetic mean to

$$(14.1) \qquad \hat{N}_{i,j,t} = \nu_{i,j}[(0.5 + \varepsilon)F_{i,t} + (0.5 - \varepsilon)M_{j,t}],$$

and the geometric mean to

$$(14.2) \qquad \hat{N}_{i,j,t} = \nu_{i,j}F_{i,t}^{0.5+\varepsilon}M_{j,t}^{0.5-\varepsilon}.$$

If it turns out that $\varepsilon > 0$, we will consider that females are more determining, if $\varepsilon < 0$, that males are more determining.

From another point of view, the estimates of nuptiality for the more recent date can be regarded as a projection of the nuptiality at the earlier date, using as an index the marriage function based on the available males and females at the two dates:

$$(14.3) \qquad \hat{N}_{i,j,t'} = N_{i,j,t}\frac{f(F_{i,t'}, M_{j,t'})}{f(F_{i,t}, M_{j,t})}.$$

With the weighted arithmetic mean, for example, the departure for the United States in 1967 would become

$$(14.4) \qquad d_{i,j}^{1967} = N_{i,j}^{1967} - \hat{N}_{i,j}^{1967}$$

$$= N_{i,j}^{1967} - N_{i,j}^{1963}\left[\frac{(0.5 + \varepsilon)F_i^{1967} + (0.5 - \varepsilon)M_j^{1967}}{(0.5 + \varepsilon)F_i^{1963} + (0.5 - \varepsilon)M_j^{1963}}\right].$$

Table III shows with the United States data the three kinds of average of the $d_{i,j}$, for values of ε from -0.5 to 0.5 at intervals of 0.1, and an enlargement of the arithmetic mean formula for the interval 0.1 to 0.2. On the whole, ε is clearly

TABLE III

DEPARTURE OF OBSERVED FROM CALCULATED FIRST MARRIAGES
The calculated first marriages are based on arithmetic and geometric weighted
means, with weights ε from −0.5 to +0.5 and three measures of departure
ranging from mean square to mean absolute value, United States 1963 and 1967
in three age groups.
Asterisks indicate minimum points.

Values of ε	$[\sum d^2/9]^{1/2}$	$[\sum |d|^{3/2}/9]^{2/3}$	$\sum |d|/9$
Arithmetic mean			
−0.5	18860	16498	13642
−0.4	17680	15414	12673
−0.3	16638	14416	11744
−0.2	15719	13489	10899
−0.1	14933	12631	10012
0	14316	11896	9069
0.1	13923	11506*	8805*
0.2	13830*	11584	9087
0.3	14127	12187	9997
0.4	14907	13149	10999
0.5	16256	14465	12079
Geometric mean			
−0.5	18860	16498	13642
−0.4	17745	15381	12607
−0.3	16736	14314	11554
−0.2	15865	13323	10484
−0.1	15166	12458	9397
0	14678	11874	8608*
0.1	14436*	11873*	9009
0.2	14468	12242	9749
0.3	14785	12822	10507
0.4	15387	13572	11283
0.5	16256	14465	12079
Enlargement for arithmetic mean			
0.1	13923	11506	8805
0.11	13899	11484	8778
0.12	13878	11466	8750
0.13	13860	11452	8722
0.14	13845	11444	8694
0.15	13834	11442*	8666*
0.16	13826	11458	8748
0.17	13821*	11482	8832
0.18	13821*	11511	8916
0.19	13823	11545	9001
0.2	13830	11584	9087

positive, showing a tendency to female dominance. The data are very skimpy—
we can hardly expect to learn much from only three age groups.

The somewhat more detailed ages for Sweden resulted in Table IV, showing ε
at 0.13 for the mean square and at 0.10 and 0.11 for the other two averages of
the $d_{i,j}$, all based on the arithmetic mean. The geometric mean is less consistent,
with ε ranging from 0.21 down to 0.10, depending on which average of the $d_{i,j}$
is taken. In both parts of Table IV, however, the ε is positive for best fit, and

TABLE IV

DEPARTURES OF ACTUAL FROM CALCULATED FIRST MARRIAGES
The calculated first marriages are based on arithmetic and geometric weighted
means, Sweden 1959 and 1963 in six age groups.
Asterisks indicate minimum points.

Values of ε	$[\sum d^2/36]^{1/2}$	$[\sum |d|^{3/2}/36]^{2/3}$	$\sum |d|/36$
Arithmetic mean			
0.09	288.36	198.83	118.97
0.10	288.24	198.79*	118.76
0.11	288.16	198.82	118.54*
0.12	288.11	199.01	118.97
0.13	288.10*	199.31	119.69
0.14	288.12	199.68	120.44
Geometric mean			
0.09	291.30	197.64	113.16
0.10	290.81	197.28	113.05*
0.11	290.36	196.97	113.10
0.12	289.96	196.70	113.16
0.13	289.60	196.48	113.21
0.14	289.28	196.30	113.26
0.15	289.00	196.17	113.31
0.16	288.77	196.09	113.37
0.17	288.59	196.06*	113.43
0.18	288.45	196.10	113.48
0.19	288.36	196.22	113.54
0.20	288.31	196.54	114.27
0.21	288.31*	197.01	115.58
0.22	288.35	197.56	116.50

this is the most solid evidence so far attained of the tendency to female marriage dominance.

One would like to see clearer minima than are exhibited in Tables III and IV. Presumably the curves showing departure of observed from expected as functions of ε would rise more sharply on either side of the minimum if the disequilibrium of the numbers single of the two sexes was more extreme, a circumstance that may show itself for the years about 1970. A more sharply defined minimum would also appear if more age groups were used. One confirmation that an ε on the female dominant side at least has the right sign comes from English data of 1891 and 1961 (P. R. Cox [1]). Cox finds a higher correlation between marriages and the supply of nonmarried women than between marriages and the supply of nonmarried men, which confirms the tendency to female dominance.

This presentation cannot but end on the need for further testing. Until the same calculation is made on a variety of times and places, no one can be certain that it is the inequality of available males and females that results in the asymmetry of the marriage function found here. The same marriage function need not apply to the two years being compared if circumstances have changed. One is tempted to complicate the marriage function by introducing into it other variables than the single males and single females present, by analogy to proceeding from zero order correlation to partial correlation in the familiar linear model. Unfortunately, in our problem it is not obvious what variables ought to be partialled out to obtain the pure effect of availabilities of single men and single women. Failing some knowledge or at least suspicion of possible extraneous variables, we can only seek further data of the kind used here. Insofar as the disturbing variables are unspecifiable and all disturbances have to be regarded merely as noise, the recourse is to perform the same calculation on the most varied populations for which data are to be had.

15. A least square estimate for ε

Richard Cohen suggests a way of reducing our problem of estimating ε to classical least squares. He linearizes (14.2) by taking logarithms, and finds

(15.1) $\log \hat{N}_{i,j,t} = \log \nu_{i,j} + (0.5 + \varepsilon) \log F_{i,t} + (0.5 - \varepsilon) \log M_{j,t}.$

The problem is now to find the ε that minimizes

(15.2) $\sum \left[-\log \hat{N}_{i,j,t} + \log \nu_{i,j} + (0.5 + \varepsilon) \log F_{i,t} + (0.5 - \varepsilon) \log M_{j,t} \right]^2.$

With the United States data of 1963 and 1967, Cohen obtains $\varepsilon = 0.1035$.

16. Conclusion

While we would like to experiment with more countries and more years, and certainly wish that more ages could be recognized than three for the United States and six for Sweden, yet the present materials strongly suggest that the degree of female dominance is $\varepsilon = 0.1$ or more. This means that number of marriages is some constant times $F_i^{0.6} M_j^{0.4}$, where F_i is the number of females aged i and M_j the number of males aged j at any time.

The 0.6 and 0.4 will be recognized as elasticities of marriages for females and males, respectively. If single females increase by one per cent marriages go up by 0.6 per cent. If single males increase by one per cent marriages go up by 0.4 per cent. Pending further data, we conclude that at the margin marriages depend at least 60 per cent on the number of women and at most 40 per cent on the number of men. Should the nonlinearity of such a geometric function prove awkward, an almost equally good fit can be obtained from the arithmetic and linear $\nu_{i,j} (0.6 F_i + 0.4 M_j)$.

Once the marriage function $\nu_{i,j}(F_i^{0.6} M_j^{0.4})$ (or some other) is ascertained, then given childbearing rates by age of father and of mother, and given mortality specific by age for single and married persons of each sex, we are at last in a position to make statements on the two-sex model corresponding to any that are possible on the one-sex model. An authentic projection can be made into the future that generalizes the standard one-sex projection. Over each finite time period, we can calculate age by age and for each sex the number of marriages. Recognizing the single and the never married, we apply life tables to find the number of survivors, and fertility tables for the number of births. If this applies over any particular time interval, it applies over all together, and so provides the asymptotic ultimate values.

The projection in its turn permits examination of the effect of change in any specific rate on the ultimate rate of increase and age distribution. The effects would probably not be very different from those given by the simpler one-sex model for any question that can be asked both of the one-sex model and the age-sex-marriage model. However, the latter permits altogether new questions—effects of changes in age specific marriage rates, for example. It also could show the effect of constantly changing proportions of the two sexes, including, for example, how the growth of a population would be affected if its birth rate oscillated about a given mean, so that it experienced an endless succession of marriage squeezes.

Among other benefits of a marriage function, it tells how to calculate the marriage rate. To answer the question asked earlier, whether the marriage rate for persons 20–24 in the United States went up or down between 1963 and 1967, we would note that in relation to the weighted geometric mean $F_i^{0.6}M_j^{0.4}$, the rate was

$$(16.1) \quad \frac{207{,}211}{(1{,}339{,}000)^{0.6}(2{,}355{,}000)^{0.4}} = 0.1235$$

in 1963 and

$$(16.2) \quad \frac{315{,}650}{(2{,}183{,}000)^{0.6}(3{,}379{,}000)^{0.4}} = 0.1214$$

in 1967. The last word based on this argument is that the rate went down from 0.1235 to 0.1214, a decline of 1.7 per cent.

Where we cannot count on the relative permanence of marriage, or where a large fraction of births are illegitimate, we will have to drop marriage from the model and use birth rates to the whole population by age of father and of mother. In the resulting simpler and cruder two-sex model, a birth function would take the place of the marriage function, and one could still perform the projection and other inferences. Presumably the birth function would be asymmetric; in the extreme case of promiscuous mating it would be weighted heavily towards the female side.

◇   ◇   ◇   ◇   ◇

My thanks are due to Richard Cohen, Griffith Feeney, A. G. Fredrickson, Louis Henry, Jan Hoem, David McFarland, Beresford Parlett, Prithwis Das Gupta, and Robert Traxler for helpful discussions and access to unpublished materials.

REFERENCES

[1] P. R. Cox, "Sex differences in age at marriage," *J. Biosocial Sci.*, Suppl. 2 (1970), pp. 73–84.

[2] P. Das Gupta, "On two-sex models leading to stable populations," *Theor. Pop. Biol.* in press.

[3] G. M. Feeney, "Suggestions for a demographic theory of marriage phenomena," unpublished manuscript, Department of Demography, University of California, Berkeley, 1971.

[4] W. Feller, *An Introduction to Probability Theory and Its Applications*, New York, Wiley, 1957 (2nd edition).

[5] H. von Foerster, "Some remarks on changing populations," *The Kinetics of Cellular Proliferation*, F. Stohlman (editor), New York, Grune & Stratton, 1959, pp. 382–407.

[6] A. G. Fredrickson, "A mathematical theory of age structure in sexual populations: random mating and monogamous marriage models," *Math. Biosci.*, Vol. 10 (1971), pp. 117–143.

[7] L. A. Goodman, "Population growth of the sexes," *Biometrics*, Vol. 9 (1953), pp. 212–225.

[8] ———, "On the age-sex composition of the population that would result from given fertility and mortality conditions," *Demography*, Vol. 4 (1967), pp. 423–441.

[9] J. Hajnal, "Age at marriage and proportions marrying," *Population Studies*, Vol. 7 (1953), pp. 111–136.

[10] L. Henry, "Schémas de nuptialité: déséquilibre des sexes et age au mariage," *Population*, Vol. 24 (1969), pp. 1067–1122.

[11] ———, "Nuptiality," unpublished manuscript, 1969.

[12] C. Hirschman and J. Matras, "A new look at the marriage market and nuptiality rates, 1915–1958," *Demography*, Vol. 8 (1971), pp. 549–569.

[13] J. M. Hoem, "Concepts of a bisexual theory of marriage formation," *Särtryck ur Statistisk Tidskrift*, Vol. 4 (1969), pp. 295–300.

[14] P. H. Karmel, "The relation between male and female reproduction rates," *Population Studies*, Vol. 1 (1947), pp. 249–274.

[15] D. G. Kendall, "Stochastic processes and population growth," *J. Roy. Statist. Soc. Ser. B*, Vol. 2 (1949), pp. 230–264.

[16] N. Keyfitz, *Introduction to the Mathematics of Population*, Reading, Addison-Wesley, 1968.

[17] P. H. Leslie, "On the use of matrices in certain population mathematics," *Biometrika*, Vol. 33 (1945), pp. 183–212.

[18] G. MacDonald, "The dynamics of helminth infections, with special reference to schistosomes," *Trans. Roy. Soc. Trop. Med. Hygiene*, Vol. 59 (1965), pp. 489–506.

[19] J. McDonald, "Effects on family size and sex ratio of sex-of-child preferences when parents can influence the sex of their children," unpublished manuscript, 1971.

[20] D. D. McFarland, "Effects of group size on the availability of marriage partners," *Demography*, Vol. 7 (1970), pp. 411–415.

[21] ———, "Availability of marriage partners under conditions of sexual imbalance," unpublished manuscript, 1971.

[22] ———, "On the extinction of families: some extensions of the Galton-Watson analysis," presented to the Fourth Conference on the Mathematics of Population, Honolulu, 1971.

[23] ———, "A model of the marriage market, with implications for two-sex population growth," unpublished Ph.D. dissertation, Department of Sociology, University of Michigan, 1971.

[24] R. Parke, Jr. and P. C. Glick, "Prospective changes in marriage and the family," *J. Marriage and the Family*, Vol. 29 (1967), pp. 249–256.

[25] J. H. Pollard, "A discrete-time two-sex age-specific stochastic population program incorporating marriage," *Demography*, Vol. 6 (1969), pp. 185–221.

[26] ———, "Mathematical models of marriage," presented to the Fourth Conference on the Mathematics of Population, Honolulu, 1971.

MEASUREMENT OF DIVERSITY: MULTIPLE CELL CONTENTS

F. N. DAVID

UNIVERSITY OF CALIFORNIA, RIVERSIDE

1. Introduction

In a previous paper [1], we discussed the distribution of a score, representing a diversity index, when a number of different colored balls are randomly dropped into $M(=mn)$ identical compartments, one ball only permitted per compartment. We now generalize and at the same time simplify the previous setup by allowing more than one ball per box.

2. Notation

A box of $m \times n = M$ compartments is supposed. There will be $(m-1)(n-1)$ crossover points each of which will be surrounded by four compartments. Denote these crossover points by (ij), $i = 1, 2, \cdots, m-1$, $j = 1, 2, \cdots, n-1$. Let there be K_1 balls in s colors with k_ℓ the number of balls of the ℓth color and

$$(2.1) \qquad \sum_{\ell=1}^{s} k_\ell = K_1.$$

These K_1 balls are supposedly dropped randomly into the M compartments, with no limitation on the individual compartment capacity. Consider the (ij)th crossover point. Let T_{ij} be the total number of balls in the four compartments surrounding (ij). Let $t_{ij\ell}$ be the total number of balls of the ℓth color in the same four compartments so that

$$(2.2) \qquad T_{ij} = \sum_{\ell=1}^{s} t_{ij\ell}.$$

The number of joins between balls of like and unlike colors will be, omitting the factor of one half,

$$(2.3) \qquad T_{ij}^{(2)} = \sum_{\ell=1}^{s} t_{ij\ell}^{(2)} + \sum_{\ell \neq h} t_{ij\ell} t_{ijh},$$

for the four boxes. Summed for all values of i and j, we have

$$(2.4) \qquad \sum_{i=1}^{m-1} \sum_{j=1}^{n-1} T_{ij}^{(2)} = \sum_{i=1}^{m-1} \sum_{j=1}^{n-1} \sum_{\ell=1}^{s} t_{ij\ell}^{(2)} + \sum_{i=1}^{m-1} \sum_{j=1}^{n-1} \sum_{\ell \neq h} t_{ij\ell} t_{ijh}.$$

This investigation was partially supported by USPHS Research Grant No. GM-10525-0 8 National Institutes of Health, Public Health Service.

Let us write this as $S_T = S_W + S_B$, a break up of the joins scores reminiscent of the classical analysis of variance setup. Clearly, S_W represents a measure of the within color joins, while S_B gives the between color joins. Accordingly, S_W may be used as a measure of aggregation (or clumping), while S_B may be used to measure segregation (or affinity). A modification of S_B is suggested below.

3. Conditional means

The restriction that there is no limit on the individual compartment capacity means that, for any four boxes considered, the number in these four boxes of any one given color will be a positive binomial variable with index k_ℓ, $\ell = 1, 2, \cdots, s$, and probability $p = 4/M$. The restriction is not very important and the procedure can be modified if desired by placing an upper content limit on each box. The supposition that the balls are randomly dropped implies an independence between and within color content for the four boxes, but because of the method of scoring S_W and S_B will be correlated. Conditional on the numbers k_ℓ, $\ell = 1, 2, \cdots, s$, and K_1, we have

$$
\begin{aligned}
(3.1) \quad & \mathcal{E}(S_T) = (m-1)(n-1)K_1^{(2)}p^2, \\
& \mathcal{E}(S_W) = (m-1)(n-1)K_2 p^2, \\
& \mathcal{E}(S_B) = (m-1)(n-1)[K_1^{(2)} - K_2]p^2,
\end{aligned}
$$

where, following our previous notation,

$$
(3.2) \qquad K_r = \sum_{\ell=1}^{s} k_\ell^{(r)}.
$$

When $n = 1$, that is, when the boxes are in a line, the score will be taken for each of two connected boxes, p will be $2/m$ and

$$
(3.3) \qquad \mathcal{E}(S_T) = (m-1)K_1^{(2)}p^2
$$

with the S_W and S_B similarly modified. It may also be noted that for three dimensions there will be a three dimensional lattice formed by the intersections of the box edges. The score will be calculated from the contents of the eight boxes surrounding the (ijw) node, p will be equal to $8/M$ where $M = m \times n \times w$, w being the number of boxes in the third dimension. Accordingly, for three dimensions,

$$
(3.4) \qquad \mathcal{E}(S_T) = (m-1)(n-1)(w-1)K_1^{(2)}p^2
$$

with similar expressions for the other two sums.

4. Unconditional means

Biologically measures conditional on the $\{k_\ell\}$ seem to be those sought after. However the k may themselves have arisen from a larger set and so the unconditional moments may be of interest. Suppose free multinomial sampling with

(4.1)
$$P\left\{\prod_{\ell=1}^{s} k_\ell\right\} = \frac{K_1!}{\prod_{\ell=1}^{s} k_\ell!} \prod_{\ell=1}^{s} p_\ell^{*k_\ell},$$

and write

(4.2)
$$P_r = \sum_{\ell=1}^{s} p_\ell^{*r}, \qquad\qquad P_1 = 1.$$

Then we have

(4.3)
$$\mathcal{E}(S_W) = (m-1)(n-1)K_1^{(2)}P_2 p^2,$$
$$\mathcal{E}(S_B) = (m-1)(n-1)p^2 K_1^{(2)}(1-P_2),$$

with

(4.4)
$$\mathcal{E}(S_T) = (m-1)(n-1)p^2 K_1^{(2)}$$

as before. The modifications for one or three dimensions instead of the two dimensional result above are easily written down.

Instead of multinomial sampling, we may wish to suppose a multiple Pólya urn model. Let there be an urn containing N balls of s different colors with R_ℓ balls of the ℓth color, $\ell = 1, 2, \cdots, s$. A ball is drawn, the color noted, and it is returned to the urn together with Δ balls of the same color. Writing $\delta = \Delta/N$, $p_\ell^* = R_\ell/N$, we have

(4.5)
$$P(\{k_\ell\}) = \binom{K_1}{k_1 \cdots k_s} \frac{\displaystyle\prod_{\ell=1}^{s} \prod_{h=1}^{k_\ell} (p_\ell^* + (h-1)\delta)}{\displaystyle\prod_{a=1}^{K_1} (1 + (a-1)\delta)}.$$

If the sampling is of this type and if

(4.6)
$$P_r = \sum_{\ell=1}^{s} \frac{p_\ell^*(p_\ell^* + \delta) \cdots (p_\ell^* + (r-1)\delta)}{1(1+\delta) \cdots (1 + (r-1)\delta)},$$

then the expectations are formally as above.

5. Conditional variances (two dimensions)

As in our previous paper it proved advantageous to evaluate the second crude moment and to split the evaluation into four different steps. Thus, we have

(5.1)
$$S_W^2 = \sum_i \sum_j \sum_r \sum_s \left\{\sum_\ell t_{ij\ell}^{(2)} t_{rs\ell}^{(2)} + \sum_{\ell \neq h} t_{ij\ell}^{(2)} t_{rsh}^{(2)}\right\}.$$

Case (i): $i = r, j = s$; $(m-1)(n-1)$ *terms.*

(5.2)
$$\sum_\ell (t_{ij\ell}^{(2)})^2 = \sum_\ell [t_{ij\ell}^{(4)} + 4t_{ij\ell}^{(3)} + 2t_{ij\ell}^{(2)}],$$

which has expectation

(5.3)
$$K_4 p^4 + 4K_3 p^3 + 2K_2 p^2.$$

Again,

(5.4)
$$\sum_{\ell \neq h} t_{ij\ell}^{(2)} t_{ijh}^{(2)} = p^4 \sum_{\ell \neq h} k_\ell^{(2)} k_h^{(2)} = p^4 \{K_2^2 - K_4 - 4K_3 - 2K_2\},$$

so that the total contribution is

$$(5.5) \qquad p^4[K_2^2 - 4K_3 - 2K_2] + 4p^3K_3 + 2p^2K_2.$$

Case (ii): $r = i + 1$, $j = s$ or $i = r$, $s = j + 1$; $2(m - 2)(n - 1)$ *or* $2(m - 1)(n - 2)$ *terms.* The total contribution is

$$(5.6) \qquad p^4[K_2^2 - 4K_3 - 2K_2] + 2p^3K_3 + \tfrac{1}{2}p^2K_2.$$

Case (iii): $r = i + 1$, $s = j + 1$; $4(m - 2)(n - 2)$ *terms.* The total contribution is

$$(5.7) \qquad p^4[K_2^2 - 4K_3 - 2K_2] + p^3K_3 + \tfrac{1}{8}p^2K_2.$$

Case (iv): $|i - r| \geqq 2$, $|j - s| \geqq 2$; $[(m - 1)^2(n - 1)^2 - (3m - 5)(3n - 5)]$ *terms.* The total contribution is

$$(5.8) \qquad p^4[K_2^2 - 4K_3 - 2K_2].$$

Collecting terms, we have

$$(5.9) \quad \mathcal{E}(S_W^2) = (m - 1)^2(n - 1)^2p^4[K_2^2 - 4K_3 - 2K_2] \\ + 4p^3K_3(2m - 3)(2n - 3) + \tfrac{1}{2}p^2K_2(3m - 4)(3n - 4)$$

with

$$(5.10) \quad \mathrm{Var}\, S_W = -(m - 1)^2(n - 1)^2p^4(4K_3 + 2K_2) \\ + 4p^3K_3(2m - 3)(2n - 3) + \tfrac{1}{2}p^2K_2(3m - 4)(3n - 4).$$

Similarly,

$$(5.11) \quad \mathrm{Var}\, S_T = -(m - 1)^2(n - 1)^2p^4(4K_1^{(3)} + 2K_1^{(2)}) \\ + 4p^3K_1^{(3)}(2m - 3)(2n - 3) + \tfrac{1}{2}p^2K_1^{(2)}(3m - 4)(3n - 4),$$

$$(5.12)$$
$$\mathrm{Var}\, S_B \\ = -(m - 1)^2(n - 1)^2p^4[4K_1^{(3)} + 2K_1^{(2)} + (4K_3 + 2K_2) - 4K_2(2K_1 - 3)] \\ + 4(2m - 3)(2n - 3)p^3[K_1^{(3)} + K_3 - 2K_2(K_1 - 2)] \\ + \tfrac{1}{2}p^2(3m - 4)(3n - 4)[K_1^{(2)} - K_2],$$

and

$$(5.13) \quad \mathrm{Cov}\, S_W S_B \\ = 4[K_3 - K_2(K_1 - 2)][p^4(m - 1)^2(n - 1)^2 - p^3(2m - 3)(2n - 3)].$$

6. Conditional variances (one and three dimensions)

Remembering that $p = 2/m$ for one dimension,

$$(6.1) \quad \mathrm{Var}\, S_W = -(m - 1)^2p^4(4K_3 + 2K_2) + 4p^3K_3(2m - 3) + p^2K_2(3m - 4)$$

with similar modifications for the others, namely,

$$(6.2) \quad \mathrm{Var}\, S_B = -(m - 1)^2p^4(4K_1^{(3)} + 4K_3 - 8K_2K_1 + 14K_2 + 2K_1^{(2)}) \\ + 4p^3(2m - 3)[K_1^{(3)} + K_3 - 2K_2K_1 + 4K_2] \\ + p^2(3m - 4)[K_1^{(2)} - K_2],$$

$$(6.3) \quad \mathrm{Cov}\, (S_W S_B) = 4[K_3 - K_2(K_1 - 2)][p^4(m - 1)^2 - p^3(2m - 3)].$$

For three dimensions m, n and w, we have that $p = 8/m \cdot n \cdot w$. The functions of K remain as before with suitable modifications of the multiplying factors.

7. Unconditional variances (two dimensions)

The unconditional variances follow along lines similar to those for the means. With free multinomial sampling, we have

(7.1) $\mathcal{E}(S_W^2) = K_1^{(4)} P_2^2 p^4 (m-1)^2 (n-1)^2$
$$+ 4K_1^{(3)} P_3 p^3 (2m-3)(2n-3) + \tfrac{1}{2}K_1^{(2)} P_2 p^2 (3m-4)(3n-4),$$

giving

(7.2) $\mathrm{Var}\, S_W = -(4K_1^{(3)} + 2K_1^{(2)}) P_2^2 p^4 (m-1)^2 (n-1)^2$
$$+ 4K_1^{(3)} P_3 p^3 (2m-3)(2n-3) + \tfrac{1}{2}K_1^{(2)} P_2 p^2 (3m-4)(3n-4).$$

Similarly,

(7.3) $\mathrm{Var}\, S_B = -(4K_1^{(3)} + 2K_1^{(2)})(1 - P_2)^2 p^4 (m-1)^2 (n-1)^2$
$$+ 4K_1^{(3)} p^3 (2m-3)(2n-3)[(P_3 - 2P_2 + 1)$$
$$+ \tfrac{1}{2}K_1^{(2)} p^2 (3m-4)(3n-4)(1-P_2)],$$
$$\mathrm{Cov}\, S_W S_B = -(4K_1^{(3)} + 2K_1^{(2)}) P_2 (1 - P_2) p^4 (m-1)^2 (n-1)^2$$
$$+ 4K_1^{(3)} p^3 (2m-3)(2n-3)[-P_3 + P_2].$$

The Pólya second order moments may be calculated from first principles but are possibly more simply achieved from the k-function technique of the next section.

8. Augmented factorial monomial symmetric procedure

As previously written, k_ℓ stands for the number of the ℓth kind to be distributed. The suffix is, however, not important and in cases where there is no possibility of confusion it may be omitted, following the usual symmetric function procedure. For the sake of example, let us suppose we are interested in the sum of the rth factorial powers of all the k. We may write this sum as follows:

(8.1) $$\sum_{\ell=1}^{s} k_\ell^{(r)} = [k_r].$$

Again, we may write

(8.2) $$\sum_{\ell=1}^{s} \sum_{h=1}^{s} k_\ell^{(r)} k_h^{(r)} = [k_r^2].$$

Accordingly for the first moments of S_W and S_B, respectively, we may write

(8.3) $\mu'_{10} = (m-1)(n-1)p^2 K_2 = (m-1)(n-1)p^2 [k_2],$
$\mu'_{01} = (m-1)(n-1)p^2 [K_1^{(2)} - K_2]p^2 = (m-1)(n-1)p^2 [k_1^2],$

since

(8.4) $[k_1^2] = \sum_{\ell \neq h} k_\ell k_h = (\sum k_\ell)^2 - \sum k_\ell^2 = K_1^2 - [\sum k_\ell^{(2)} + \sum k_\ell]$

$= K_1^{(2)} - K_2.$

This notation enables complicated multiplications to be carried out quickly and lessens the risk of error. Thus, we have, for two dimensions,

$$(8.5) \quad \mu_{20} = p^4(m-1)^2(n-1)^2[-4[k_3] - 2[k_2]] \\ + 4p^3(2m-3)(2n-3)[k_3] + \tfrac{1}{2}p^2(3m-4)(3n-4)[k_2],$$

$$(8.6) \quad \mu_{11} = 4[k_2k_1][-p^4(m-1)^2(n-1)^2 + p^3(2m-3)(2n-3)],$$

$$(8.7) \quad \mu_{02} = p^4(m-1)^2(n-1)^2[-4[k_2k_1] - 4[k_1^3] - 2[k_1^2]] \\ + 4p^3(2m-3)(2n-3)[[k_2k_1] + [k_1^3]] + \tfrac{1}{2}p^2(3m-4)(3n-4)[k_1^2],$$

giving as a check

$$(8.8) \quad \text{Var } S_T = -p^4(m-1)^2(n-1)^2\{4[[k_3] + 3[k_2k_1] + [k_1^3]] + 2[[k_2] + [k_1^2]]\} \\ + 4p^3(2m-3)(2n-3)\{[k_3] + 3[k_2k_1] + [k_1^3]\} \\ + \tfrac{1}{2}p^2(3m-4)(3n-4)\{[k_2] + [k_1^2]\},$$

or

$$(8.9) \quad \text{Var } S_T = -p^4(m-1)^2(n-1)^2\{4K_1^{(3)} + 2K_1^{(2)}\} \\ + 4p^3(2m-3)(2n-3)K_1^{(3)} + \tfrac{1}{2}p^2(3m-4)(3n-4)K_1^{(2)}$$

as before.

In a previous paper [1] when I introduced these k-functions I demonstrated how the augmented monomial symmetric function tables ([2] or [3]) could, formally, be used to evaluate the k-functions in terms of the K-functions, and gave expressions for the products of the K-functions corresponding to the products of the usual augmented monomial symmetrics. From these tables (see Table IV for illustrations), we read off the K-functions from the k experssions and writing for brevity,

$$(8.10) \quad \begin{array}{lll} X = K_3, & Y = K_2(K_1 - 2), & Z = K_1^{(3)}, \\ x = K_2, & y = K_1^{(2)}; \end{array}$$

we have, as already demonstrated,

$$(8.11) \quad \mu'_{10} = (m-1)(n-1)p^2 \cdot x, \qquad \mu'_{01} = (m-1)(n-1)p^2[y-x],$$

$$(8.12) \quad \mu_{20} = -p^4(m-1)^2(n-1)^2[4X + 2x] \\ + 4p^3(2m-3)(2n-3)X + \tfrac{1}{2}p^2(3m-4)(3n-4)x,$$

$$(8.13) \quad \mu_{11} = -4[-p^4(m-1)^2(n-1)^2 + p^3(2m-3)(2n-3)][X - Y],$$

$$(8.14) \quad \mu_{02} = -p^4(m-1)^2(n-1)^2[4(X - 2Y + Z) - 2(x-y)] \\ + 4p^3(2m-3)(2n-3)[X - 2Y + Z] \\ + \tfrac{1}{2}p^2(3m-4)(3n-4)[-(x-y)].$$

9. Conditional third moments (two dimensions)

Using the k-function technique and writing

$$(9.1) \quad \begin{array}{lll} \alpha = K_4, & \beta = K_3(K_1 - 3), & \gamma = K_2(K_2 - 2) - 4K_3, \\ & \delta = K_2(K_1 - 2)^{(2)}, & \varepsilon = K_1^{(4)} \end{array}$$

with X, Y, Z, x, and y as defined above, we may construct Table I.

TABLE I

CONDITIONAL THIRD MOMENTS

Notation:

$$\mu_{30} = \mathcal{E}(S_W - \mathcal{E}(S_W))^3, \ \mu_{21} = \mathcal{E}(S_W - \mathcal{E}(S_W))^2(S_B - \mathcal{E}(S_B)), \ \mu_{12} = \mathcal{E}(S_W - \mathcal{E}(S_W))(S_B - \mathcal{E}(S_B))^2, \ \mu_{03} = \mathcal{E}(S_B - \mathcal{E}(S_B))^3$$

$$\alpha = K_4, \ \beta = K_3(K_1 - 3), \ \gamma = K_2(K_2 - 2), \ \delta = K_2(K_1 - 2)^{(2)}, \ \varepsilon = K_1^{(4)}$$

$$X = K_3, \ Y = K_2(K_1 - 2), \ Z = K_1^{(3)}$$

$$x = K_2, \ y = K_1^{(2)}$$

Multipliers of Tabular Entries

Central Moments	$p^6(m - 1)^3(n - 1)^3$	$p^5(m - 1)(n - 1)(2m - 3)(2n - 3)$	$p^4(m - 1)(n - 1)(3m - 4)(3n - 4)$
μ_{30}	$40\alpha + 64X + 8x$	$-72\alpha - 72X$	$-6X - 3x$
μ_{21}	$-40\alpha + 32\beta + 8\gamma + 16(-X + Y)$	$72\alpha - 56\beta - 16\gamma + 16(X + Y)$	$2(X - Y)$
μ_{12}	$40\alpha - 64\beta - 16\gamma + 40\delta - 32(X - Y)$	$-72\alpha + 112\beta + 32\gamma - 72\delta + 40(X - Y)$	$2(X - Y)$
μ_{03}	$-40\alpha + 96\beta + 24\gamma - 120\delta + 40\varepsilon$ $+ 80X - 144Y + 64Z + 8(-x + y)$	$72\alpha - 168\beta - 48\gamma + 216\delta - 72\varepsilon$ $- 96X + 168Y - 72Z$	$-6X + 12Y - 6Z + 3(x - y)$
μ_{3T}	$40\varepsilon + 64Z + 8y$	$-72\varepsilon - 72Z$	$-6Z - 3y$

Multipliers of Tabular Entries

Central Moments	$p^4(8m - 15)(8n - 15)$	$p^4(4m - 7)(4n - 7)$	$p^3(3m - 5)(3n - 5)$	$p^3(5m - 8)(5n - 8)$	$p^2(5m - 8)(5n - 8)$
μ_{30}	6α	8α	$24X$	$2X$	x
μ_{21}	$-6\alpha + 4\beta + 2\gamma$	$-8\alpha + 8\beta$	$-8(X - Y)$	—	—
μ_{12}	$6\alpha - 8\beta - 4\gamma + 6\delta$	$8\alpha - 16\beta + 8\delta$	$-8(X - Y)$	$-2(X - Y)$	—
μ_{03}	$-6\alpha + 12\beta + 6\gamma - 18\delta + 6\varepsilon$	$-8\alpha + 24\beta - 24\delta + 8\varepsilon$	$24X - 48Y - 24Z$	$4X - 6Y + 2Z$	$-(x - y)$
μ_{3T}	6ε	8ε	$24Z$	$2Z$	y

TABLE II

NUMBERS OF TERMS IN THE EXPANSION OF EXPRESSIONS SUCH AS $\left[\sum_i \sum_j \alpha_{ij}\right]^3$

	i^3	$i^2(i+1)$	i^2r	$i(i+1)(i+2)$	$i(i+1)r$	ihr	Total
j^3	$(m-1)(n-1)$	$6(m-2)(n-1)$	$3(m-2)^{(2)}(n-1)$	$6(m-3)(n-1)$	$6(m-3)^{(2)}(n-1)$	$(m-3)^{(3)}(n-1)$	$(m-1)^3(n-1)$
$j^2(j+1)$	$6(m-1)(n-2)$	$36(m-2)(n-2)$	$18(m-2)^{(2)}(n-2)$	$36(m-3)(n-2)$	$36(m-3)^{(2)}(n-2)$	$6(m-3)^{(3)}(n-2)$	$6(m-1)^3(n-2)$
j^2s	$3(m-1)(n-2)^{(2)}$	$18(m-2)(n-2)^{(2)}$	$9(m-2)^{(2)}(n-2)^{(2)}$	$18(m-3)(n-2)^{(2)}$	$18(m-3)^{(2)}(n-2)^{(2)}$	$3(m-3)^{(3)}(n-2)^{(2)}$	$3(m-1)^3(n-2)$
$j(j+1)(j+2)$	$6(m-1)(n-3)$	$36(m-2)(n-3)$	$18(m-2)^{(2)}(n-3)$	$36(m-3)(n-3)$	$36(m-3)^{(2)}(n-3)$	$6(m-3)^{(3)}(n-3)$	$6(m-1)^3(n-3)$
$j(j+1)s$	$6(m-1)(n-3)^{(2)}$	$36(m-2)(n-3)^{(2)}$	$18(m-2)^{(2)}(n-3)^{(2)}$	$36(m-3)(n-3)^{(2)}$	$36(m-3)^{(2)}(n-3)^{(2)}$	$6(m-3)^{(3)}(n-3)^{(2)}$	$6(m-1)^3(n-3)^{(2)}$
jhs	$(m-1)(n-3)^{(3)}$	$6(m-2)(n-3)^{(3)}$	$3(m-2)^{(2)}(n-3)^{(3)}$	$6(m-3)(n-3)^{(3)}$	$6(m-3)^{(2)}(n-3)^{(3)}$	$(m-3)^{(3)}(n-3)^{(3)}$	$(m-1)^3(n-3)^{(3)}$
Total	$(m-1)(n-1)^3$	$6(m-2)(n-1)^3$	$3(m-2)^{(2)}(n-1)^3$	$6(m-3)(n-1)^3$	$6(m-3)^{(2)}(n-1)^3$	$(m-3)^{(3)}(n-1)^3$	$(m-1)^3(n-1)^3$

No new principle is involved in finding these third order moments and so I have not reproduced the algebraic detail. The numbers of terms involved is not without interest and so they are given in Table II. Each cell, however, will need to be split again according to the permutations of the suffices under consideration.

10. Product of k-functions

In finding the central third moments given in Table I, I found it convenient to derive the crude moments and then reduce them. This meant some algebraic manipulations became rather heavy, with transforming k-functions to K-functions and conversely. Accordingly, it proved profitable to tabulate products of the Augmented Factorial Monomial Symmetric Functions (AFMSF's). Thus, for example,

$$(10.1) \quad [k_3 k_1][k_1^2] = \left(\sum_{\ell \neq h} k_\ell^{(3)} k_h^{(1)} \right) \left(\sum_{u \neq v} k_u k_v \right)$$

$$= 2 \sum_{\ell \neq h} (k_\ell^{(3)} k_\ell)(k_h^2) + 2 \sum_{\ell \neq h \neq u} (k_\ell^{(3)} k_\ell)(k_h)(k_u)$$

$$+ 2 \sum_{\ell \neq h \neq u} (k_\ell^{(3)})(k_h^2)(k_u) + \sum_{\ell \neq h \neq u \neq v} (k_\ell^{(3)})(k_h)(k_u)(k_v)$$

$$= 2[k_4 k_2] + \{6[k_3 k_2] + 2[k_4 k_1]\} + \{6[k_3 k_1]\}$$

$$+ 2[k_4 k_1^2] + \{6[k_3 k_1^2]\} + 2[k_3 k_2 k_1] + \{2[k_3 k_1^2]\}$$

$$+ [k_3 k_1^3].$$

Table AI of the Appendix gives the expression of the products of all separates of weight 6, 5, 4, 3, 2, in terms of the AFMSF's. This table enables any reduction from crude moments to central moments to be made reasonably quickly.

11. Unconditional moments

Expression of the moments in terms of the AFMSF's calls for the minimum of manipulation when we turn from the conditional to the unconditional case. With free multinomial sampling

$$(11.1) \quad \mathcal{E}[k_a k_b k_c \cdots] = \sum_{\ell_1 \neq \ell_2 \neq \ell_3} k_{\ell_1}^{(a)} k_{\ell_2}^{(b)} k_{\ell_3}^{(c)} \cdots$$

$$= K_1^{(a+b+c+\cdots)} \sum_{\ell_1 \neq \ell_2 \neq \ell_3 \neq \cdots} p_{\ell_1}^{*a} p_{\ell_2}^{*b} p_{\ell_3}^{*c} \cdots ,$$

with the reduction of the last summation following from the AMSF's of [2]. With Pólya sampling of the type delineated earlier, writing

$$(11.2) \quad p_\ell^{*[a]_\delta} = p_\ell^*[p_\ell^* + \delta][p_\ell^* + 2\delta] \cdots [p_\ell^* + (a-1)\delta],$$

we have

$$(11.3) \quad \mathcal{E}[k_a k_b k_c \cdots] = \frac{K_1^{(a+b+c+\cdots)}}{1^{[a+b+c\cdots]_\delta}} \sum_{\ell_1 \neq \ell_2 \neq \ell_3 \cdots} p_{\ell_1}^{*[a]_\delta} p_{\ell_2}^{*[b]_\delta} p_{\ell_3}^{*[c]_\delta} \cdots .$$

Thus, for example, conditionally,

$$(11.4) \quad \mu'_{20} = p^4(m-1)^2(n-1)^2\{[k_4] + [k_2^2]\}$$
$$+ 4p^3(2m-3)(2n-3)[k_3] + \tfrac{1}{2}p^2(3m-4)(3n-4)[k_2].$$

If the contents of the $m \times n$ squares have supposedly arisen from sampling from a multiple Pólya urn scheme, then unconditionally

(11.5)

$$\mu'_{20} = p^4(m-1)^2(n-1)^2 \frac{K_1^{(4)}}{1(1+\delta)(1+2\delta)(1+3\delta)}$$

$$\left\{ \sum_{l=1}^{s} p_l^*(p_l^* + \delta)(p_l^* + 2\delta)(p_l^* + 3\delta) + \sum_{l \neq h} p_l^*(p_l^* + \delta)p_h^*(p_h^* + \delta) \right\}$$

$$+ 4p^3(2m-3)(2n-3)\frac{K_1^{(3)}}{1(1+\delta)(1+2\delta)}\left\{ \sum_{l=1}^{s} p_l^*(p_l^* + \delta)(p_l^* + 2\delta) \right\}$$

$$+ \frac{1}{2}p^2(3m-4)(3n-4)\frac{K_1^{(2)}}{1(1+\delta)}\left\{ \sum_{l=1}^{s} p_l^*(p_l^* + \delta) \right\}.$$

Here $\delta = 0$ gives the multinomial result, $\delta = -1/N$ gives the "no replacement" result. Generally,

$$(11.6) \quad \mu'_{20} = p^4(m-1)^2(n-1)^2 \frac{K_1^{(4)}}{(1+\delta)(1+2\delta)(1+3\delta)}$$

$$\{P_2^2 + \delta(4P_3 + 2P_2) + \delta^2(10P_2 + 1) + 6\delta^3\}$$

$$+ 4p^3(2m-3)(2n-3)\frac{K_1^{(3)}}{(1+\delta)(1+2\delta)}\{P_3 + 3P_2\delta + 2\delta^2\}$$

$$+ \frac{1}{2}p^2(3m-4)(3n-4)\frac{K_1^{(2)}}{(1+\delta)}\{P_2 + \delta\}$$

with

$$(11.7) \quad \mu'_{10} = p^2(m-1)(n-1)\frac{K_1^{(2)}}{1+\delta}\{P_2 + \delta\}.$$

No general simplification appears possible for the central moments, except in the multinomial case. For this latter case, we have

$$(11.8) \quad \mu'_{30} = p^6(m-1)^3(n-1)^3 K_1^{(6)} P_2^3$$
$$+ 12p^5(m-1)(n-1)(2m-3)(2n-3)K_1^{(5)}P_3P_2$$
$$+ \tfrac{3}{2}p^4(m-1)(n-1)(3m-4)(3n-4)K_1^{(4)}P_2^2$$
$$+ p^4[6(8m-15)(8n-15) + 8(4m-7)(4n-7)]P_4K_1^{(4)}$$
$$+ p^3[24(3m-5)(3n-5) + 2(5m-8)(5n-8)]K_1^{(3)}P_3$$
$$+ p^2(5m-8)(5n-8)K_1^{(2)}P_2.$$

For brevity, let

$$(11.9) \quad \begin{aligned} K_1^{(6)} - 3K_1^{(4)}K_1^{(2)} + 2(K_1^{(2)})^3 &= F, \\ K_1^{(5)} - K_1^{(3)}K_1^{(2)} &= G, \\ K_1^{(4)} - (K_1^{(2)})^2 &= H. \end{aligned}$$

Then

(11.10) $\mu_{30} = p^6(m-1)^3(n-1)^3P_2^3F$

$\qquad +p^5(m-1)(n-1)(2m-3)(2n-3)12P_3P_2G$

$\qquad + \frac{3}{4}p^4(m-1)(n-1)(3m-4)(3n-4)P_2^2H$

$\qquad + p^4[6(8m-15)(8n-15) + 8(4m-7)(4n-7)P_4K_1^{(4)}$

$\qquad + p^3[24(3m-5)(3n-5) + 2(5m-8)(5n-8)]P_3K_1^{(3)}$

$\qquad + p^2(5m-8)(5n-8)P_2K_1^{(2)},$

(11.11) $\mu_{21} = p^6(m-1)^3(n-1)^3P_2^2(1-P_2)F$

$\qquad + 4p^5(m-1)(n-1)(2m-3)(2n-3)[-3P_2P_3 + 2P_2^2 + P_3]G$

$\qquad + \frac{1}{2}p^4(m-1)(n-1)(3m-4)(3n-4)P_2(1-P_2)H$

$\qquad + 2p^4(8m-15)(8n-15)K_1^{(4)}(-3P_4 + P_2^2 + 2P_3)$

$\qquad + 8p^4(4m-7)(4n-7)K_1^{(4)}[-P_4 + P_3]$

$\qquad + 8p^3(3m-5)(3n-5)K_1^{(3)}(-P_3 + P_2),$

(11.12)

$\mu_{12} = p^6(m-1)^3(n-1)^3P_2(1-P_2)^2F$

$\qquad + 4p^5(m-1)(n-1)(2m-3)(2n-3)[3P_2P_3 - 2P_3 - 4P_2^2 + 3P_2]G$

$\qquad + \frac{1}{2}p^4(m-1)(n-1)(3m-4)(3n-4)P_2(1-P_2)H$

$\qquad + 2p^4(8m-15)(8n-15)K_1^{(4)}(3P_4 - 2P_2^2 - 4P_3 + 2P_2)$

$\qquad + 8p^4(4m-7)(4n-7)K_1^{(4)}[P_4 - 2P_3 + P_2]$

$\qquad + p^3[8(3m-5)(3n-5) + 2(5m-8)(5n-8)K_1^{(3)}[-P_3 + P_2],$

(11.13)

$\mu_{30} = p^6(m-1)^3(n-1)^3(1-P_2)^3F$

$\qquad + 12p^5(m-1)(n-1)(2m-3)(2n-3)G(1-P_2)(P_3 - 2P_2 + 1)$

$\qquad + \frac{3}{2}p^4(m-1)(n-1)(3m-4)(3n-4)(1-P_2)^2H$

$\qquad + 6p^4(8m-15)(8n-15)K_1^{(4)}[(1-P_2)^2 - (P_4 - 2P_3 + P_2)]$

$\qquad + 8p^4(4m-7)(4n-7)K_1^{(4)}[1 - 3P_2 + 3P_3 - P_4]$

$\qquad + 24\,p^3(3m-5)(3n-5)K_1^{(3)}(1 - 2P_2 + P_3)$

$\qquad + 2p^3(5m-8)(5n-8)K_1^{(3)}[1 - 2P_2 + P_3]$

$\qquad + p^2(5m-8)(5n-8)(1-P_2)K_1^{(2)}.$

It remains to note that $F = 40K_1^{(4)} + 64K_1^{(3)} + 8K_1^{(2)}$ with similar reductions for the others.

12. Distribution of S_W and S_B

In order to reduce S_W or S_B to a diversity index, it was suggested in [1] that for an observed score S_0 it would be appropriate to calculate $P\{S \leq S_0\}$ and use this quantity as a measure of aggregation, or segregation, in diversity. It will however be recognized that this requires the distribution of S and this is difficult to obtain except possibly for the case of one dimension. Such random sampling experiments as we have done indicates that both S_W and S_B have distributions which look like χ^2 (or χ) and we would accordingly suggest that a suitable approximating function to these distributions may be χ^2, keeping the normal approximation for use when β_1 is very small. Thus, we write

$$(12.1) \qquad \mathcal{E}(S) - A = af, \qquad \text{Var } S = 2a^2f, \qquad \mu_3(S) = 8a^3f,$$

so that

$$(12.2) \qquad a = \frac{\mu_3}{4\mu_2}, \qquad f = \frac{8}{\beta_1}, \qquad A = \mathcal{E}(S) - \frac{2\mu_2^2}{\mu_3}.$$

This will usually mean that f, the degrees of freedom, are fractional, and interpolation into the χ^2 tables will be necessary. On the whole, such sampling results as we have indicate that for reasonable sized chessboards and with K_1 not very different from $M = mn$ the χ^2 approximation is adequate. For one dimension as indicated below the start may be fixed at one half below the first possible frequency of S and the first two moments only will then yield values of a and f. It will not escape notice that the numerical calculation of μ_3 will be heavy arithmetically and we have in fact written a program for it.

12.1. *One dimension.* The distribution of S_W for five balls of the same color in five boxes arranged in a line is as in Table III.

The momental constants are

$$(12.3) \qquad \begin{array}{lll} \mu_1' = 12.8, & \mu_2 = 28.032, & \sigma = 5.294525 \\ \beta_1 = 1.4288, & \beta_2 = 4.7768. \end{array}$$

For the $(\beta_1\beta_2)$ point to lie on the Type III line, we should have $2\beta_2 - 3\beta_1 - 6 = 0$, or for given β_1, we have $\beta_2 = 5.1432$.

The true $(\beta_1\beta_2)$ point accordingly lies in the Type I area but it is not far off the Type III line.

If A, a, and f have the meanings of the previous section then $A = 3.94136$, $a = 1.5822$, $f = 5.5989$. We use the χ^2 tables and obtain $\chi^2_{0.05} = 11.9832$; thus, the frequency beyond $a\chi^2_{0.05}$ is 183 which is 5.86 per cent. The $\chi^2_{0.01} = 16.1216$; thus the frequency beyond $a\chi^2_{0.01}$ is 33 or 1.056 per cent. This example takes an extreme case and the approximation using $\chi^2_{0.05}$ may be expected to become better as the number of balls and/or boxes increases. For instance, suppose we drop five balls of one color and four balls of another color in five boxes arranged in a line. The distribution of S_W is shown in Table IV.

The momental constants are:

$$(12.4) \qquad \begin{array}{llll} \mu_1' = 20.48, & \mu_2 = 43.008, & \sigma = 6.5580, & \beta_1 = 0.7673, \\ A = 5.50656, & f = 10.42615+, & a = 1.43614. \end{array}$$

The $\chi^2_{0.05}$ point cuts off 4.6 per cent from the upper tail and the $\chi^2_{0.01}$, 1.1 per cent.

If β_1 is of negligible proportions, which implies that f, the degrees of freedom of the χ^2 are large, the normal curve may be used. For small degrees of freedom, as above, the use of the normal curve may be misleading. Thus, $1.6449 \times 6.5580 + 20.48 = 31.26$. The actual percentage frequency beyond 31.26 is 7.39 per cent.

TABLE III

DISTRIBUTION OF S_W FOR FIVE BALLS OF THE SAME COLOR IN FIVE BOXES ARRANGED IN A LINE

S_W	4	6	8	10	12	14	16	18	20	22	24	26	28	30	32	34	36	38	40	Total
Frequency	30	220	520	640	430	540	110	220	212	20	90	20	40	·	30	·	·	·	3	3125

TABLE IV

DISTRIBUTION OF S_W FOR FIVE BALLS OF ONE COLOR AND FOUR BALLS OF ANOTHER COLOR IN FIVE BOXES ARRANGED IN A LINE

S_W	6	8	10	12	14	16	18	20	22	24	26	28	30	32	34
Frequency	720	9420	47880	127860	21560	258000	270760	235480	197008	155776	136650	88322	65716	54500	25424
S_W	36	38	40	42	44	46	48	50	52	54	56	58	60	62	64
Frequency	25794	16388	8710	5052	4110	1884	1008	924	330	36	126	72	·	·	9

Total 1953125

The complete enumeration of S for two dimensions called for extensive computations, given any realistic set of numbers. Accordingly, we resorted to random sampling. Given $m = 4$, $n = 5$, $k_1 = 10$, $k_2 = 8$, $k_3 = 5$, $k_4 = 4$, (that is, $K_1 = 27$), the 27 points were put down randomly on the 4×5 chessboard and S_W and S_B calculated. In all, this process was carried out 500 times. The distributions obtained are shown in Table V. The observed value of β_2 is 3.88. The

TABLE V

DISTRIBUTION OF S_W IN 500 SAMPLES
$m = 4$, $n = 5$, $k_1 = 10$, $k_2 = 8$, $k_3 = 5$, $k_4 = 4$

S_W	Frequency	S_W	Frequency	S_W	Frequency
36	1	88	20	140	1
38	—	90	14	142	2
40	—	92	22	144	—
42	—	94	15	146	—
44	2	96	12	148	—
46	4	98	12	150	1
48	—	100	16	152	1
50	6	102	11	154	—
52	3	104	6	156	—
54	10	106	5	158	—
56	9	108	12	160	—
58	10	110	10	162	—
60	10	112	8	164	—
62	15	114	5	166	—
64	10	116	1	168	—
66	17	118	6	170	—
68	22	120	7	172	1
70	11	122	6	174	1
72	21	124	3	176	1
74	20	126	3		
76	31	128	1	Total	500
78	19	130	3		
80	17	132	1		
82	12	134	1		
84	22	136	3		
86	15	138	—		

condition for the Type III line is $2\beta_2 - 3\beta_1 - 6 = 0$, which will give for the theoretical β_2 (if the Type III assumption is justified) a value of 3.87. It is clear that a Type III may be a suitable approximating function, although the $(\beta_1\beta_2)$ point might suggest the inverse of the Type III, that is, the Type V. Using Type III and the χ^2 tables with fractional degrees of freedom, we obtain the values of S_W, in both the observed and theoretical cases, which should cut off 50 per cent, 5 per cent, and 1 per cent from the right tail of the distribution (Table VI). These values are then used on the actual sampling distribution of S_W to obtain the true percentage tail content. The results are given in Table VII. For the case we are considering $20(= 5 \times 4)$ cells and 27 objects the agreement between the estimated percentage points and the true 5 per cent points would appear

TABLE VI

MOMENTAL CONSTANTS FOR DISTRIBUTION OF S_W

	μ_1	μ_2	μ_3	β_1
Observed	85.424	486.4042	7550.01	0.495
Theoretical	85.44	457.4336	7457.88	0.581

TABLE VII

PERCENTAGE POINTS FOR S_W USING CONSTANTS
OF TABLE VI AND THE TYPE III DISTRIBUTION

	A	a	f	Nominal points 50%	5%	1%
Observed	22.75	3.881	16.151	49.8	4.2	1.2
Theoretical	29.33	4.076	13.767	49.8	4.2	1.2

reasonably good. With a larger chessboard, and thus a lessening of the part played by the edge effects, the agreement should be closer.

For S_B we have the following distribution in the 500 samples shown in Tables VIII, IX, and X.

The values of the momental constants are in reasonably close agreement. Using the assumption that $S_B/2$ is distributed as $a\chi^2$ the nominal 50 per cent, 5 per cent, and 2.5 per cent points were found in each case and the actual percentages were calculated for these points from the sampling distribution.

12.2. *Two dimensions (Pielou's examples)*. Pielou ([4], p. 180) gives two examples of spatial patterns which she has created in order to illustrate specific points. We use her data here to illustrate the application of the various criteria proposed. Two species only are considered. We denote these by A and C. The areas were gridded by us into 10×8 cells and the count per cell was determined. The counts for Pattern 1 are shown in Table XI.

We note that A and C together have a random pattern; A and C are segregated (that is, tend not to occur together). We have as observed moments

$$\begin{aligned}
&S_T = 2246, &\bar{S}_T &= 2325.015, &\text{Var } S_T &= 28835.906275,\\
(12.5) \quad &S_W = 1664, &\bar{S}_W &= 1349.775, &\text{Var } S_W &= 12551.642875,\\
&S_B = 582, &\bar{S}_B &= 975.24, &\text{Var } S_B &= 7906.4874,\\
& & & &\text{Cov } S_W S_B &= 4188.888.
\end{aligned}$$

Calculation of the third moments show the skewness to be negligible. Consequently from normal tables,

(12.6)

$$P\{S_T \leqq S_{T_0}\} = 0.309, \quad P\{S_W \leqq S_{W_0}\} = 0.998, \quad P\{S_B \leqq S_{B_0}\} = 0.231.$$

TABLE VIII

DISTRIBUTION OF $S_B/2$ IN 500 SAMPLES
$m = 4, n = 5, k_1 = 10, k_2 = 8, k_3 = 5, k_4 = 4$

$S_B/2$	Frequency	$S_B/2$	Frequency	$S_B/2$	Frequency	$S_B/2$	Frequency
70	1	113	5	156	3	199	—
71	—	114	7	157	2	200	—
72	—	115	1	158	1	201	—
73	—	116	12	159	8	202	—
74	—	117	9	160	—	203	—
75	—	118	5	161	2	204	—
76	1	119	10	162	4	205	—
77	—	120	7	163	1	206	—
78	1	121	10	164	4	207	—
79	2	122	7	165	4	208	1
80	2	123	8	166	1	209	—
81	2	124	7	167	7	210	—
82	2	125	6	168	2	211	—
83	4	126	11	169	3	212	—
84	1	127	6	170	—	213	—
85	—	128	10	171	2	214	—
86	3	129	8	172	1	215	—
87	2	130	6	173	1	216	1
88	3	131	4	174	1	217	—
89	2	132	5	175	—	218	—
90	2	133	5	176	2	219	—
91	3	134	5	177	—	220	—
92	4	135	5	178	—	221	—
93	7	136	3	179	—	222	—
94	9	137	8	180	2	223	—
95	2	138	8	181	1	224	—
96	4	139	1	182	—	225	—
97	6	140	5	183	2	226	—
98	6	141	4	184	1	227	—
99	2	142	6	185	—	228	—
100	8	143	4	186	1	229	—
101	4	144	8	187	1	230	—
102	6	145	3	188	2	231	—
103	4	146	4	189	1	232	—
104	6	147	8	190	1	233	—
105	10	148	3	191	—	234	—
106	12	149	3	192	—	235	1
107	9	150	5	193	—	236	—
108	6	151	11	194	—	237	1
109	10	152	3	195	—		
110	5	153	6	196	—	Total	500
111	12	154	7	197	—		
112	11	155	4	198	—		

TABLE IX

DISTRIBUTION OF $S_B/2$ IN 500 SAMPLES
Momental Constants

	μ_1'	μ_2	μ_3	β_1
Observed	126.146	673.5287	11516.5453	0.43
Theoretical	125.76	655.7792	11485.8965	0.47

TABLE X

PERCENTAGE POINTS FOR $S_B/2$ USING THE CONSTANTS
OF TABLE IX AND THE TYPE III DISTRIBUTION

	Mean	S.D.	50%	Nominal 5%	2.5%
Observed	126.146	25.95	49.0%	3.8%	2.0%
Theoretical	125.760	25.61	50.6%	4.0%	2.2%

TABLE XI

COUNTS FOR PATTERN 1

A's										C's									
2	2	0	0	0	1	2	1	1	0	0	0	2	1	0	0	0	0	0	0
1	1	0	0	0	4	2	1	2	2	0	0	2	1	3	0	0	0	1	3
1	2	2	0	0	1	1	2	0	0	0	0	0	0	2	0	0	0	0	2
2	0	2	0	2	0	4	0	0	0	0	0	0	0	0	0	0	1	2	1
1	0	0	1	2	1	2	0	0	0	0	1	1	0	0	0	0	1	4	1
2	2	0	2	2	3	1	1	0	0	0	0	2	0	0	0	0	0	0	0
1	1	0	1	2	1	0	1	2	2	0	1	2	2	0	0	0	0	0	0
0	2	1	1	2	2	2	2	1	1	0	0	0	0	0	0	0	0	0	0

Total A's: 86   Total C's: 36

Since the correlation between the within and between scores is high ($\rho = +0.4205$) and S_W is large, it would seem appropriate to modify S_B by calculating the quantity

$$(12.7) \qquad \frac{1}{(1 - \rho^2)^{1/2}} \left(\frac{S_B - \bar{S}_B}{\sigma_{S_B}} - \rho \frac{S_W - \bar{S}_W}{\sigma_{S_W}} \right) = S_B^* \qquad \text{(say).}$$

From unit normal tables S_B^* cuts off 0.017 from the left tail. It is clear that if the $86 + 36 = 122$ are put down randomly on the 10×8 chessboard, then the ideal randomness score will give a value of 0.5 for $P\{S_T \leqq S_{T_0}\}$. If the observed value S_{T_0} is large, then this will imply clumping of the combined values; if it is small, then we would suspect there was regularity in the positioning of the A's and the

C's. The fact that S_W is large indicates that the A's and the C's tend to be clumped among themselves. A glance at the counts shows this indeed to be the case. The small value of S_B^* indicates that A tends not to occur with C, which is again the case.

TABLE XII

COUNTS FOR PATTERN 2

A's										C's									
0	0	1	1	2	2	4	0	0	0	0	0	0	1	1	1	1	1	0	0
0	0	0	3	3	1	2	0	0	0	0	0	0	2	0	0	2	0	0	0
0	0	0	2	2	2	0	0	0	0	0	0	0	1	1	1	0	0	0	0
0	0	0	0	0	0	0	0	0	0	0	0	0	0	0	0	0	0	0	1
0	0	0	0	0	0	0	1	1	3	0	0	0	0	0	0	0	0	3	0
0	2	2	0	0	0	2	1	2	0	0	3	0	0	0	0	1	0	0	1
0	3	2	0	0	0	0	3	0	3	0	2	1	0	0	0	0	1	1	0
0	1	0	0	0	0	2	2	3	0	0	0	0	0	0	0	1	1	1	1

| Total A's: 58 | Total C's: 30 |

The counts for Pattern 2 are shown in Table XII. Here we note a two species population in which the plants have clumped patterns but the species are unsegregated (that is, tend to occur together).

We have as observed moments

$$(12.8) \quad \begin{array}{lll} S_T = 2216, & \bar{S}_T = 1205.82, & \text{Var } S_T = 12020.2071, \\ S_W = 1132, & \bar{S}_W = 657.72, & \text{Var } S_W = 4869.2856, \\ S_B = 1084, & \bar{S}_B = 548.10, & \text{Var } S_B = 3776.5395, \\ & & \text{Cov } S_B S_W = 1687.1910. \end{array}$$

The indices for S_T, S_W, S_B and S_{B*} are all unity to five decimal places. Thus, neither the species, considered together or separately have a random pattern and A and C are not random with respect to their juxtaposition.

Table XIII shows the counts for Pattern 3, which is a random arrangement of

TABLE XIII

COUNTS FOR PATTERN 3

A's										C's									
3	0	1	2	1	2	1	0	1	1	1	0	2	0	2	0	0	0	0	1
0	0	0	1	1	1	0	1	2	1	1	1	0	0	1	0	2	0	0	1
1	0	3	4	0	2	1	0	2	1	0	0	0	1	1	1	0	1	0	0
0	2	1	1	2	0	0	1	1	3	0	2	0	0	2	1	0	1	1	0
0	4	1	1	1	0	1	0	1	1	0	1	0	0	0	1	0	0	0	0
2	0	1	2	0	2	1	1	1	1	0	0	1	1	0	1	0	0	0	0
1	1	1	0	0	0	0	0	2	2	0	0	0	0	0	0	0	2	1	0
1	2	0	3	1	2	0	3	1	1	0	1	0	0	1	1	0	0	1	1

Pattern 1. In fact the 86 A's and 36 C's of Pattern 1 were put down randomly using a random number table.

We have the observed

$$
\begin{aligned}
S_T &= 2134, \\
S_W &= 1170, \\
S_B &= 964,
\end{aligned}
$$

(12.9)

with indices S_T: 0.130, S_W: 0.054, and S_B: 0.450, and

(12.10)
$$
\begin{aligned}
S_W(A) &= 996, \\
S_W(C) &= 174,
\end{aligned}
$$

observed separately, with indices $S_W(A)$: 0.072 and $S_W(C)$: 0.244.

Although the letters were put down randomly there is a suspicion of the antithesis of clumping as evidenced by the low value of the index for S_W. We break up S_W into the two parts of the contribution for A and the contribution for C, calculate the separate means and variances and calculate an index for each. The indications are that there is a suspicion of nonrandomness among those "random" numbers used to put down the A's.

13. Discussion

The spatial pattern of points representing objects belonging to different categories has been examined in a series of papers relating to the distribution of the chromosomes in the human cell in mitosis. The material algebra for these investigations was given in Barton and David [5]. The essence of the method is to recognize that the plotted centromeres (that is, the central points of the chromosomes) will most likely not be spatially random, but the numbers attached to the chromosomes might be. Accordingly, it was suggested that the variance of two like numbers be compared with the overall variance.

There is no doubt that this randomization test could be extended and applied to this present problem, but there is an essential difference. Given several species of plants (A, B, C, D, $\cdots$), it is hypothesized that the spatial points representing these plants are randomly distributed over the area. (In the chromosome case we were reasonably certain that they were not, and we were principally interested in whether the like pairs tended to lie too close together.) Under the hypothesis alternate to randomness we ask do the plants of the same species tend to cluster together (possibly in many clusters) and is there any tendency for there to be a segregation of the different species?

It is recognized that the method used—that of gridding the area—may lead to a loss of information, and certainly the optimum number of cells to use for the chessboard is a matter for investigation. Intuitively, one feels that an average of one observation per cell should be aimed at, but only the specification of suitable alternate hypotheses could decide this. Further, and more importantly, the scoring for the four cells surrounding each node is flexible. For example, if there are t_{ijl} plants of the lth kind and t_{ijh} of the hth kind in the four cells surrounding the (ij)th node, then the contribution towards aggregation has been taken as $t_{ijl}^{(2)} + t_{ijh}^{(2)}$ and the contribution towards segregation as $t_{ijl} \times t_{ijh}$. A different system, suggested in [1] might be to exclude contributions which are only joined by a diagonal line. For example, consider the sets of four cells in Figure 1. Under the system of scoring of this present paper, we would count 6, 3, 1, 1, respectively. But if we adopt a nondiagonal system of scoring, we would count 4, 2, 1, 0. Again, only the specification of an alternate hypothesis would make a decision possible as to which was the optimum procedure.

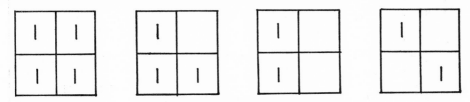

FIGURE 1

Sets of four cells

14. Previous work

As mentioned in the last paragraph, the basic work on one aspect of spatial randomization tests was given in [1]. A suggestion of gridding and counting joins will be found in Pielou [4], although not the scoring system. The first of these present papers was done independently of Dr. Pielou's work which leads one to the hope that we may be on the right lines. A paper by Mandel and [6] concerned with the clustering of cases of a disease, also using "joins," appeared in a recent journal, but seems different from the present approach.

◊   ◊   ◊   ◊   ◊

The material discussed here arose from problems presented to the writer by the scientific staff of the Pacific-Southwest Range and Experiment Station, U.S.D.A.

◊   ◊   ◊   ◊   ◊

APPENDIX

Table AI gives the products of all separates of weight for the k-functions in terms of the AFMSF's.

Table AII gives the K-functions in terms of the AFMSF's and *vice versa*. Equations (A.1) and (A.2) illustrate the notation:

(A.1)
$$[k_3 k_2 k_1] = \sum_{a \neq b \neq c} k_a^{(3)} k_b^{(2)} k_c^{(1)},$$

(A.2)
$$K_r = \sum_a k_a^{(r)}.$$

TABLE AI

Products of Separates up to Weight 6 for *k*-Functions in Terms of the Augmented Monomial Symmetric Functions

	[k₆]	[k₅k₁]	[k₄k₂]	[k₄k₁²]	[k₃²]	[k₃k₂k₁]	[k₃k₁³]	[k₂³]	[k₂²k₁²]	[k₂k₁⁴]	[k₁⁶]	[k₅]	[k₄k₁]	[k₃k₂]	[k₃k₁²]	[k₂²k₁]	[k₂k₁³]	[k₁⁵]
[k₆]	1																	
[k₅][k₁]	1	1										5						
[k₄k₁][k₁]		1	1	1		1	1						5					
[k₃k₂][k₁]		1	1		1	2		1						5				
[k₃k₁²][k₁]				1	1	2	1		1	1					5			
[k₂²k₁][k₁]						1		1	1	3						5		
[k₂k₁³][k₁]							1		3	5							5	
[k₁⁵][k₁]										1	5							5
[k₄k₂]	1		1			1												
[k₃k₁][k₂]		1	2		1	1	2	1	1				6	2	4	4		
[k₂²][k₂]								2		1				8				
[k₂k₁²][k₂]				2		2	1	2	1	1					4	8	8	
[k₄][k₁²]		2		2		4			4	4		8	2	6	8	12	8	8
[k₃k₁][k₁²]						4			12	8					4	12	24	8
[k₂²k₁][k₁²]											1							
[k₅]²	1	1		1		1	1	2	1	1	1	9	6	3	9	5	9	9
[k₂k₁][k₃]				3	1	2		1	1				6		4			
[k₃][k₃]				1	1	6		3	3	9			1	8	6	12	36	
[k₂k₁²][k₃]						6	3	6	18	9	1	11				18		
[k₃k₁²][k₃]																		
[k₄][k₁²]²	1	1	1	1		1	1	1	1	1		9	9	5	9	5		9
[k₃][k₂][k₁]	1	1	2	2	2	3	1	1	1			11	6	9	11	12		
[k₃k₁][k₂][k₁]	2	2	2	3		2	1						9	6		18		
[k₃][k₂²][k₁]	2	3	3	4		6	1	1	1	1		12	16	12				
[k₂]³	1			1		4	1	1	3	1			16	8	4	8	11	
[k₂]²[k₁²]	2	2	1	1	1	3	1	1	3	1			9	13	4	7	12	
[k₃k₁][k₂][k₁]			3	3		6	4	2	3	1		4			21	12	11	
[k₂][k₁³][k₁]	1	2	3	4		8	4	2	4	1		4	4	20	28	20	12	

TABLE AI (Continued)

	$[k_4]$	$[k_3k_1]$	$[k_2^2]$	$[k_2k_1^2]$	$[k_1^4]$	$[k_3]$	$[k_2k_1]$	$[k_1^3]$	$[k_2]$	$[k_1^2]$	$[k_1]$
$[k_6]$											
$[k_5][k_1]$											
$[k_4k_1][k_1]$											
$[k_3k_2][k_1]$											
$[k_3k_1^2][k_1]$											
$[k_2^2k_1][k_1]$											
$[k_2k_1^3][k_1]$											
$[k_1^5][k_1]$											
$[k_4][k_2]$	12	6	4	2							
$[k_3k_1][k_2]$		6									
$[k_2^2][k_2]$			8	10							
$[k_2k_1^2][k_2]$					12						
$[k_4][k_1^2]$	18	6				6		6			
$[k_3k_1][k_1^2]$		4	6	2			2				
$[k_2^2][k_1^2]$				12							
$[k_2k_1^2][k_1^2]$				18	18						
$[k_1^4][k_1^2]$											
$[k_3]^2$											
$[k_2k_1][k_3]$											
$[k_1^3][k_3]$						18					
$[k_2k_1]^2$											
$[k_2k_1^2][k_1^3]$											
$[k_1^3]^2$											
$[k_4][k_1]^2$	16	6									
$[k_3k_2][k_1][k_1]$	30	16	6	2		32	8		4		
$[k_3k_1][k_1^2][k_1]$		24	8	2			6				
$[k_2^2][k_1^2][k_1]$		28	10	24							
$[k_2]^3$	38	18									
$[k_2]^2[k_1^2]$											
$[k_2k_1][k_2][k_1]$											
$[k_2][k_1^3][k_1]$											
$[k_2][k_1^2]^2$		20	16	34			16				

TABLE AI (Continued)

	$[k_1^5]$	$[k_2 k_1^3]$	$[k_2^2 k_1]$	$[k_3 k_1^2]$	$[k_3 k_2]$	$[k_4 k_1]$	$[k_5]$
$[k_2 k_1][k_1^2][k_1]^3$	9	11	26	18	20	2	
$[k_2 k_1^2][k_1]^2$	11	9	18	6			
$[k_1^4][k_1]^2$	12	36	54	12	24	24	12
$[k_1^3][k_1^2][k_1]$		66	96	24	12	17	13
$[k_1^2]^3$		84		12	23	19	7
$[k_3][k_1]^3$	13	12	9	4	22	22	
$[k_2 k_1^2][k_1]^2$	12	13	29	24	29	4	
$[k_2 k_1][k_1]^3$		104	30	36	49		14
$[k_1^2][k_2^2][k_1]^2$		84	126	56	56	42	15
$[k_1^2]^2[k_1]$	14	14	72	36	84	28	1
$[k_3][k_1]^3$	15	126	42	42	150	75	1
$[k_2][k_1]^4$		150	168	98			1
$[k_1^2][k_1]^4$			225	150		1	
$[k_1]^6$	1	1	1	1	1	2	1
$[k_5]$	1	1	1	1	1	1	
$[k_4][k_1]$	1	1	1	1	2	2	
$[k_3][k_2]$			2	3	2	1	1
$[k_3][k_1^2]$			2	2	3	1	
$[k_3 k_1][k_1]^2$		4	3	1	4		
$[k_3][k_1]^2$	1	6	6	3		2	
$[k_2^2][k_1]$	1	7	6	7	4		1
$[k_2 k_1^2][k_2]$	1	3	4	7	6	2	
$[k_2 k_1][k_1^2][k_1]$	1	9	12	10	10	5	
$[k_2][k_1]^3$	1	10	15	10			

	$[k_1^6]$	$[k_2 k_1^4]$	$[k_2^2 k_1^2]$	$[k_2^3]$	$[k_3 k_1^3]$	$[k_3 k_2 k_1]$	$[k_3^2]$	$[k_4 k_1^2]$	$[k_4 k_2]$	$[k_5 k_1]$	$[k_6]$
$[k_2 k_1][k_1^2][k_1]^3$	1	1	5	2	3	10	2	2	2	3	1
$[k_2 k_1^2][k_1]^2$	1	1	5	2	2	6	2	1		2	1
$[k_1^4][k_1]^2$		9	12	6	4	12				1	
$[k_1^3][k_1^2][k_1]$	1	11	24	8	6	24	4	3	3	2	
$[k_1^2]^3$	1	12	30		8	3	1	1	3		1
$[k_3][k_1]^3$			1	1	1	4	2	3	4	2	
$[k_2 k_1^2][k_1]^2$	1	1	6	3	3	13	3	5	4		
$[k_2 k_1][k_1]^3$	1	13	5	2	4	12	2	4	4	6	1
$[k_1^2][k_2^2][k_1]^2$		12	34	10	12	32	4	3	4		
$[k_1^2]^2[k_1]$	1	1	27	6	10	18		6	7	4	1
$[k_3][k_1]^3$	1	14	6	3	4	16	4	9	8	2	1
$[k_2][k_1]^4$	1	15	39	12	16	44	6	15	15	6	1
$[k_1^2][k_1]^4$			45	15	20	60	10				

TABLE AI (Continued)

	$[k_4]$	$[k_3k_1]$	$[k_2^2]$	$[k_2k_1^2]$	$[k_1^4]$	$[k_3]$	$[k_2k_1]$	$[k_1^3]$	$[k_2]$	$[k_1^2]$	$[k_1]$
$[k_2k_1][k_1^2][k_1]$											
$[k_2k_1^2][k_1]^2$											
$[k_1^4][k_1]^2$				28							
$[k_1^3][k_1^2][k_1]$				16							
$[k_1^2]^3$		12		66							
$[k_3][k_1]^3$		8	20	120			12				
$[k_2]^2[k_1]^2$		37	36	2			24				
$[k_2k_1][k_1]^3$		33	20	37	16		12				
$[k_2][k_1^2][k_1]^2$		37	9	44	30		27	18			
$[k_1^2]^2[k_1]^2$	37	59	26	291	30		34	32			
$[k_1^3][k_1]^3$	46	33	66	111	46	27	58	46		4	
$[k_2][k_1]^4$	28	110	55	55	37	46	65	27	8	8	
$[k_1^2][k_1]^4$	55	110	110	380	55	65	130	65	16	16	
$[k_1]^6$	65	260	195	495	65	90	270	90	31	31	1
$[k_4][k_1]$											
$[k_3][k_2]$											
$[k_3][k_1^2]$											
$[k_3k_1][k_1]$											
$[k_2^2][k_1]$											
$[k_2k_1][k_2]$											
$[k_2k_1^2][k_1]$											
$[k_2k_1][k_1^2]$											
$[k_2][k_1^3]$											
$[k_2k_1][k_1]^2$		6									
$[k_2][k_1^2][k_1]$		4		6							
$[k_2]^2[k_1]$		7	4	6							
$[k_2][k_1]^3$		4	2	4			2				
$[k_1^4][k_1]$		4	4	7			2				
$[k_1^3][k_1^2]$	4	2	4	9			4				
$[k_1^3][k_1]^2$	6	7	7	12	4	6	9	1			
$[k_1^2]^2[k_1]$	7	18	9	21	6	9	19	9			
$[k_1^2][k_1]^3$	8	4	12	26	7	14	16	8		4	
$[k_1^2][k_1]^3$	9	18	18	45	2	19	38	19	8	8	
$[k_1]^5$	10	40	30	60	9	25	75	25	15	15	1

TABLE AI (Continued)

	$[k_4]$	$[k_3k_1]$	$[k_2^2]$	$[k_2k_1^2]$	$[k_1^4]$	$[k_3]$	$[k_2k_1]$	$[k_1^3]$	$[k_2]$	$[k_1^2]$	$[k_1]$
$[k_4]$	1					3			2		
$[k_3][k_1]$	1	1				4	4				
$[k_2]^2$	1		1				3				
$[k_2][k_1^2]$		2				5	5		4		
$[k_2k_1][k_1]$	1	1	1	1			4				
$[k_3][k_1]^2$		2	1	1		6	8		7	2	
$[k_1^3][k_1]$				3	1	1	18	3			
$[k_1^2]^2$		2	2	4	1	1		4		2	
$[k_1^2][k_1]^2$		4	2	5	1			5			
$[k_1]^4$	1		3	6	1			6			
$[k_3]$						1	1	1	2	7	
$[k_2][k_1]$							2	1	3	2	1
$[k_2^2][k_1]$							3		1	3	
$[k_1]^3$									1	1	1
$[k_2]$									1		
$[k_1]^2$										1	1

TABLE AII

K-Functions in Terms of the AFMSF's and *Vice Versa*

Weight 6	$[k_6]$	$[k_5k_1]$	$[k_4k_2]$	$[k_4k_1^2]$	$[k_3^2]$	$[k_3k_2k_1]$	$[k_3k_1^3]$	$[k_2^3]$	$[k_2^2k_1^2]$	$[k_2k_1^4]$	$[k_1^6]$
K_6	1	-1	-1	2	-1	2	-6	2	-6	24	-120
$K_5(K_1 - 5)$	1	1		-2		-1	6	-3	4	-24	144
$K_4(K_2 - 12) - 8K_5$	1		1	-1		-1	3		5	-18	90
$K_4(K_1 - 4)^{(2)}$	1	2	1	1			-3		-1	12	-90
$K_3(K_3 - 6) - 9(K_5 + 2K_4)$	1				1	-1	2	1	2	-8	40
$(K_3(K_2 - 6) - 6K_4)(K_1 - 5)$	1	1	3		1	1	-3	1	-4	20	-120
$K_3(K_1 - 3)^{(3)}$	1	3	3	3	1	3	1			-4	40
$K_2(K_2 - 2)(K_2 - 4) - 12K_3(K_2 - 2) + 40(K_4 + K_3)$	1					4		3	-1	3	-15
$(K_2(K_2 - 2) - 4K_3)(K_1 - 4)^{(2)}$	1	2	3	1	2	16	4	1	1	-6	45
$K_2(K_1 - 4)^{(4)}$	1	4	7	16	4	60	20	3	6	1	-15
$K_1^{(6)}$	1	6	15	15	10	60	20	15	45	15	1

To express K-functions in terms of the AFMSF's, read horizontally up to and including the heavy type diagonal; for example,

(A.3) $(K_3(K_2 - 6) - 6K_4)(K_1 - 5) = [k_6] + [k_5k_1] + [k_4k_2] + [k_3^2] + [k_3k_2k_1]$.

To express the AFMSF's in terms of the K-functions, read vertically downward including the heavy type diagonal; for example,

(A.4)
$$[k_3k_2k_1] = 2K_6 - K_5(K_1 - 5) - [K_4(K_2 - 12) - 8K_5]$$
$$- [K_3(K_3 - 6) - 9(K_5 + 2K_4)] + [K_3(K_2 - 6) - 6K_4][K_1 - 5].$$

REFERENCES

[1] F. N. DAVID, "Measurement of diversity," *Proceedings of the Sixth Berkeley Symposium on Mathematical Statistics and Probability*, Berkeley and Los Angeles, University of California Press, Vol. 1, 1972, pp. 631–648.

[2] F. N. DAVID and M. G. KENDALL, "Tables of symmetric functions," *Biometrika*, Vol. 36 (1950), pp. 431–449.

[3] F. N. DAVID, M. G. KENDALL, and D. E. BARTON, *Symmetric Function and Allied Tables*, Cambridge, Cambridge University Press, 1967.

[4] E. C. PIELOU, *An Introduction to Mathematical Ecology*, New York, Wiley-Interscience, 1969.

[5] D. E. BARTON and F. N. DAVID, "Randomisation bases for multivariate tests," *Proc. I.S.I.*, *32nd Session* (1961), pp. 44–51.

[6] N. MANTEL and J. C. BAILAR, "A class of permutational and multinomial tests," *Biometrics*, Vol. 26 (1971), pp. 687–700.

MODELS AND APPROXIMATIONS FOR SYNCHRONOUS CELLULAR GROWTH

W. A. O'N. WAUGH
UNIVERSITY OF TORONTO

1. Introduction

To recall the notion of a synchronous culture, it will suffice to reproduce one of the many graphs in the literature illustrating the results of experiments with such cultures. Figure 1 is from Mitchison and Vincent [6], reprinted with permission of Mitchison, and shows cell numbers in a synchronous culture prepared by a technique of density gradient centrifugation. Alongside this figure we may place an idealization (Figure 2).

In common with many other authors, in evaluating their technique for preparing synchronous cultures, Mitchison and Vincent refer to the "degree of synchrony" it produces. Leaving aside the question of numerical measurement of this degree, "perfect synchrony" would be represented by Figure 2, while "asyn-

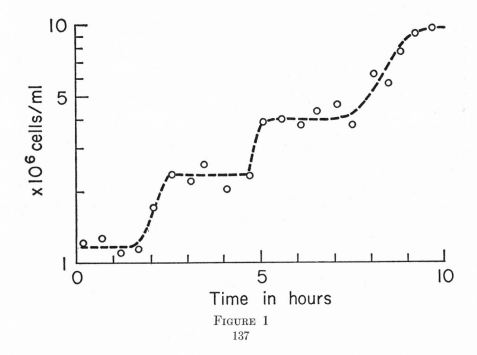

FIGURE 1

137

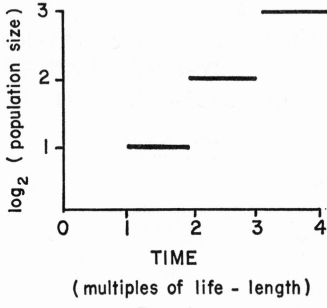

FIGURE 2

chronous growth" is linear growth of the logarithm of the population size. Growth such as is actually observed, as in Figure 1, is called "parasynchronous."

Stochastic effects ensure that experiments always lead to parasynchronous growth. Some of these may be termed "accidental" such as errors of observation and unavoidable fluctuations in conditions. These are not the subject of the present paper. We shall consider at least two stochastic effects as "essential": (i) stochastic fluctuations in the life lengths of individuals, (ii) random values of the ages of the individual or individuals present at the beginning of observation (time $t = 0$) which will lead to different probabilities for fission at later times.

A common situation is that a synchronizing event (for example, environmental shock or selection of newly born cells) is followed by a period during which the population grows parasynchronously according to some growth process.

A mathematical model of a synchronous culture must contain counterparts to these two features of the experiment. The first part of this paper contains a proposed classification of models according to the way they are specified. This classification is analogous to the well-known classification of queueing models according to the input process, service time distribution, and number of servers. It will be applied to models set up by various authors and will also be used to discuss the relationships of simpler models (as approximations) to more realistic but mathematically less tractable ones. Some examples of one type of approximation will be given.

2. Specification of the growth mechanism

Almost any mathematical model that has been proposed for the growth and reproduction of cellular populations could be used for this part of the complete model. General models would allow the reproduction probabilities to depend on the population size and the age of each individual, and would include correlations between mother and daughter or between sisters. More special models allow more complete solutions, and such models as branching and renewal processes are commonly considered. For later reference we shall call these B and R, respectively, and refer to the general model as G. The model may be Markovian M in which case the life lengths are negative exponential. An opposite extreme is provided by the "clock models" C in which the life length distributions are degenerate; they give probability one to a certain fixed life length.

In specifying the growth mechanism, a second classification is also useful. The process may be handled in terms of expectations, as in actuarial practice, perhaps because the population can be considered as large at all times. We shall refer to this as A. An alternative is a stochastic model S in which the population may be small (starting perhaps with 1 at $t = 0$), leading to calculations with distributions of ages and other variables.

3. Specification of the starting conditions

We shall suppose that a procedure to induce synchrony takes place up to or at time $t = 0$. This means that the growth mechanism already specified develops out of an initial state determined by a probability distribution $I(t)$ (the "initial state distribution" of Engelberg and Hirsch [4]). We have

(3.1) $P\{$individual alive at time 0 undergoes fission by time $t\} = I(t)$.

A general distribution G could be arbitrarily adopted. However, $I(t)$ may also be derived from more basic assumptions about the age distribution at $t = 0$ and about life lengths conditional upon ages.

The age distribution may be stable for the conditions prevailing before $t = 0$, or it may consist of such a distribution with some age class deleted or modified, and referred to as D. It is convenient again to consider degenerate distributions F, giving fixed ages at the start. An environmental shock may be modelled E by taking the age distribution resulting from one growth process as initial state for another.

The conditional life length distributions for the starting generation may involve age dependent fission probabilities. In this case they may be the same A as prevail throughout the whole subsequent growth scheme or they may be modified, referred to as A mod, say due to viability being changed by the induction. They may also be degenerate as in the clock model C.

4. Specification of time scale and structure

Time may be treated as discrete Δ or continuous Γ. Most models involve time homogeneous growth mechanisms h, but Engelberg and Hirsch, for example, postulate fission probabilities that fluctuate cyclically with time as a model for forced synchrony. This gives a nonhomogeneous growth model n.

5. Classification of models: examples

Summing up Sections 1 through 4, we shall classify models by means of a sequence of symbols representing: growth mechanism|"acturial" or "stocastic"|initial state|time structure.

The proposed symbols for use in this sequence may be summarized under the corresponding four headings in Table I.

TABLE I

CLASSIFICATION OF MODELS

Growth mechanism		Nature of process		Initial state		Time structure	
Branching	B	"Actuarial"		General	G	Discrete	Δ
Renewal	R	(mean		Stable	S	Continuous	Γ
General	G	growth)	A	Deletion of age class	D	Homogeneous	h
"Clock"	C	"Stochastic"	S	Fixed age at start	F	Nonhomogenous	n
				Environmental shock	E		
				Age dependent life length distributions same for first and later generations	A		
				Age dependent life length distributions in first generation modified relative to others	A mod		
				Fixed life length for first generation ("clock")	C		

Some examples follow.

EXAMPLE 5.1. Engelberg and Hirsch [4] study $G|A|G|\Delta, h$ and briefly $G|A|G|\Delta, n$, in an essay on general models of synchrony.

EXAMPLE 5.2. Burnett-Hall and Waugh [2] attempted to quantify the decay of synchrony in branching processes with age dependent birth rates. Synchrony was supposed to arise through the individuals at the start being of zero age, and the population was considered in terms of its expected growth with time, leading to a model $B|A|F, A|\Gamma, h$. Sankoff [7] considers the same problem and model.

EXAMPLE 5.3. Selection synchrony such as sizing methods or filtration will lead to models of the form $-|-|D|-$ (here a dash indicates an unspecified component). If the selection is for a fixed age (in fact for a narrow age class), then $-|-|F|-$ will be appropriate. (See, for example, Terasima and Tolmach [8].) This will also be true for blocking techniques by which a culture is brought effectively into a single age class and subsequently released. Labelling experiments lead to a labelled subpopulation which has been effectively synchronized by selection. MacDonald [5] examines the fraction labelled mitoses curve by means of $B|S|D|\Gamma$, h and Bartlett [1] obtains large-time approximations to the moments of the total population and, hence, also approximations for grain counts using $G|G|F|\Gamma$, h (the starting condition being one cell of age zero). Radiation and chemotherapy also produce synchronous populations by selection of the cells which survive treatment.

EXAMPLE 5.4.   Shifts and shocks are generally applied to cultures which are in a steady state. Their effect is to take the steady state distribution for the growth mechanism before shock as initial state for a different age dependent growth mechanism which leads to models of the forms G (or B, and so forth) $|-|G, A|-$.

One or two shifts can be treated by taking the state induced, after a period, by one shift, as the initial state for the next.

6. Models with branching growth mechanism: clock approximations

For the remainder of this paper, we shall consider models $B|S|D$ or $E|\Gamma$, h and clock models $C|S|D$ or $E|\Gamma$, h. Note that clock models can still involve stochastic effects in their initial states. Suppose the coefficient of variation of the initial state distribution is large relative to that of the life lengths in the growth mechanism. Then it is clear that stochastic variations at least in the first few generations will predominantly come from the variability of the initial state, and a clock model may be a good approximation to a stochastic branching model. The question of the "truth" of a clock model is sometimes discussed in the biological literature, but it seems desirable to replace such discussion by considerations of the goodness of the approximation.

7. Synchronization by selection: a model $B|S|D|\Gamma$, h

As indicated by the first symbol, we are considering a model in which the reproductive mechanism is a continuous time age dependent branching process. Specifically, we shall suppose this process develops by binary fission, and the life length distribution is $G(\cdot)$. For the starting conditions, let us suppose that the population was growing, before $t = 0$, according to the same branching process for long enough to establish the corresponding stable age distribution $A(\cdot)$. Selection means that there is a probability $q(u)$ that an individual of age u is retained in the new starting population. Thus, we can consider the population after time zero as commencing with a single individual whose age X has a distribution $A_0(\cdot)$ given by

(7.1) $$P(X \leqq x) = A_0(x)$$

$$= \frac{\int_0^x q(u) A \{du\}}{\int_0^\infty q(u) A \{du\}}.$$

The residual life length R of the initial individual will depend on its age X. We shall consider all conditions as being unchanged by the selection so that the conditional distribution $H(\cdot|\cdot)$ of R will be

(7.2) $$P(R \leqq r|X = x) = H(r|x)$$

$$= \frac{G(r + x) - G(x)}{1 - G(x)}.$$

If $G(x) = 1$, we shall put $P(R = 0|X = x) = 1$. Thus specified, the growth mechanism is a branching process with random start such as has been treated by Weiner [9]. The process is considered in terms of the family tree of a single individual at time $t = 0$, whence it is categorized S. Equation (7.1) provides the "deletion" D and we have already referred to the continuous time and fixed conditions of growth, giving homogeneity.

8. Synchronization by selection: a clock model $C|S|D|\Gamma, h$

The reproductive mechanism will again be a continuous time binary fission branching process, but we suppose that the distribution $G(\cdot)$ is degenerate, giving probability one to the fixed life length ℓ. This can never lead to a stable age distribution, but considering the limit of a branching process with mean life length ℓ and variance of life length tending to zero, we obtain the density

(8.1) $$\frac{d}{dt} A(t) = \begin{cases} (2\ell^{-1} \log 2) 2^{-t/\ell} & \text{for } 0 \leqq t \leqq \ell, \\ 0 & \text{otherwise,} \end{cases}$$

which is usually adopted in this situation (see, for example, Campbell [3]). The age distribution $A_0(\cdot)$ after selection will be obtained from $A(\cdot)$ just as in (7.2). Modelling unchanged conditions as in Section 7, the residual life length will simply be

(8.2) $$R = \begin{cases} \ell - x & \text{for } 0 \leqq x \leqq \ell, \\ 0 & \text{otherwise.} \end{cases}$$

The rest of the categorization of this model is the same as that in Section 7. This model can be regarded as an approximation to the former (which might be considered more realistic) as mentioned in Section 6.

9. First and subsequent fissions: synchrony in the first wave of reproduction

Let us refer to the model of Section 7 as $B/-$ and that of section 8 as $C/-$ for brevity. In both models the first fission will occur at time R. Suppose the (unconditional) distribution of R is $P(R \leqq r) = F(r)$. In a parasynchronous population starting with a number of individuals selected as in (7.1), there will be a tendency for the first wave of reproduction to occur about the time $t = E(R)$. This wave will be more concentrated (show a higher degree of synchrony) for smaller values of the standard deviation $SD(R)$. If, in the model $B/-$, the coefficient of variation of the life length distribution $G(\cdot)$ is small, we can expect a negligible contribution to the first wave of reproduction from fissions in the second and later generations. In the model $C/-$, the first wave of reproduction must occur before time $t = \ell$ and so this contribution will be zero. In $B/-$, later waves of reproduction will become blurred through the effect of generation overlap (decay of synchrony), which will not occur in $C/-$. Since in the presence of decay of synchrony, the first wave is the most coherent, its timing and effect on the transient age distribution, and so forth, are of interest if the purpose is to work with a culture in the closest available state of synchrony.

Explicit solutions for the transient or short term behavior of $B/-$ are not readily available for general life length distributions $G(\cdot)$. In this section, we shall consider the waves of reproduction in $C/-$, and in the following sections, we will examine the corresponding time dependent fluctuations in the age distribution.

Let the population size be $Z(t)$, with $Z(0) = 1$. Write $m(t) = E\{Z(t)\}$. Since the jth doubling occurs at $R + (j - 1)\ell$ for $j = 0, 1, \cdots$, we get

$$(9.1) \qquad P\{Z(t) = 2^j\} = F(t - j\ell + \ell) - F(t - j\ell).$$

Hence,

$$(9.2) \qquad m(t) = 1 + \sum_{j=0}^{\infty} 2^j F(t - j\ell),$$

where, for fixed t, only finitely many terms are nonzero. Since $R = \ell - X$, we have $F(r) = 1 - A_0(\ell - r)$ so long as the life length distributions are continuous, whence

$$(9.3) \qquad m(t) = 1 + \sum_{j=0}^{\infty} 2^j[1 - A_0\{(j + 1)\ell - t\}].$$

The first wave of fission occurs before $t = \ell$, and thus for mean growth $m^*(t)$ over the first wave, we get

$$(9.4) \qquad m^*(t) = 2 - A_0(\ell - t),$$

where $0 \leq t \leq \ell$.

10. First fission: time varying age distribution during the first wave of reproduction

Still considering the model $C/-$, let the age of a randomly chosen member of the population, at time t, be X_t, with distribution function $A_t(\cdot)$. We can determine $A_t(\cdot)$ by considering the population commencing with a single individual. For the age of this individual at $t = 0$, we have $X_0 = X$ as in preceding sections, and its distribution function is $A_0(\cdot)$. There are two cases:

(i) the first fission occurs after time t, that is, $R > t$; in such case $X_t = X + t$;

(ii) the first fission occurs before time t, and the second occurs after t, that is, $R \leq t$ and $R + \ell > t$; in such case $X = t - R$.

Thus, at least for $0 \leq t \leq \ell$, we have

$$(10.1) \quad A_t(x) = P\{R > t, X + t \leq x\} + P\{R \leq t, t - R \leq x\}$$
$$= P\{X < \min(\ell - t, x - t)\} + P\{\ell - t \leq X \leq \ell - t + x\}.$$

In (10.1) if $x < t$, we have $P\{X < \min(\ell - t, x - t)\} = 0$ so that

$$(10.2) \quad A_t(x) = A_0(\ell - t + x) - A_0(\ell - t).$$

If $x > t$, we have certainly $X \leq \ell < \ell + x - t$ so

$$(10.3) \quad A_t(x) = P\{X < x - t\} + P\{\ell - t \leq X\}.$$

Supposing that all distributions are continuous, this gives

$$(10.4) \quad A_t(x) = A_0(x - t) + 1 - A_0(\ell - t).$$

11. Synchronization by deletion of an early age group

A common feature of experiments involving partial destruction of a cellular population is that a brief incident such as irradiation kills some of the cells, frequently the younger ones. We shall consider in model $C/-$ synchrony by complete deletion of the age group $(0, k)$. In (7.1), we can take

$$(11.1) \quad q(u) = \begin{cases} 0 & \text{for } 0 \leq u < k, \\ 1 & \text{for } k \leq u < \ell. \end{cases}$$

Then

$$(11.2) \quad A_0(x) = \begin{cases} 0 & \text{for } 0 \leq x < k, \\ \dfrac{A(x) - A(k)}{1 - A(k)} & \text{for } k \leq x < \ell. \end{cases}$$

Referring to (8.1), this gives

$$(11.3) \quad A_0(x) = \begin{cases} 0 & \text{for } 0 \leq x < k, \\ \dfrac{2^{-k/\ell} - 2^{-x/\ell}}{2^{-k/\ell} - 1} & \text{otherwise,} \end{cases}$$

a negative exponential truncated on the left at k and on the right at ℓ. Hence, from (9.4), mean growth over the first wave of reproduction is given by

$$(11.4) \quad m^*(t) = \begin{cases} \dfrac{2 - 2^{-k/\ell} - 2^{-(\ell-t)/\ell}}{1 - 2^{-k/\ell}} & \text{for } 0 \leq t \leq \ell - k, \\ 2 & \text{for } t > \ell - k. \end{cases}$$

The time dependent behavior of the age density is given by

$$(11.5) \quad A_t(x) = \begin{cases} \dfrac{2^{-(\ell-t)/\ell} \log 2}{\ell(1 - 2^{-k/\ell})} 2^{-x/\ell} & \text{for } 0 \leq x \leq t, \\ \dfrac{2^{-1} \log 2}{\ell(1 - 2^{-k/\ell})} 2^{-x/\ell} & \text{for } t \leq x \leq \ell. \end{cases}$$

Finally, we will apply these results to determine an optimum policy if the destruction of cells in the young age group is the desired purpose, as in cancer chemotherapy. We can suppose that k is small relative to ℓ. Consideration of (10.1), (10.2), and (10.4) shows that the development of $A_t(x)$ with time is simply an interchange of age groups. For $x < t$ and time zero, consider the individuals in the age group $(\ell - t, \ell - t + x)$. At time t they have moved into (or, equivalently, been replaced by their offspring in) the age group $(0, x)$. The same applies to $x > t$. Thus, (10.2) and (10.4) can be treated as periodic in t of period ℓ, though the approximation is of course satisfactory only for fairly small t. With the truncated distribution (11.2), we see that at time $\ell - k$ the age distribution is just the original $A_0(x)$ translated by $\ell - k$. Furthermore, since the density $A_0(x)$ is monotone decreasing where it is nonzero, the magnitude of the age group $(0, k)$ reaches a local maximum at time $\ell - k$, and this is the optimum epoch to repeat the destructive treatment for maximum effect. The results of two successive "attacks" of this kind appear in Table II.

TABLE II

DELETION OF AN EARLY AGE GROUP
p_i = proportion killed at ith step for $i = 1, 2$.
q_i = proportion of total population killed
up to and including ith step.

k	Step no. i	p_i	q_i
0.05	1	0.07	0.07
	2	0.07	0.13
0.10	1	0.13	0.13
	2	0.14	0.26
0.15	1	0.20	0.20
	2	0.22	0.38

The increased effectiveness if the age group destroyed is broader is clear but such deletion would, in any case, require numerous repetitions to eliminate the population, especially as the blurring of the age groups corresponding to the decay of synchrony would act to make elimination less effective.

REFERENCES

[1] M. S. BARTLETT, "Distributions associated with cell populations," *Biometrika*, Vol. 56 (1969), pp. 391–400.
[2] D. G. BURNETT-HALL and W. A. O'N. WAUGH, "Indices of synchrony in cellular cultures," *Biometrics*, Vol. 23 (1967), pp. 693–715.
[3] A. CAMPBELL, "The theoretical basis of synchronization by shifts in environmental conditions," *Synchrony in Cell Division and Growth* (edited by E. Zeuthen), New York, Interscience, 1964, pp. 469–484.

[4] J. ENGELBERG and H. R. HIRSCH, "On the theory of synchronous cultures," *Cell Synchrony* (edited by I. L. Cameron and G. M. Padilla), New York, Academic Press, 1966, pp. 14–37.

[5] P. D. M. MACDONALD, "Statistical inference from the fraction labelled mitoses curve," *Biometrika*, Vol. 57 (1970), pp. 489–593.

[6] J. M. MITCHISON and W. S. VINCENT, "A method of making synchronous cultures by density gradient centrifugation," *Cell Synchrony* (edited by I. L. Cameron and G. M. Padilla), New York, Academic Press, 1966, pp. 328–331.

[7] D. SANKOFF, "Duration of detectable synchrony in a binary branching process," *Biometrika*, Vol. 58 (1971), pp. 77–81.

[8] T. TERASIMA and L. J. TOLMACH, "Growth and nucleic acid synthesis in synchronously dividing populations of HeLa cells," *Exp. Cell. Res.*, Vol. 30 (1963), pp. 344–362.

[9] H. J. WEINER, "Application of the age distribution in age dependent branching processes," *J. Appl. Probability*, Vol. 3 (1966), pp. 179–201.

A TIME DEPENDENT SIMPLE STOCHASTIC EPIDEMIC

GRACE L. YANG
UNIVERSITY OF MARYLAND
and
CHIN LONG CHIANG
UNIVERSITY OF CALIFORNIA, BERKELEY

1. Introduction

Since the pioneer work of A. M. McKendrick in 1926, many authors have contributed to the advancement of the stochastic theory of epidemics, including Bartlett [4], Bailey [1], D. G. Kendall [12], Neyman and Scott [13], Whittle [16], to name a few. Mathematical complexity involved in some of the epidemic models has aroused the interest of many others. For example, the general stochastic epidemic model where a population consists of susceptibles, infectives, and immunes (see [2], p. 39), has motivated Kendall to suggest an ingenious device. Other authors also have investigated various aspects of the problem. (See, for example, Daniels [8], Downton [9], Gani [11] and Siskind [15].) The model discussed in the present paper deals with a closed population without removal of infectives, a special case of which has been studied very extensively by Bailey [3]. Following Bailey, we label it "a time dependent simple stochastic epidemic."

In a simple stochastic epidemic model, a population consists of two groups of individuals: susceptibles and infectives; there are no removals, no deaths, no immunes, and no recoveries from infection. At the initial time $t = 0$, there are N susceptibles and 1 infective. For each time t, for $t > 0$, there are a number of infectives denoted by $Y(t)$ and a number of uninfected susceptibles $X(t)$, with $Y(t) + X(t) = N + 1$, the total population size remaining unchanged. Our primary purpose is to derive an explicit solution for the probability distribution of the random variable $Y(t)$,

$$(1) \qquad P_{1n}(0, t) = Pr\{Y(t) = n | Y(0) = 1\}, \qquad n = 1, \cdots, N + 1.$$

For each interval (τ, t), $0 \leq \tau \leq t < \infty$, and for each n, we assume the existence of a nonnegative continuous function $\beta_n(\tau)$ such that

$$(2) \qquad \frac{\partial}{\partial t} P_{n,m}(\tau, t) \Big|_{t=\tau} = \begin{cases} -\beta_n(\tau) & \text{for } m = n, \\ \beta_n(\tau) & \text{for } m = n + 1, \\ 0 & \text{otherwise.} \end{cases}$$

Under the assumption of homogeneous mixing of the population, we let

147

(3) $\beta_n(\tau) = n(N + 1 - n)\beta(\tau) = a_n\beta(\tau),$

where

(4) $a_n = n(N + 1 - n).$

The quantity $\beta(\tau)$, which is a function of time τ, is known as the infection rate. Thus, in this model, the intensity of spreading of disease may vary with time during an epidemic. It follows from (2) that, for each $t > 0$, the probability function $P_{1n}(0, t)$ satisfies the following system of differential equations

$$\frac{d}{dt} P_{11}(0, t) = -a_1\beta(t)P_{11}(0, t)$$

(5)

$$\frac{d}{dt} P_{1n}(0, t) = -a_n\beta(t)P_{1n}(0, t) + a_{n-1}\beta(t)P_{1,n-1}(0, t)$$

for $n = 2, \cdots, N + 1$, with the initial condition $P_{11}(0, 0) = 1$.

Equations (5) are essentially the same as those studied extensively by Bailey [1], [2], [3], except that in those publications the infection rate is assumed to be independent of time (that is, $\beta(t) = \beta$) and the random variable is $X(t)$, the number of susceptibles remaining at time t. Bailey used the Laplace transform, the generating function, and a very skillful mathematical manipulation to provide the solution. However, the computations involved are too complex. Yang has recently established a relationship between the density function of the time of infections and the probability of the number of infections to arrive at a solution [17]. In the present paper, we offer another approach to the problem.

The present solution of system (5) requires the following two lemmas.

LEMMA 1.   *Whatever may be distinct real numbers* $a_1, \cdots, a_n$,

(6) $$\sum_{i=1}^{n} \frac{1}{\prod_{\alpha=1,\alpha\neq i}^{n} (a_i - a_\alpha)} = 0.$$

Lemma 1 may be found in Pólya and Szegö [14]. Several proofs of the lemma have been given in Chiang [5], [6], pp. 126–127.

LEMMA 2.   *Whatever may be* k, *for* $1 \leq k < n$, *the probabilities in* (1) *satisfy the equality*

(7) $$P_{1n}(0, t) = \int_0^t P_{1k}(0, \tau)a_k\beta(\tau)P_{k+1,n}(\tau, t) \, d\tau.$$

Equation (7) may be easily justified. Let k be an arbitrary but *fixed* integer, $1 \leq k < n$; the $(k + 1)$th infection must take place somewhere between 0 and t. Let it take place in interval $(\tau, \tau + d\tau)$; then there are k infectives at τ, and $(n - k - 1)$ infectives occurring during (τ, t); the corresponding probability is

(8) $$P_{1k}(0, \tau)a_k\beta(\tau) \, d\tau \, P_{k+1,n}(\tau, t),$$

where $P_{k+1,n}(\tau, t)$ is the conditional probability of n infectives at t given $k + 1$ infectives at τ. Since the events corresponding to the probability (8) for different τ are mutually exclusive, we may integrate (8) from $\tau = 0$ to $\tau = t$ to obtain the required equation (7). Equation (7) holds true whatever may be $1 \leq k < n$ and regardless of whether the a_i are distinct. For a general discussion on the lemma, the reader is referred to Chiang [7].

2. Solution for the probability $P_{1n}(0, t)$

Solution of the differential equations in (5) depends on whether $n \leqq (N + 1)/2$ or $n > (N + 1)/2$. The two cases are presented separately below.

Case 1: $1 \leqq n \leqq (N + 1)/2$. For these values of n, $a_1, \cdots, a_n$ are all distinct; the differential equations in (5) have the solution

$$(9) \quad P_{1n}(0, t) = (-1)^{n-1} a_1 \cdots a_{n-1} \left[\sum_{i=1}^{n} \frac{\exp \{-a_i \lambda(t)\}}{\prod_{\alpha=1, \alpha \neq i}^{n} (a_i - a_\alpha)} \right],$$

$$n = 1, \cdots, \frac{N}{2} \text{ or } \frac{N+1}{2},$$

where

$$(10) \quad \lambda(t) = \int_0^t \beta(\tau) \, d\tau$$

is assumed to be such that $\lim_{t \to \infty} \lambda(t) = \infty$. We assume that $a_0 = 1$ and $\pi(a_i = a_\alpha) = 1$ for $n = 1$.

Solution (9), which can be verified by induction using Lemma 1, is similar to that in the pure birth process (see, for example, Feller [10] and Chiang [6], pp. 51–52), except that, in the present case, $\beta(\tau)$ is a function of time.

When $\beta(\tau) = \beta$, $\lambda(t) = \beta t$, and solution (9) becomes

$$(11) \quad P_{1n}(0, t) = (-1)^{n-1} a_1 \cdots a_{n-1} \left[\sum_{i=1}^{n} \frac{\exp \{-a_i \beta t\}}{\prod_{\alpha=1, \alpha \neq i}^{n} (a_i - a_\alpha)} \right],$$

$$n = 1, \cdots, \frac{N}{2} \text{ or } \frac{N+1}{2}.$$

For a_i defined in (4),

$$(12) \quad a_1 \cdots a_{n-1} = (n - 1)! \frac{N!}{(N + 1 - n)!},$$

$$(13) \quad \prod_{\alpha=1, \alpha \neq i}^{n} (a_i - a_\alpha) = (-1)^{n-i} \frac{(i - 1)!(n - i)!(N - i)!}{(N - 2i + 1)(N - i - n)!},$$

and solution (11) may be rewritten

$$(14)$$

$$P_{1n}(0, t) = \sum_{i=1}^{n} (-1)^{i-1} \frac{(N - 2i + 1)(n - 1)!N!(N - i - n)! \exp \{-a_i \beta t\}}{(i - 1)!(N - i)!(N + 1 - n)!(n - i)!},$$

for $n = 1, 2, \cdots, (N/2 \text{ or } (N + 1)/2)$, which is the same as that obtained by Bailey [2].

Case 2: $(N + 1)/2 < n \leqq N + 1$. Formula (9) no longer holds true when $n > (N + 1)/2$ for the reason that in this case the a_i are not all distinct, and in particular,

$$(15) \qquad a_i = i(N + 1 - i) = a_{N+1-i}.$$

However, solution of the differential equations in (5) can be obtained by using Lemma 2. In applying equality (7) to the present problem, the integer k must be chosen so that the a_i in the probability $P_{1k}(0, \tau)$ are distinct and the a_i in $P_{k+1,n}(\tau, t)$ also are distinct. When N is even, $k = N/2$; when N is odd, $k = (N + 1)/2$.

With these values of k, we apply formula (9) to the two probabilities in the integrand in equation (7) to obtain

$$(16) \qquad P_{1k}(0, \tau) = (-1)^{k-1} a_1 \cdots a_{k-1} \left[\sum_{i=1}^{k} \frac{\exp\{-a_i \lambda(\tau)\}}{\prod\limits_{\alpha=1, \alpha \neq i}^{k} (a_i - a_\alpha)} \right]$$

and

$$(17) \qquad P_{k+1,n}(\tau, t) = (-1)^{n-k-1} a_{k+1} \cdots a_{n-1} \left[\sum_{j=k+1}^{n} \frac{\exp\{-a_j[\lambda(t) - \lambda(\tau)]\}}{\prod\limits_{\delta=k+1, \delta \neq j}^{n} (a_j - a_\delta)} \right].$$

Substituting (16) and (17) in (7) gives the basic formula

$$(18) \quad P_{1n}(0, t) = (-1)^n a_1 \cdots a_{n-1}$$

$$\sum_{i=1}^{k} \sum_{j=k+1}^{n} \int_0^t \frac{\exp\{-a_i \lambda(\tau)\} \exp\{-a_j[\lambda(t) - \lambda(\tau)]\}}{\prod\limits_{\alpha=1, \alpha \neq i}^{k} (a_i - a_\alpha) \prod\limits_{\delta=k+1, \delta \neq j}^{n} (a_j - a_\delta)} \beta(\tau) \, d\tau.$$

The integral in (18) depends on the values of a_i and a_j. According to the definition of $\lambda(t)$ in (10),

$$(19) \quad \int_0^t \exp\{-a_i \lambda(\tau)\} \exp\{-a_j[\lambda(t) - \lambda(\tau)]\} \beta(\tau) \, d\tau$$

$$= \frac{-1}{a_i - a_j} [\exp\{-a_i \lambda(t)\} - \exp\{-a_j \lambda(t)\}], \qquad a_i \neq a_j,$$

and

$$(20) \quad \int_0^t \exp\{-a_i \lambda(\tau)\} \exp\{-a_j[\lambda(t) - \lambda(\tau)]\} \beta(\tau) \, d\tau$$

$$= \lambda(t) \exp\{-a_i \lambda(t)\}, \qquad a_j = a_i.$$

There are $(n - k)$ terms where $a_i = a_j$ with $i + j = 2k + 1$ when $N = 2k$, and $i + j = 2k$ when $N = 2k - 1$; they are

$$(21) \qquad a_{2k+1-n} = a_n, a_{2k+2-n} = a_{n-1}, \cdots, a_k = a_{k+1},$$

for $N = 2k$, and

$$(22) \qquad a_{2k-n} = a_n, a_{2k+2-n} = a_{n-1}, \cdots, a_{k-1} = a_{k+1},$$

for $N = 2k - 1$. The probabilities $P_{1n}(0, t)$ assume slightly different forms for $N = 2k$ and for $N = 2k - 1$.

(i) *N is even*: $N = 2k$. Substituting (19) and (20) in (18) gives the desired formula for the probability

$$(23) \quad P_{1n}(0, t) = (-1)^{n-1} a_1 \cdots a_{n-1} \left[- \sum_{i=2k+1-n}^{k} \frac{\lambda(t) \exp\{-a_i \lambda(t)\}}{\prod\limits_{\alpha=1, a_\alpha \neq a_i}^{n} (a_i - a_\alpha)} \right.$$

$$\left. + \sum_{i=1}^{k} \sum_{\substack{j=k+1 \\ a_i \neq a_j}}^{n} \frac{\exp\{-a_i \lambda(t)\} - \exp\{-a_j \lambda(t)\}}{(a_i - a_j) \prod\limits_{\alpha=1, \alpha \neq i}^{k} (a_i - a_\alpha) \prod\limits_{\delta=k+1, \delta \neq j}^{n} (a_j - a_\delta)} \right],$$

for $n = k + 1, \cdots, N$, where $k = N/2$.

Note that in the product $\prod_{\alpha=1}^{n} (a_i - a_\alpha)$ in formula (23) there are two values of α for which $a_\alpha = a_i$; namely, a_i and a_{N+1-i}; they are both excluded from the product.

The probability $P_{1,N+1}(0, t)$ may be computed from

$$(24) \quad P_{1,N+1}(0, t) = \int_0^t P_{1,N}(0, \tau) a_N \beta(\tau) \, d\tau$$

$$= a_1 \cdots a_N \left[\sum_{i=1}^{k} \frac{\int_0^t \lambda(\tau) \exp\{-a_i \lambda(\tau)\} \beta(\tau) \, d\tau}{\prod\limits_{\alpha=1, a_\alpha \neq a_i}^{N} (a_i - a_\alpha)} \right.$$

$$\left. - \sum_{i=1}^{k} \sum_{j=k+1}^{N} \frac{\int_0^t [\exp\{-a_i \lambda(\tau)\} - \exp\{-a_j \lambda(\tau)\}] \beta(\tau) \, d\tau}{\prod\limits_{\alpha=1}^{k} (a_i - a_\alpha) \prod\limits_{\delta=k+1}^{N} (a_j - a_\delta)(a_i - a_j)} \right].$$

The first integral of (24) is evaluated to give

$$(25) \quad \int_0^t \lambda(\tau) \exp\{-a_i \lambda(\tau)\} \beta(\tau) \, d\tau = \frac{1}{a_i^2} - \frac{\exp\{-a_i \lambda(t)\}}{a_i^2} - \frac{\lambda(t) \exp\{-a_i \lambda(t)\}}{a_i}.$$

Thus, the first term inside the brackets in (24) becomes

$$(26)$$

$$\sum_{i=1}^{k} \frac{1}{\prod\limits_{\alpha=1, a_\alpha \neq a_i}^{N} (a_i - a_\alpha) a_i^2} - \sum_{i=1}^{k} \frac{\exp\{-a_i \lambda(t)\}}{\prod\limits_{\alpha=1, a_\alpha \neq a_i}^{N} (a_i - a_\alpha) a_i^2} - \sum_{i=1}^{k} \frac{\lambda(t) \exp\{-a_i \lambda(t)\}}{\prod\limits_{\alpha=1, a_\alpha \neq a_i}^{N} (a_i - a_\alpha) a_i}.$$

The second integral in (24) is

$$(27) \quad \int_0^t [\exp\{-a_i \lambda(\tau)\} - \exp\{-a_j \lambda(\tau)\}] \beta(\tau) \, d\tau$$

$$= -\frac{a_i - a_j}{a_i a_j} - \left[\frac{\exp\{-a_i \lambda(t)\}}{a_i} - \frac{\exp\{-a_j \lambda(t)\}}{a_j} \right],$$

and the second term inside the brackets in (24) becomes

$$(28) \quad \sum_{i=1}^{k} \sum_{\substack{j=k+1 \\ a_i \neq a_j}}^{N} \frac{1}{\prod\limits_{\alpha=1}^{k} (a_i - a_\alpha) \prod\limits_{\delta=k+1}^{N} (a_j - a_\delta) a_i a_j}$$

$$+ \sum_{i=1}^{k} \sum_{\substack{j=k+1 \\ a_i \neq a_j}}^{N} \frac{[\exp\{-a_i \lambda(t)\}/a_i] - [\exp\{-a_j \lambda(t)\}/a_j]}{\prod\limits_{\alpha=1, \alpha \neq i}^{k} (a_i - a_\alpha) \prod\limits_{\delta=k+1, \delta \neq j}^{N} (a_j - a_\delta)(a_i - a_j)}$$

Combining the two constant terms in (26) and (28), and using Lemma 1, we have

$$(29) \quad \sum_{i=1}^{k} \frac{1}{\prod\limits_{\alpha=1, a_\alpha \neq a_i}^{N} (a_i - a_\alpha) a_i^2} + \sum_{i=1}^{k} \sum_{\substack{j=k+1 \\ a_i \neq a_j}}^{N} \frac{1}{\prod\limits_{\alpha=1}^{k} (a_i - a_\alpha) \prod\limits_{\delta=k+1}^{N} (a_j - a_\delta) a_i a_j}$$

$$= \left[\sum_{i=1}^{k} \frac{1}{\prod\limits_{\alpha=1}^{k} (a_i - a_\alpha) a_i} \right]^2 = \left[\frac{1}{\prod\limits_{i=1}^{k} (-a_i)} \right]^2 = \frac{1}{\prod\limits_{i=1}^{N} a_i}.$$

In the second term in (28), the running indices i and j are interchangeable, so that

$$(30) \quad \sum_{i=1}^{k} \sum_{\substack{j=k+1 \\ a_i \neq a_j}}^{N} \frac{[\exp\{-a_i\lambda(t)\}/a_i] - [\exp\{-a_j\lambda(t)\}/a_j]}{\prod\limits_{\alpha=1}^{k} (a_i - a_\alpha) \prod\limits_{\delta=k+1}^{N} (a_j - a_\delta)(a_i - a_j)}$$

$$= 2 \sum_{i=1}^{k} \sum_{\substack{j=k+1 \\ a_i \neq a_j}}^{N} \frac{\exp\{-a_i\lambda(t)\}}{\prod\limits_{\alpha=1}^{k} (a_i - a_\alpha) \prod\limits_{\delta=k+1}^{N} (a_j - a_\delta)(a_i - a_j) a_i}.$$

With the simplifications in (29) and (30), we substitute (26) and (28) in (24) to obtain the formula

$$(31) \quad P_{1,N+1}(0, t)$$

$$= 1 - a_1 \cdots a_N \left[\sum_{i=1}^{k} \frac{\lambda(t) \exp\{-a_i\lambda(t)\}}{\prod\limits_{\alpha=1, a_\alpha \neq a_i}^{N} (a_i - a_\alpha) a_i} + \sum_{i=1}^{k} \frac{\exp\{-a_i\lambda(t)\}}{\prod\limits_{\alpha=1, a_\alpha \neq a_i}^{N} (a_i - a_\alpha) a_i^2} \right.$$

$$\left. - 2 \sum_{i=1}^{k} \sum_{\substack{j=k+1 \\ a_i \neq a_j}}^{N} \frac{\exp\{-a_i\lambda(t)\}}{\prod\limits_{\alpha=1, \alpha \neq i}^{k} (a_i - a_\alpha) \prod\limits_{\delta=k+1, \delta \neq j}^{N} (a_j - a_\delta)(a_i - a_j) a_i} \right],$$

where $k = N/2$ and $\lambda(t) = \int_0^t \beta(\tau) \, d\tau$.

(ii) *N is odd: $N = 2k - 1$.* The essential difference between this case and the preceding one is in the limits of the summations and the value of a_k (that is, $a_{(N+1)/2}$) which is now distinct from all other a_i. Keeping these differences in mind, we again substitute (19) and (20) in (18) to obtain the probabilities

$$(32) \quad P_{1n}(0, t) = (-1)^{n-1} a_1 \cdots a_{n-1} \left[- \sum_{i=2k-n}^{k-1} \frac{\lambda(t) \exp\{-a_i\lambda(t)\}}{\prod\limits_{\alpha=1, a_\alpha \neq a_i}^{n} (a_i - a_\alpha)} \right.$$

$$\left. + \sum_{i=1}^{k} \sum_{\substack{j=k+1 \\ a_i \neq a_j}}^{n} \frac{\exp\{-a_i\lambda(t)\} - \exp\{-a_j\lambda(t)\}}{\prod\limits_{\alpha=1, \alpha \neq i}^{k} (a_i - a_\alpha) \prod\limits_{\delta=k+1, \delta \neq j}^{n} (a_j - a_\delta)(a_i - a_j)} \right],$$

for $n = k + 1, \cdots, N$; with $k = (N + 1)/2$, and

$$(33) \quad P_{1,N+1}(0, t) = 1 - a_1 \cdots a_N \left[\sum_{i=1}^{k-1} \frac{(\lambda(t) + a_i^{-1}) \exp\{-a_i\lambda(t)\}}{\prod_{\alpha=1}^{N} (a_i - a_\alpha)a_i} \right.$$

$$\left. + \sum_{i=1}^{k} \sum_{\substack{j=k+1 \\ a_i \neq a_j}}^{N} \frac{[\exp\{-a_i\lambda(t)\}/a_i] - [\exp\{-a_j\lambda(t)\}/a_j]}{\prod_{\alpha=1,\alpha \neq i}^{k} (a_i - a_\alpha) \prod_{\delta=k+1,\delta \neq j}^{N} (a_i - a_\delta)(a_i - a_j)} \right].$$

In formulas (9), (23), and (32) of the probabilities $P_{1n}(0, t)$, every term contains a factor $\exp\{-a_i\lambda(t)\}$ with $a_i > 0$. Therefore, as $t \to \infty$, $P_{1n}(0, t) \to 0$, for $n = 1, \cdots, N$; whereas formulas (31) and (33) show that $P_{1,N+1}(0, t) \to 1$ as $t \to \infty$. This means that in the simple epidemic model considered here, all the N susceptibles will be infected sooner or later; and the epidemic is said to be complete (see Bailey [2]).

3. Infection time and duration of the epidemic

The length of time elapsed till the occurrence of the nth infection is a continuous random variable taking on nonnegative real numbers. Let it be denoted by T_n, for $1 < n \leq N + 1$, with $T_1 = 0$. When $n = N + 1$, T_{N+1} is the duration of the epidemic. The purpose of this section is to derive explicit formulas for the density $f_n(t)$, the distribution function $F_n(t)$, the expectation and variance of T_n.

The density function $f_n(t)$ has a close relationship with the probability $P_{1,n-1}(0, t)$ of $n - 1$ infectives at time t. By definition, $f_n(t) dt$ is the probability that the random variable T_n will assume values in the interval $(t, t + dt)$. This means that at time t there are $n - 1$ infectives and the nth infection takes place in interval $(t, t + dt)$; the probability of the occurrence of these events is $P_{1,n-1}(0, t)a_{n-1}\beta(t) dt$. Therefore, we have the density function

$$(34) \qquad f_n(t) dt = P_{1,n-1}(0, t)a_{n-1}\beta(t) dt,$$

and, hence, the distribution function

$$(35) \qquad F_n(t) = \int_0^t P_{1,n-1}(0, \tau)a_{n-1}\beta(\tau) d\tau, \qquad n = 2, \cdots, N.$$

Using the formulas of the probabilities $P_{1,n-1}(0, t)$ in the preceding section, we can write down explicit functions for $f_n(t)$ and $F_n(t)$ for each n. We give two examples below.

EXAMPLE 1: $n \leq (N + 1)/2$. We substitute formula (9) in (34) and (35) to obtain the density function

$$(36) \qquad f_n(t) dt = (-1)^{n-2}a_1 \cdots a_{n-1} \left[\sum_{i=1}^{n-1} \frac{\beta(t) \exp\{-a_i\lambda(t)\}}{\prod_{\alpha=1,\alpha \neq i}^{n-1} (a_i - a_\alpha)} \right] dt,$$

and the distribution function

$$(37) \qquad F_n(t) = (-1)^{n-2}a_1 \cdots a_{n-1} \sum_{i=1}^{n-1} \frac{1 - \exp\{-a_i\lambda(t)\}}{\prod_{\alpha=1,\alpha \neq i}^{n-1} (a_i - a_\alpha)a_i}$$

for $n = 2, \cdots, N/2$ or $(N + 1)/2$, and $0 < t < \infty$. As $t \to \infty$, $f_n(t) \to 0$ and

$$(38) \qquad F_n(\infty) = (-1)^{n-2} a_1 \cdots a_{n-1} \sum_{i=1}^{n-1} \frac{1}{\prod\limits_{\alpha=1, \alpha \neq i}^{n-1} (a_i - a_\alpha) a_i} = 1,$$

since Lemma 1 implies that

$$(39) \qquad \sum_{i=1}^{n-1} \frac{1}{\prod\limits_{\alpha=1, \alpha \neq i}^{n-1} (a_i - a_\alpha) a_i} = - \frac{1}{\prod\limits_{i=1}^{n-1} (-a_i)}.$$

EXAMPLE 2: *the duration of epidemic* T_{N+1}, *when* $N = 2k$. In this case formula (23) for $n = N$ is used in (34) and (35). The density function and the distribution function for T_{N+1} are, respectively,

(40)

$$f_{N+1}(t) \, dt = (-1) a_1 \cdots a_N \left[- \sum_{i=1}^{k} \frac{\lambda(t) \exp\{-a_i \lambda(t)\}}{\prod\limits_{\alpha=1, a_\alpha \neq a_i}^{N} (a_i - a_\alpha)} \right.$$

$$\left. + \sum_{i=1}^{k} \sum_{\substack{j=k+1 \\ a_i \neq a_j}}^{N} \frac{\exp\{-a_i \lambda(t)\} - \exp\{-a_j \lambda(t)\}}{\prod\limits_{\alpha=1, \alpha \neq i}^{k} (a_i - a_\alpha) \prod\limits_{\delta=k+1, \delta \neq j}^{N} (a_j - a_\delta)(a_i - a_j)} \right] \beta(t) \, dt,$$

where $k = N/2$, and

$$(41) \quad F_{N+1}(t) = (-1) a_1 \cdots a_N \left[\sum_{i=1}^{k} \frac{1}{\prod\limits_{\alpha=1, a_\alpha \neq a_i}^{N} (a_i - a_\alpha)} \right.$$

$$\left\{ \frac{\lambda(t)}{a_i} \exp\{-a_i \lambda(t)\} - \frac{1 - \exp\{-a_i \lambda(t)\}}{a_i^2} \right\}$$

$$+ \sum_{i=1}^{k} \sum_{\substack{j=k+1 \\ a_i \neq a_j}}^{N} \frac{1}{(a_i - a_j) \prod\limits_{\alpha=1, \alpha \neq i}^{k} (a_i - a_\alpha) \prod\limits_{\delta=k+1, \delta \neq j}^{N} (a_j - a_\delta)}$$

$$\left. \left\{ \frac{1 - \exp\{-a_i \lambda(t)\}}{a_i} - \frac{1 - \exp\{-a_j \lambda(t)\}}{a_j} \right\} \right]$$

for $0 < t < \infty$. As $t \to \infty$, $f_{N+1}(t) \to 0$ and $F_{N+1}(t) \to 1$. To prove the last assertion, we take the limit of (41) as $t \to \infty$,

$$(42) \quad F_{N+1}(\infty) = (-1) a_1 \cdots a_N \left[\sum_{i=1}^{k} \frac{1}{\prod\limits_{\alpha=1, a_\alpha \neq a_i}^{N} (a_i - a_\alpha)} \left(-\frac{1}{a_i^2} \right) \right.$$

$$\left. - \sum_{i=1}^{k} \sum_{\substack{j=k+1 \\ a_i \neq a_j}}^{N} \frac{1}{\prod\limits_{\alpha=1, \alpha \neq i}^{k} (a_i - a_\alpha) a_i \prod\limits_{\delta=k+1, \delta \neq j}^{N} (a_j - a_\delta) a_j} \right].$$

Since $a_j = a_{N+1-j}$ and $k = N/2$, the limits of j (in the summation) and δ (in the product) in (42) may be changed from $(k + 1, N)$ to $(k, 1)$, and (42) may be rewritten

$$(43) \qquad F_{N+1}(\infty) = a_1 \cdots a_N \left[\sum_{i=1}^{k} \frac{1}{\prod\limits_{\alpha=1,\alpha\neq i}^{k} (a_i - a_\alpha)a_i} \right]^2,$$

where $k = N/2$,

$$(44) \qquad a_1 \cdots a_N = (a_1 \cdots a_k)^2,$$

and, in light of Lemma 1,

$$(45) \qquad \sum_{i=1}^{k} \frac{1}{\prod\limits_{\alpha=1,\alpha\neq i}^{k} (a_i - a_\alpha)a_i} = \frac{-1}{\prod\limits_{i=1}^{k} (-a_i)}.$$

Substituting (44) and (45) in (43) yields

$$(46) \qquad F_{N+1}(\infty) = 1.$$

In the same manner, it can be shown that whatever may be $n = 2, \cdots, N + 1$, $f_n(t) \to 0$ and $F_n(t) \to 1$ as $t \to \infty$, and the corresponding random variables T_n are all proper.

The expectation and variance of T_n can be computed directly from

$$(47) \qquad E(T_n) = \int_0^\infty t f_n(t) \, dt$$

and

$$(48) \qquad \sigma_{T_n}^2 = \int_0^\infty [t - E(T_n)]^2 f_n(t) \, dt.$$

For the duration of epidemic T_{N+1} with $N = 2k$, for example, we substitute (40) in (47) to obtain the expectation

$$(49) \quad E(T_{N+1}) = (-1)a_1 \cdots a_N \left[-\sum_{i=1}^{k} \frac{\int_0^\infty t\lambda(t) \exp\{-a_i\lambda(t)\}\beta(t) \, dt}{\prod\limits_{\alpha=1,a_\alpha\neq a_i}^{N} (a_i - a_\alpha)} \right.$$

$$\left. + \sum_{i=1}^{k} \sum_{j=k+1}^{N} \frac{\int_0^\infty t(\exp\{-a_i\lambda(t)\} - \exp\{-a_j\lambda(t)\})\beta(t) \, dt}{\prod\limits_{\alpha=1,\alpha\neq i}^{k} (a_i - a_\alpha) \prod\limits_{\delta=k+1,\delta\neq j}^{N} (a_j - a_\delta)(a_i - a_j)} \right].$$

Obviously, explicit formulas of $E(T_n)$ and $\sigma_{T_n}^2$ depend upon the infection rate $\beta(t)$. When the infection rate is independent of time so that $\beta(t) = \beta$, the corresponding formulas may be obtained by an alternative method.

The length of time elapsed till the occurrence of the nth infection may be divided into two periods: a period of length T_{n-1} up to the occurrence of the $(n-1)$th infection and a period of length W_n between the occurrence of the $(n-1)$th and the nth infections. The sum of the two periods is equal to the entire length of time, or

$$(50) \qquad T_n = T_{n-1} + W_n.$$

Equality (50) can be easily verified. When $\beta(t) = \beta$, T_{n-1} and W_n are independently distributed nonnegative random variables. The density functions of T_{n-1} and W_n can be derived from (34); they are

$$(51) \qquad f_{n-1}(t) = P_{1,n-2}(0, t)a_{n-2}\beta$$

and

$$(52) \qquad g_n(t) = P_{n-1,n-1}(0, t)a_{n-1}\beta,$$

respectively. According to (50), the distribution of T_n is the convolution of the distributions of T_{n-1} and W_n. Therefore, the corresponding density functions satisfy the relationship

$$(53) \qquad f_n(t) = \int_0^t f_{n-1}(\tau)g_n(t - \tau) \, d\tau.$$

To prove (53), we recall identity (7) in Lemma 2,

$$(54) \qquad P_{1,n-1}(0, t) = \int_0^t P_{1,n-2}(0, \tau)a_{n-2}\beta P_{n-1,n-1}(\tau, t) \, d\tau,$$

and multiply both sides of (54) by $a_{n-1}\beta$ to obtain

$$(55) \qquad P_{1,n-1}(0, t)a_{n-1}\beta = \int_0^t [P_{1,n-2}(0, \tau)a_{n-2}\beta][P_{n-1,n-1}(\tau, t)a_{n-1}\beta] \, d\tau,$$

which, in light of (34), (51), and (52), is identical to (53), proving (50). Equation (50) is a special case of a general equality, for which the reader is referred to [6], p. 110.

Now, the probability in (52) is

$$(56) \qquad P_{n-1,n-1}(0, t) = \exp\{-a_{n-1}\beta t\};$$

therefore, the random variable W_n has an exponential distribution with the density function

$$(57) \qquad g_n(t) = a_{n-1}\beta \exp\{-a_{n-1}\beta t\}.$$

The expectation and the variance of W_n, thus, are given by

$$(58) \qquad E(W_n) = \frac{1}{a_{n-1}\beta}$$

and

$$(59) \qquad \sigma_{W_n}^2 = \frac{1}{a_{n-1}^2\beta^2},$$

respectively.

Equation (50) can be easily extended. Let

$$(60) \qquad W_i = T_i - T_{i-1}, \qquad\qquad i = 2, \cdots, N + 1,$$

be the length of time elapsed between the $(i - 1)$th and the ith infections. Using the arguments in proving (50), we can show that

$$(61) \qquad T_n = W_2 + \cdots + W_n, \qquad\qquad n = 2, \cdots, N + 1,$$

where the W_i are independently distributed random variables, and each has an exponential distribution (see equation (57)) with

$$(62) \qquad E(W_i) = \frac{1}{a_{i-1}\beta}, \qquad \sigma^2_{W_i} = \frac{1}{a^2_{i-1}\beta^2}, \qquad i = 2, \cdots, N+1.$$

It follows that the expectation and variance of T_n are

$$(63) \qquad E(T_n) = \sum_{i=1}^{n-1} \frac{1}{a_i\beta}, \qquad \sigma^2_{T_n} = \sum_{i=1}^{n-1} \frac{1}{a_i^2\beta^2}, \qquad n = 2, \cdots, N+1.$$

For the duration of the epidemic T_{N+1}, we may use the relationship $a_i = a_{N+1-i}$ to have

$$(64) \qquad E(T_{N+1}) = 2\sum_{i=1}^{k} \frac{1}{a_i\beta}, \qquad \sigma^2_{T_{N+1}} = 2\sum_{i=1}^{k} \frac{1}{a_i^2\beta^2},$$

when N is even with $k = N/2$, and

$$(65) \qquad E(T_{N+1}) = 2\sum_{i=1}^{k-1} \frac{1}{a_i\beta} + \frac{1}{a_k\beta}, \qquad \sigma^2_{T_{N+1}} = 2\sum_{i=1}^{k-1} \frac{1}{a_i^2\beta^2} + \frac{1}{a_k^2\beta^2},$$

when N is odd with $k = (N+1)/2$. They are the same as those derived from the cumulant generating function in [2], p. 47.

REFERENCES

[1] N. T. J. BAILEY, "A simple stochastic epidemic," *Biometrika*, Vol. 37 (1950), pp. 193–202.

[2] ———, *The Mathematical Theory of Epidemics*, London, Charles Griffin, 1957.

[3] ———, "The simple stochastic epidemic: a complete solution in terms of known functions," *Biometrika*, Vol. 50 (1963), pp. 235–240.

[4] M. S. BARTLETT, "Deterministic and stochastic models of recurrent epidemics," *Proceedings of the Third Berkeley Symposium on Mathematical Statistics and Probability*, Berkeley and Los Angeles, University of California Press, 1956, Vol. 4, pp. 81–109.

[5] C. L. CHIANG, "A stochastic model of competing risks of illness and competing risks of death," *Stochastic Models in Medicine and Biology* (edited by J. Gurland), Madison, University of Wisconsin Press, 1964, pp. 323–354.

[6] ———, *Introduction to Stochastic Processes in Biostatistics*, New York, Wiley, 1968.

[7] ———, "An equality in stochastic processes," *Proceedings of the Sixth Berkeley Symposium on Mathematical Statistics and Probability*, Berkeley and Los Angeles, University of California Press, 1972, Vol. 4, pp. 187–196.

[8] H. E. DANIELS, "The distribution of the total size of an epidemic," *Proceedings of the Fifth Berkeley Symposium on Mathematical Statistics and Probability*, Berkeley and Los Angeles, University of California Press, 1965, Vol. 4, pp. 281–293.

[9] F. DOWNTON, "A note on the ultimate size of a general stochastic epidemic," *Biometrika*, Vol. 54 (1967), pp. 314–316.

[10] W. FELLER, *An Introduction to Probability Theory and Its Applications*, Vol. 2, New York, Wiley, 1965.

[11] J. GANI, "On a partial differential equation of epidemic theory," *Biometrika*, Vol. 52 (1965), pp. 617–620.

[12] D. G. KENDALL, "Deterministic and stochastic epidemics in a closed population," *Proceedings of the Third Berkeley Symposium on Mathematical Statistics and Probability*, Berkeley and Los Angeles, University of California Press, 1956, Vol. 4, pp. 149–165.

[13] J. NEYMAN and E. L. SCOTT, "A stochastic model of epidemics," *Stochastic Models in*

Medicine and Biology (edited by J. Gurland), Madison, University of Wisconsin Press, 1964, pp. 45–83.

[14] G. Pólya and G. Szegö, *Aufgaben und Lehrsätze aus der Analysis*, Vol. 2, Berlin, Springer-Verlag, 1964.

[15] V. Siskind, "A solution of the general stochastic epidemic," *Biometrika*, Vol. 52 (1965), pp. 613–616.

[16] P. Whittle, "The outcome of a stochastic epidemic," *Biometrika*, Vol. 42 (1955), pp. 116–122.

[17] G. L. Yang, "On the probability distributions of some stochastic epidemic models," TR 70-141, Department of Mathematics, University of Maryland, 1970.

GALTON-WATSON PROCESSES
WITH GENERATION DEPENDENCE

DEAN H. FEARN

CALIFORNIA STATE COLLEGE, HAYWARD

1. Introduction

A Galton-Watson process Z_n can be thought of in the following way. There is one cell alive in generation zero. This cell dies and gives birth to a random number Z_1 of baby cells in the first generation. Each of these cells dies and gives birth to a random number of cells in the second generation. The number of cells in the second generation is Z_2. The process continues; Z_n is the number of cells in the nth generation. The number of daughters born to a cell is allowed to be a random variable whose distribution depends upon the generation of the cell in question. In this paper the following questions are answered under certain conditions.

(i) What are the mean and variance of Z_n?

(ii) Does $Z_n/E(Z_n)$ converge to a nonzero and nonconstant random variable W?

(iii) If the answer to (ii) is yes, what are the mean and variance of W?

(iv) What is the behavior of $P(Z_n \neq 0)$ for large n?

If X and Y are random variables and A and B denote events, then $E(X)$ is mean of X, Var (X) is the variance of X, $E(X|Y)$ is the conditional mean of X given Y, $P(A)$ is the probability that A happens, and $P(A|B)$ is the conditional probability that A happens, given that B occurs. This paper is the first chapter of [1].

2. Definition of Z_n, the probability generating function of Z_n, and the Markov nature of Z_n

First, Z_n is defined inductively. Let $X_{n,k}$, for $n = 0, 1, 2, \cdots, k = 1, 2, \cdots$, be a family of independent nonnegative integer valued random variables such that, for n fixed, $X_{n,k}, k = 1, 2, \cdots$, are identically distributed. Define $Z_0 = 1$, and having defined Z_n, define

(1)
$$Z_{n+1} = \begin{cases} \sum_{k=1}^{Z_n} X_{n,k} & \text{if } Z_n \geq 1, \\ 0 & \text{if } Z_n = 0. \end{cases}$$

This definition may be expressed more simply by allowing the equation

$$(2) \qquad \sum_{k=1}^{0} a_k = 0$$

to be true for any sequence a_k. This convention will be followed throughout the rest of this paper. With this convention,

$$(3) \qquad Z_{n+1} = \sum_{k=1}^{Z_n} X_{n,k}, \qquad\qquad Z_n \geqq 0,$$

for $n = 0, 1, 2, \cdots$.

In the rest of this paper, s will denote an arbitrary number such that $0 \leqq s \leqq 1$. Let

$$(4) \qquad f_n(s) = \sum_{j=0}^{\infty} P(X_{n,1} = j)s^j$$

for $n = 0, 1, 2, \cdots$. Then $f_n(s)$ is called the probability generating function of $X_{n,1}$. The probability generating function of Z_n will now be determined. Let

$$(5) \qquad f^0(s) = s, \qquad f^{n+1}(s) = f^n(f_n(s)).$$

PROPOSITION 1.   *The probability generating function of Z_n is $f_n(s)$.*

PROOF.   Let $\bar{f}_n(s)$ be the probability generating function of Z_n. Evidently Proposition 1 is true when $n = 0$. Assume Proposition 1 is true when $n = k$:

$$(6) \qquad \bar{f}^{k+1}(s) = E(s^{Z_{k+1}})$$

$$= \sum_{m=0}^{\infty} E\left(s^{\sum_{i=1}^{m} X_{k,i}} \Big| Z_k = m\right) P(Z_k = m).$$

Now since the $X_{k,j}$ are independent of Z_k,

$$(7) \qquad \bar{f}^{k+1}(s) = \sum_{m=0}^{\infty} E\left(s^{\sum_{i=1}^{m} X_{k,i}}\right) P(Z_k = m).$$

Since the $X_{k,j}$ are themselves independent,

$$(8) \qquad \bar{f}^{k+1}(s) = \sum_{m=0}^{\infty} (E(s^{X_{k,1}}))^m P(Z_k = m)$$

$$= f^k(f_k(s)) = f^{k+1}(s)$$

by the induction hypothesis and (5). Thus, Proposition 1 is true. Let $Z_{n,0} = 1$, and having defined $Z_{n,k}$, let

$$(9) \qquad Z_{n,k+1} = \sum_{j=0}^{Z_{n,k}} X_{n+k,j}.$$

Now $Z_{n,k}$, for $k = 0, 1, 2, \cdots$, may be interpreted as follows. One cell is alive in the nth generation; this cell dies and gives birth to a random number, distributed as $X_{n,1}$, of baby cells. Each of these cells dies and gives birth, independently of one another, to a random number, distributed as $X_{n+1,1}$, of baby cells. This process continues for k generations, giving rise to $Z_{n,k}$ $(n + k)$th generation cells, having started with one nth generation cell. Notice that $Z_{0,k}$ is the same as Z_k.

For $n = 0, 1, 2, \cdots$, let $f_n^{0+n}(s) = s$, and having defined $f_n^{n+k}(s)$, let

(10) $$f_n^{k+1+n}(s) = f_n^{k+n}(f_{k+n}(s)).$$

PROPOSITION 2. *The probability generating function of $Z_{n,k}$ is $f_n^{n+k}(s)$.*

PROOF. The proof of this proposition is practically the same as for Proposition 1.

PROPOSITION 3. *Let $Z_{n,k,j}$, $j = 1, 2, \cdots$, be independent and identically distributed random variables, distributed like $Z_{n,k}$ and independent of $Z_n, Z_{n-1}, \cdots$, Z_1, Z_0. Then Z_{n+k} is distributed like*

(11) $$\sum_{j=0}^{Z_n} Z_{n,k,j},$$

or, what amounts to the same thing, for each nonnegative integer k,

(12) $$f^n(f_n^{n+k}(s)) = f^{n+k}(s), \qquad n = 0, 1, 2, \cdots.$$

PROOF. Certainly (12) is evident when $k = 0$. Assume (12) is true when $k = \ell$. Then, by (10),

(13) $$f^n(f_n^{n+\ell+1}(s)) = f^n[f_n^{n+\ell}(f_{n+\ell}(s))].$$

By the induction assumption,

(14) $$f^n[f_n^{n+\ell}(f_{n+\ell}(s))] = f^{n+\ell}(f_{n+\ell}(s)).$$

By the definition of $f^{n+\ell+1}(s)$,

(15) $$f^{n+\ell}(f_{n+\ell}(s)) = f^{n+\ell+1}(s).$$

Thus, (12) is true for $k = 0, 1, 2, \cdots$.

COROLLARY 1. *The branching process Z_n is a Markov chain.*

PROOF. Let $n_1, \cdots, n_j$ be less than n, and let

(16) $$n_j = \max_{0 \le i \le j} \{n_i\}.$$

By Proposition 3,

(17) $\quad P(Z_n = \ell_n | Z_{n_1} = \ell_{n_1}, \cdots, Z_{n_j} = \ell_{n_j})$

$$= P\left(\sum_{i=1}^{Z_{n_j}} Z_{n_j, n-n_j, i} = \ell_n | Z_{n_1} = \ell_{n_1}, \cdots, Z_{n_j} = \ell_{n_j}\right)$$

$$= P\left(\sum_{i=1}^{Z_{n_j}} Z_{n_j, n-n_j, i} = \ell_n | Z_{n_j} = \ell_{n_j}\right),$$

since the $Z_{n_j, n-n_j, i}$, $i = 1, 2, \cdots$, are independent of $Z_{n_1}, Z_{n_2}, \cdots, Z_{n_j}$. So Corollary 1 is true.

Note that Z_n is not necessarily a stationary Markov chain. It would be stationary if the $X_{n,k}$ were identically distributed for all n and all k, in addition to being independent; however, in that case, Z_n would be the ordinary Galton-Watson process studied in [2] and in [3].

3. The mean and variance of Z_n; the convergence of Z_n/EZ_n

In the rest of this paper, products of the form

$$(18) \qquad a_0 a_1 \cdots a_n = \prod_{j=0}^{n} a_j$$

will frequently be used. For simplicity, the convention

$$(19) \qquad \prod_{j=0}^{-1} a_j = 1$$

will be adopted for all sequences a_n.

Much of the theory concerning the asymptotic behavior of Z_n (as $n \to \infty$) will now be developed, frequently using the methods in [2]. Let

$$(20) \qquad m_n = E(X_{n,1}), \qquad\qquad n = 0, 1, 2, \cdots,$$

and suppose from now on $m_n < \infty$.

PROPOSITION 4. *The expectation*

$$(21) \qquad EZ_n = \prod_{j=0}^{n-1} m_j$$

and

$$(22) \qquad EZ_{n,k} = \prod_{j=n}^{n+k-1} m_j$$

for $k = 0, 1, 2, \cdots$.

PROOF. Equation (21) will be proved. The proof of (22) is very much the same. When $n = 1$, equation (21) is true because

$$(23) \qquad E(Z_0) = E1 = 1.$$

Now assume (21) is true when $n = k$. Then

$$(24) \qquad E(Z_{k+1}) = E\left(\sum_{j=1}^{Z_k} X_{k,j} \right) = E(Z_k)E(X_{k,1}),$$

since Z_k is independent of the $X_{k,j}$. Thus, Proposition 4 holds.

Let

$$(25) \qquad W_n = \frac{Z_n}{E(Z_n)}, \qquad\qquad n = 0, 1, 2, \cdots.$$

Here and from now on it is assumed the $m_n > 0$.

PROPOSITION 5. *The random variable W_n is a martingale.*

PROOF. By (21),

$$(26) \qquad E(W_{n+k}|W_n) = \frac{E(Z_{n+k}|Z_n)}{\displaystyle\prod_{j=0}^{n+k-1} m_j}.$$

Thus, by Proposition 3,

$$(27) \qquad E(W_{n+k}|W_n) = \frac{E\left(\sum_{j=0}^{Z_n} Z_{n,k,j}|Z_n\right)}{\prod_{j=0}^{n+k-1} m_j}$$

$$= \frac{Z_n E(Z_{n,k,1})}{\prod_{j=0}^{n+k-1} m_j}.$$

Thus, by (21) and (22),

$$(28) \qquad E(W_{n+k}|W_n) = \frac{Z_n}{E(Z_n)} = W_n.$$

Moreover, by Corollary 1, W_n is a Markov chain; hence,

$$(29) \qquad E(W_{n+k}|W_n, W_{n-1}, \cdots, W_0) = E(W_{n+k}|W_n).$$

So W_n is a martingale, which was to be proven.

COROLLARY 2. *The random variable W_n approaches a random variable W almost surely as $n \to \infty$; moreover, $EW < \infty$.*

PROOF. For all n,

$$(30) \qquad E|W_n| = EW_n = 1.$$

The martingale convergence theorem (see, for example [5], p. 396) may now be applied to W_n to yield Corollary 2.

Unfortunately, it is possible for W to reduce to zero almost surely. For example, this is the case if the $X_{n,k}$ are independent and identically distributed with mean less than or equal to one (see [2], pp. 7–8; in this vein, also see [2], p. 14).

Now, necessary and sufficient conditions will be developed for the convergence of W_n to W in quadratic mean as $n \to \infty$. These conditions will then be easily seen to guarantee that W is not almost surely equal to zero.

Let

$$(31) \qquad \sigma_n^2 = \operatorname{Var} X_{n,1}, \qquad\qquad n = 0, 1, 2, \cdots.$$

It will be assumed from now on that $\sigma_n^2 < \infty$.

PROPOSITION 6. *The variance*

$$(32) \qquad \operatorname{Var} Z_n = \left(\prod_{j=0}^{n-1} m_j\right)^2 \sum_{k=0}^{n-1} \frac{\sigma_k^2}{m_k^2 \prod_{j=0}^{k-1} m_j}, \qquad n = 0, 1, 2, \cdots.$$

PROOF. First, formulas will be determined for the first and second derivatives $f^{n'}(s)$ and $f^{n''}(s)$, respectively, of $f^n(s)$:

$$(33) \qquad f^{n'}(s) = f^{n-1'}(f_{n-1}(s))f'_{n-1}(s),$$

$$(34) \qquad f^{n''}(s) = f^{n-1''}(f_{n-1}(s))(f'_{n-1}(s))^2 + f^{n-1'}(f_{n-1}(s))f''_{n-1}(s).$$

Now if X is a nonnegative integer valued random variable with probability generating function g,

$$(35) \qquad EX = g'(1),$$

$$(36) \qquad \operatorname{Var} X = g''(1) + g'(1) - (g'(1))^2$$

whenever the quantities on either side of these equations are finite.

Due to the finiteness of m_n and σ_n^2, it can be seen inductively that the quantities in (33) and (34) are finite. Upon substituting $s = 1$ in (34) and using (21), (35), and (36), it is seen that for $n = 1, 2, \cdots$,

$$(37) \quad \operatorname{Var} Z_n = \left(\operatorname{Var} Z_{n-1} - \prod_{j=0}^{n-2} m_j + \left(\prod_{j=0}^{n-2} m_j \right)^2 \right) m_{n-1}^2$$

$$+ (\sigma_n^2 - m_{n-1} + m_{n-1}^2) \prod_{j=0}^{n-2} m_j + \prod_{j=0}^{n-1} m_j - \left(\prod_{j=0}^{n-1} m_j \right)^2.$$

So, upon simplifying this equation,

$$(38) \qquad \operatorname{Var} Z_n = m_{n-1}^2 \operatorname{Var} (Z_{n-1}) + \sigma_{n-1}^2 \prod_{j=0}^{n-2} m_j.$$

Thus,

$$(39) \qquad \frac{\operatorname{Var} Z_n}{\prod_{j=0}^{n-1} m_j} = \frac{\operatorname{Var} Z_{n-1}}{\prod_{j=0}^{n-2} m_j} + \frac{\sigma_{n-1}^2}{m_{n-1}^2 \prod_{j=0}^{n-2} m_j}.$$

Hence, since $\operatorname{Var} Z_0 = 0$, summing both sides of this equation yields

$$(40) \qquad \frac{\operatorname{Var} Z_n}{\left(\prod_{j=0}^{n-1} m_j \right)^2} = \sum_{k=1}^{n} \frac{\sigma_k^2}{m_{k-1}^2 \prod_{j=0}^{k-2} m_j}.$$

Finally,

$$(41) \qquad \operatorname{Var} Z_n = \left(\prod_{j=0}^{n-1} m_j \right)^2 \sum_{k=0}^{n-1} \frac{\sigma_k^2}{m_k^2 \prod_{j=0}^{k-1} m_j},$$

which was to be proven.

COROLLARY 3. *The variance*

$$(42) \qquad \operatorname{Var} W_n = \sum_{k=0}^{n-1} \frac{\sigma_k^2}{m_k^2 \prod_{j=0}^{k-1} m_j}.$$

PROOF.

$$(43) \qquad \operatorname{Var} W_n = \operatorname{Var} \frac{Z_n}{\prod_{j=0}^{n-1} m_j} = \frac{\operatorname{Var} Z_n}{\left(\prod_{j=0}^{n-1} m_j \right)^2}$$

and Corollary 3 follows from Proposition 6.

LEMMA 1. *The expected squared difference*

$$(44) \qquad E((W_{n+k} - W_n)^2) = E(W_{n+k}^2) - E(W_n^2).$$

PROOF. We know

(45) $\quad E((W_{n+k} - W_n)^2) = E(W_{n+k}^2) - 2E(W_{n+k}W_n) + E(W_n^2).$

Now

(46) $\quad\quad\quad\quad E(W_{n+k}W_n) = E(E(W_{n+k}W_n|W_n)).$

So by Proposition 5 and Corollary 1,

(47) $\quad\quad\quad E(W_{n+k}W_n) = E(E(W_n^2|W_n)) = E(W_n^2).$

Thus Lemma 1 is true.

The following theorem is a consequence of Corollary 3 and Lemma 1.

THEOREM 1. *The following statements are equivalent:*

(i) W_n *converges in quadratic mean to* W*, with* $EW = 1$ *and*

(48) $$\text{Var } W = \sum_{k=0}^{\infty} \frac{\sigma_k^2}{m_k \prod_{j=0}^{k-1} m_j} < \infty ;$$

(ii)

(49) $$\lim_{n \to \infty} \text{Var } W_n = \sum_{k=0}^{\infty} \frac{\sigma_k^2}{m_k^2 \prod_{j=0}^{k-1} m_j} < \infty.$$

PROOF. Statement (i) certainly implies (ii). Assume now that (ii) is true. Then by Corollary 4 and Lemma 1, W_n converges in quadratic mean to a random variable W^* with $E(W^{*2}) < \infty$, using the L_2 completeness theorem (see, for example [5], p. 161). Thus, there is a subsequence $W_{n'}$ of W_n such that $W_{n'}$ converges almost surely to W^*. But it is known from Corollary 2 that $W_{n'}$ approaches W almost surely as $n \to \infty$. Hence, W and W^* coincide almost surely. The mean and variance of W will now be determined. By the triangle inequality,

(50) $\quad\quad EW_n - E|W_n - W| \leq EW \leq EW_n + E|W_n - W|.$

Thus, $EW = 1$, since $EW_n = 1$ for all n, and the L_2 convergence of W_n implies the L_1 convergence of W_n (see, for example [5], p. 164). By the Minkowski inequality,

(51) $\quad (\text{Var } W_n)^{1/2} + [E((W_n - W)^2)]^{1/2}$
$\quad\quad\quad\quad\quad \geq (\text{Var } W)^{1/2} \geq (\text{Var } W_n)^{1/2} - [E((W_n - W)^2)]^{1/2}.$

Notice that the finiteness of the left side for n sufficiently large follows from the facts that $\text{Var } W_n < \infty$ and $E((W_n - W)^2) \to 0$ as $n \to \infty$. Thus, it is valid to apply Minkowski's inequality for n sufficiently large. By letting $n \to \infty$ and squaring in (51), it is seen from Corollary 3 that

(52) $$\text{Var } W = \sum_{k=0}^{\infty} \frac{\sigma_k^2}{m_k^2 \prod_{j=0}^{k-1} m_j} < \infty$$

which was to be proven.

COROLLARY 4. *If* (ii) *in Theorem 1 is true, then W is not almost surely equal to zero. Moreover, if in addition, $\sigma_n^2 > 0$ for some n, then W is not a constant almost surely.*

PROOF. If (ii) is true, then $EW = 1$, so W cannot be equal to zero almost surely. If in addition $\sigma_n^2 > 0$ for some n, then Var $W > 0$, so W cannot be a constant almost surely.

4. Rate of convergence of Z_n to zero in probability when $m_n \to 1$ as $n \to \infty$

In what follows, it will be assumed that the series in (ii) of Theorem 1 diverges, that is Var $W_n \to \infty$ as $n \to \infty$. Sufficient conditions on the $f_n(s)$ will be determined to allow

$$(53) \qquad \frac{(1 - f^{n+1}(s))^{-1} - \left((1 - s) \prod_{j=0}^{n} m_j\right)^{-1}}{\text{Var } W_{n+1}} \to \frac{1}{2} \quad \text{as} \quad n \to \infty$$

uniformly in s, for $0 \leqq s < 1$.

The methods used to establish (53) will be the same as those in [2] (see pp. 20–21), except that some preliminary lemmas will be needed. Also the assumption of a third moment (that is $f_n'''(1) < \infty$) is dropped. Equation (53) is analogous to Lemma 10.1, equation 10.1 of [2] (see p. 20). Presumably, the methods in [4] (see p. 515) can also be modified to yield (53) under appropriate conditions. In [4] the condition that $f_n'''(1) < \infty$ was dropped. Under the conditions imposed on $f_n(s)$, it will then easily be seen that $P(Z_n \neq 0)$ behaves like $2/\text{Var } W_n$ as $n \to \infty$. Thus, Corollary 4 is about as good as can be expected, as far as the nondegeneracy of W is concerned.

The conditions on $f_n(s)$ are that for some $B < \infty$ and some probability generating function $f(s)$, with $f'(1) = 1$ and $f''(1) < \infty$,

(a) $B > m_n \geqq 1$ for all n, and $m_n \to 1$ as $n \to \infty$;

(b) $B > \sigma_n^2 > 1/B$ for all n, and there is a function, $O_n(s)$, bounded on $0 \leqq s \leqq 1$ uniformly in n, where

$$(54) \qquad \frac{O_n(s)}{(1 - s)^2} \to 0$$

as s increases to 1 uniformly in n, and

$$(55) \qquad 1 - f_n(s) = m_n(1 - s) - \tfrac{1}{2}f_n''(1)(1 - s)^2 + O_n(s);$$

(c) $f_n(s) \to f(s)$ as $n \to \infty$ uniformly in s; and

(d) $1 - f_n(0) \geqq 1/B$ for all n.

THEOREM 2. *If* (a), (b), (c) *and* (d) *are true, then so is* (53).

It can be seen from the proof of Theorem 2 and the proofs of the preliminary lemmas that (a) through (d) are not the only possible set of conditions needed for (53). The basic idea of these conditions is to force $f_n(s)$ to behave eventually very much like $f(s)$.

For the rest of this paper assume (a) through (d) hold and let $f^{(k)}(s)$ be the k-fold iterate of $f(s)$.

LEMMA 2. *For each n,*

(56) $$q_n = \lim_{k \to \infty} f_n^{n+k}(0)$$

exists.

PROOF. The probability that $Z_{n,k}$ is equal to zero is $f_n^{n+k}(0)$. Evidently, from the inductive definition of $Z_{n,k}$, this probability is nondecreasing as k increases. Hence, $f_n^{n+k}(0)$ is a nondecreasing sequence in k, bounded above by 1. Hence, $\lim f_n^{n+k}(0)$ exists. Notice that q_n may be interpreted as the probability that the branching process $Z_{n,k}$ dies as $k \to \infty$. None of the assumptions (a) through (d) are needed for Lemma 2. However, under these assumptions, Theorem 2 yields the fact that $q_n = 1$ for all n. Now a weaker result will be proven using (c).

LEMMA 3. *Let $\varepsilon > 0$ be given. There is an N, independent of s such that k, $n \geq N$ implies*

(57) $$0 \leq 1 - f_n^{n+k}(s) \leq \varepsilon.$$

PROOF. For all n and k,

(58) $$1 - f_n^{n+k}(0) \geq 1 - f_n^{n+k}(s) \geq 0.$$

Thus, it suffices to establish (57) when $s = 0$. Now when $j \geq k$, for all n,

(59) $$f_n^{n+j}(0) \geq f_n^{n+k}(0)$$

as was seen in the proof of Lemma 3. By Theorem 6.1 of [2] (see p. 7), choose N_1 such that

(60) $$1 - f^{(N_1)}(0) \leq \frac{\varepsilon}{2}.$$

By the uniform continuity of $f^{(j)}(s)$ for $j = 0, 1, 2, \cdots, N_1 - 1$ and $0 \leq s \leq 1$, choose $\delta_{N_1,\varepsilon} > 0$ independently of j such that $|s - t| \leq \delta_{N_1,\varepsilon}$ implies

(61) $$|f^{(j)}(s) - f^{(j)}(t)| \leq \frac{\varepsilon}{2N_1}$$

for $j = 1, 2, \cdots, N_1; 0 \leq s, t \leq 1$. Also, from (c) choose N_2 independently of s, so large that $n \geq N_2$ implies

(62) $$|f_n(s) - f(s)| < \delta_{N_1,\varepsilon}$$

for $0 \leq s \leq 1$. Then for $n \geq N_2$,

(63) $$|f_{n+j}(f_{n+j+1}^{n+N_1}(s)) - f(f_{n+j+1}^{n+N_1}(s))| \leq \delta_{N_1,\varepsilon},$$

so

(64) $$|f^{(j)}(f_{n+j}^{n+N_1}(s)) - f^{(j+1)}(f_{n+j+1}^{n+N_1}(s))| \leq \frac{\varepsilon}{2N_1}$$

for $0 \leq s \leq 1$, $0 \leq j \leq N_1 - 1$, and $n \geq N_2$. Hence, for $n \geq N_2$,

(65) $$|f_n^{n+N_1}(0) - f^{(N_1)}(0)| = \left| \sum_{j=0}^{N_1-1} f^{(j)}(f_{n+j}^{n+N_1}(0)) - f^{(j+1)}(f_{n+j+1}^{n+N_1}(0)) \right|$$

$$\leq N_1 \frac{\varepsilon}{2N_1} = \frac{\varepsilon}{2}.$$

Thus, for $n \geqq N_2$,

(66) $1 - f_n^{n+N_1}(s) \leqq 1 - f^{(N_1)}(0) + |f_n^{n+N_2}(0) - f^{(N_1)}(0)| \leqq \varepsilon.$

Let

(67) $N = \max \{N_1, N_2\}.$

From (59) and (66) with $N_1 = k, j, n \geqq N$ implies

(68) $\varepsilon \geqq 1 - f_n^{n+j}(0) \geqq 0.$

So Lemma 3 is true.

LEMMA 4.   *There is a constant d such that for all k and for $0 \leqq s < 1$,*

(69) $\dfrac{|1 - f_k(s) - m_k(1 - s)|}{m_k(1 - s)} < d < 1.$

PROOF.   We know

(70) $\dfrac{1 - f_k(s) - m_k(1 - s)}{m_k(1 - s)} = -1 + \sum_{j=1}^{\infty} \dfrac{p_{k_j}(1 - s^j)}{m_k(1 - s)},$

where

(71) $p_{k_j} = P(X_{k,1} = j).$

Thus,

(72) $\dfrac{1 - f_k(s) - m_k(1 - s)}{m_k(1 - s)} = -1 + \sum_{j=1}^{\infty} \dfrac{p_{k_j}}{m_k} \left(\sum_{\ell=0}^{j-1} s^\ell \right)$

and the left side of this equation increases to

(73) $-1 + \dfrac{m_k}{m_k} = 0$

as s increases to 1. Hence for all k and for $0 \leqq s < 1$,

(74) $0 \geqq \dfrac{1 - f_k(s) - m_k(1 - s)}{m_k(1 - s)} > -1 + \dfrac{1 - f_k(0)}{m_k} > -1 + \dfrac{1}{B^2} > -1$

by (a), (b), and (d). So Lemma 4 is true for

(75) $d = 1 - \dfrac{1}{B^2}.$

LEMMA 5.   *If $0 \leqq s < 1$, then*

(76)

$$\frac{1}{1 - f^{n+1}(s)} = \frac{1}{(1 - s) \prod\limits_{j=0}^{n} m_j} + \sum_{k=0}^{n} \frac{a_k}{m_k \prod\limits_{j=0}^{k} m_j}$$

$$- \sum_{k=0}^{n} \frac{O_k(f_{k+1}^{n+1}(s))}{(1 - f_{k+1}^{n+1}(s))^2 m_k \prod\limits_{j=0}^{k} m_j} + \sum_{k=0}^{n} \frac{d_k(f_{k+1}^{n+1}(s))}{(1 - f_{k+1}^{n+1}(s)) m_k \prod\limits_{j=0}^{k} m_j},$$

where $a_k = f_k''(1)/2$; $d_k(s)$ is bounded uniformly in k for $0 \leqq s < 1$,

(77)
$$\frac{d_k(s)}{1-s} \to 0$$

as s increases to 1, uniformly in k, and $O_k(s)$ is as described in (b).

PROOF. By (b),

(78)
$$1 - f_k(s) = m_k(1-s) - a_k(1-s)^2 + O_k(s).$$

Thus,

(79)
$$\frac{1}{1-f_k(s)} = \left[m_k(1-s)\left(1 - \frac{a_k(1-s)}{m_k} - \frac{O_k(s)}{m_k(1-s)}\right)\right]^{-1}.$$

Or, for $0 \leq s < 1$,

(80)
$$\frac{1}{1-f_k(s)} = \frac{1 + \dfrac{a_k(1-s)}{m_k} - \dfrac{O_k(s)}{m_k(1-s)}}{m_k(1-s)} + \frac{\dfrac{d_k s}{m_k}}{m_k(1-s)},$$

where $d_k(s)$ has, as shall be seen, the required properties. Equation (80) holds since for all k,

(81)
$$\frac{\left| \dfrac{a_k(1-s)}{m_k} - O_k(s)\right|}{m_k(1-s)} = \frac{1 - f_k(s) - m_k(1-s)}{m_k(1-s)} < d < 1$$

for $0 \leq s < 1$, by Lemma 4. (Here $O_k(s)$ is as described in (b).) To see that $d_k(s)$ has the required properties, notice that

(82)
$$\frac{d_k(s)}{m_k} = \sum_{j=2}^{\infty} u^j = \frac{u^2}{1-u},$$

where

(83)
$$u = \frac{a_k(1-s)}{m_k} - \frac{O_k(s)}{m_k(1-s)} = -\frac{1-f_k(s) - m_k(1-s)}{m_k(1-s)} \geq 0.$$

Thus, for $0 \leq s < 1$,

(84)
$$\frac{d_k(s)}{1-s} \leq \frac{m_k\left(\dfrac{a_k(1-s)}{m_k} - \dfrac{O_k(s)}{m_k(1-s)}\right)^2}{(1-d)(1-s)}$$

by Lemma 4. The right side approaches zero uniformly in k as s increases to one, by (a) and (b). Moreover, these assumptions also allow the right side to be bounded uniformly for $0 \leq s < 1$ and all k.

Now, multiply both sides of (80) by $1/(\prod_{j=0}^{k-1} m_j)$, plug in $f_{k+1}^{n+1}(s)$ for s, then add the resulting equation for $k = 0, 1, 2, \cdots, n$. After cancellation, it is seen that Lemma 5 is true.

LEMMA 6. *Let A_n be the second term on the right side of* (76). *Then*

(85)
$$\frac{A_n}{\operatorname{Var} W_{n+1}} \to \frac{1}{2} \quad \text{as} \quad n \to \infty.$$

PROOF. By Corollary 3,

$$(86) \qquad \frac{A_n}{\operatorname{Var} W_{n+1}} = \frac{\operatorname{Var} W_{n+1}}{2 \operatorname{Var} W_{n+1}} + \frac{\sum_{k=0}^{n} \dfrac{m_k^2 - m_k}{m_k \prod\limits_{j=0}^{k} m_j}}{2 \operatorname{Var} W_{n+1}};$$

and the second term approaches zero as $n \to \infty$ by a special case of the Toeplitz lemma (see, for example [5], p. 238), since $\operatorname{Var} W_n \to \infty$,

$$(87) \qquad B \sum_{k=0}^{n} \left(m_k \prod_{j=0}^{k} m_j \right)^{-1} \geqq \operatorname{Var} W_{n+1} \geqq \frac{1}{B} \sum_{k=0}^{n} \left(m_k \prod_{j=0}^{k} m_j \right)^{-1}$$

by Corollary 4 and (b), and $m_k \to 1$ as $k \to \infty$ by (a). Hence, Lemma 6 holds.

LEMMA 7. *Let*

$$(88) \qquad D_n(s) = \sum_{k=0}^{n} \frac{O_k(f_{k+1}^{n+1}(s))}{m_k \prod\limits_{j=0}^{k} m_j (1 - f_{k+1}^{n+1}(s))^2} - \frac{d_k(f_{k+1}^{n+1}(s))}{1 - f_{k+1}^{n+1}(s)}.$$

Then

$$(89) \qquad \frac{D_n(s)}{\operatorname{Var} W_{n+1}} \to 0 \quad as \quad n \to \infty$$

uniformly in s, for $0 \leqq s < 1$.

PROOF. Let $\delta > 0$ be given. Choose $\varepsilon > 0$ so that $0 < 1 - s < \varepsilon$ implies

$$(90) \qquad \left| \frac{O_k(s)}{(1 - s)^2} - \frac{d_k(s)}{1 - s} \right| < \delta$$

for all k. Let N be chosen as in Lemma 3. Let $B_1 < \infty$ be an upper bound for the quantity on the left side of (90). Then, for $0 \leqq s < 1$,

$$(91) \qquad |D_n(s)| \leqq \sum_{k=0}^{N} \frac{B_1}{m_k \prod\limits_{j=0}^{k} m_j} + \sum_{k=N+1}^{n-N} \frac{\delta}{m_k \prod\limits_{j=0}^{k} m_j} + \sum_{k=n-N+1}^{n} \frac{B_1}{m_k \prod\limits_{j=0}^{k} m_j}$$

for $n \geqq 2N$. The truth of Lemma 7 now follows by dividing both sides of this inequality by $\operatorname{Var} W_{n+1}$ and letting $n \to \infty$, since $\delta > 0$ was arbitrary.

From Lemmas 5, 6, and 7, it is clear that Theorem 2 is true.

COROLLARY 5. *Under the hypotheses of Theorem 2,*

$$(92) \qquad P(Z_n \neq 0) \operatorname{Var} W_n \to 2 \quad as \quad n \to \infty,$$

$$(93) \qquad Z_n \to 0 \quad almost \ surely \ as \quad n \to \infty,$$

and $W = 0$ almost surely.

PROOF. The result (92) follows immediately from (53), upon plugging in $s = 0$. Also for every k,

$$(94) \qquad P(Z_n \to 0 \ as \ n \to \infty) \geqq P(Z_k = 0) = 1 - P(Z_k \neq 0).$$

So (93) follows from (92), since $\operatorname{Var} W_n \to \infty$ as $n \to \infty$. Also, for each k,

$$(95) \qquad P(W = 0) \geq P(Z_k = 0) = 1 - P(Z_k \neq 0),$$

so using (92) as before, $P(W = 0) = 1$.

EXAMPLE. The geometric probability generating functions

$$(96) \qquad f_{n-1}(s) = \frac{\dfrac{n}{2n+1}}{1 - \dfrac{n+1}{2n+1}\, s}, \qquad n = 1, 2, \cdots,$$

provide an example where $1 - f^n(0)$ can be computed explicitly. Assume $X_{n,1}$ has the probability generating function $f_n(s)$. Then for $n = 1, 2, \cdots$

$$(97) \qquad m_{n-1} = \frac{n+1}{n}$$

and

$$(98) \qquad \sigma_{n-1}^2 = \frac{(2n+1)(n+1)}{n^2}.$$

From [7] (see pp. 46–47), after some calculations, it can be seen that

$$(99) \qquad f^n(0) = 1 - \left(1 + \sum_{k=1}^{n} \frac{1}{\prod\limits_{j=0}^{k-1} m_j}\right)^{-1} = 1 - \left(1 + \sum_{k=1}^{n} \frac{1}{k+1}\right)^{-1}$$

for $n = 1, 2, \cdots$. Also,

$$(100) \qquad \mathrm{Var}\, W_n = \sum_{k=0}^{n-1} \frac{\sigma_k^2}{m_k^2 \prod\limits_{j=0}^{k-1} m_j} = \sum_{k=0}^{n-1} \frac{\dfrac{(2k+1)(k+1)}{k^2}}{\left(\dfrac{k+1}{k}\right)^2 k}$$

$$= \sum_{k=0}^{n-1} \frac{2k+1}{k(k+1)} = \sum_{k=1}^{n} \frac{2}{k+1} + \sum_{k=1}^{n} \frac{1}{k(k+1)}.$$

Hence, $(1 - f^n(0))\, \mathrm{Var}\, W_n \to 2$, confirming (92).

From the proof of Lemma 5, it seems as though the behavior of iterates of geometric probability generating functions really ought to determine the behavior of iterates of wide classes of probability generating functions. This suggests that the theory in [7] might play a role in proving theorems like Theorem 2. It should be pointed out that the importance of the geometric probability generating functions was also noticed in [4] (see p. 515).

It is anticipated that results concerning the limiting behavior of Z_n, given that Z_n does not approach zero as $n \to \infty$, may be determined by methods in [2] or [4]. Reference [6] also contains a good survey of these methods.

REFERENCES

[1] D. H. FEARN, "Branching processes with generation dependent birth distributions," Ph.D. thesis, University of California, Davis, 1971.
[2] T. E. HARRIS, *The Theory of Branching Processes*, Englewood Cliffs, Prentice-Hall, 1963.
[3] S. KARLIN, *A First Course in Stochastic Processes*, New York, Academic Press, 1966.

[4] H. KESTEN, P. NEY, and F. SPITZER, "Galton-Watson processes with mean one and finite variance," *Theor. Probability Appl.*, Vol. 13 (1966), pp. 513–540.
[5] M. LOÈVE, *Probability Theory*, New York, Van Nostrand, 1963 (3rd ed.).
[6] E. SENETA, "Functional equations and the Galton-Watson process," *Advances Appl. Probability*, Vol. 1 (1969), pp. 1–42.
[7] H. S. WALL, *Analytic Theory of Continued Fractions*, New York, Van Nostrand, 1948.

MARKOV CHAIN CLUSTERING
OF BIRTHS BY SEX

JEROME KLOTZ

UNIVERSITY OF WISCONSIN, MADISON

1. Introduction and summary

This paper is concerned with a simple generalization of the Bernoulli trials model to a Markov chain which has an additional parameter that measures dependence between trials. Small and large sample distribution theories are worked out for the model with a new and simple closed form expression obtained for the exact distribution of the sufficient statistics.

The model is applied to a sample of birth order data from an appropriate human population and a slight dependence of sex on that of the previous child is found to be significant.

2. Notation and model

In the Bernoulli model, denote two valued random variables by $X_i = 1$ with probability p and 0 with probability $q = 1 - p$, for $i = 1, 2, \cdots, n$. The joint distribution for a sequence of independent trials is given by

$$(2.1) \qquad P[X_1 = x_1, X_2 = x_2, \cdots, X_n = x_n] = p^s q^{n-s},$$

where $s = x_1 + x_2 + \cdots + x_n$ and $x_i = 1$ or 0. To generalize this model to permit dependence between successive trials, consider a Markov chain with symmetric conditional probabilities given by

$$(2.2) \qquad P[X_i = 1 | X_{i-1} = 1] = P[X_i = 1 | X_{i+1} = 1] = \theta p,$$

with the remaining conditional probabilities completely determined by symmetry:

$$(2.3) \qquad P[X_i = 0 | X_{i\pm 1} = 1] = 1 - \theta p,$$

$$(2.4) \qquad P[X_i = 1 | X_{i\pm 1} = 0] = \frac{P[X_i = 1, X_{i\pm 1} = 0]}{P[X_{i\pm 1} = 0]} = \frac{(1 - \theta p)p}{q},$$

$$(2.5) \qquad P[X_i = 0 | X_{i\pm 1} = 0] = 1 - \frac{(1 - \theta p)p}{q} = \frac{1 - 2p + \theta p^2}{q},$$

and unconditionally

$$(2.6) \qquad P[X_i = 1] = 1 - P[X_i = 0] = p.$$

With the partial support of the National Institutes of Health PHS. Research Grant GM-10525-08 and the National Science Foundation under Grant GP-12093.

The parameter θ is a measure of dependence. The value $\theta = 1$ gives the Bernoulli model (2.1) and independence, while values of $\theta > 1$ ($\theta < 1$) imply a tendency for pairwise clustering of like (unlike) values in the sequence of random variables. In order to avoid negative conditional probabilities (2.2) through (2.5), we restrict θ to the range $\max (0, (2p - 1)/p^2) \leqq \theta \leqq 1/p$ which contains the value 1.

The joint distribution of a sequence can be written

$$
(2.7) \quad P[X_1 = x_1, X_2 = x_2, \cdots, X_n = x_n]
$$
$$
= P[X_n = x_n | X_{n-1} = x_{n-1}, X_{n-2} = x_{n-2}, \cdots, X_1 = x_1]
$$
$$
P[X_{n-1} = x_{n-1}, X_{n-2} = x_{n-2}, \cdots, X_1 = x_1]
$$
$$
= P[X_n = x_n | X_{n-1} = x_{n-1}] P[X_{n-1} = x_{n-1} | X_{n-2} = x_{n-2}]
$$
$$
\cdots P[X_2 = x_2 | X_1 = x_1] P[X_1 = x_1],
$$

repeatedly using the Markov dependence assumption. Using (2.2) through (2.6) and $x_i = 1$ or 0, we can write

$$
(2.8) \quad P[X_i = x_i | X_{i-1} = x_{i-1}]
$$
$$
= (\theta p)^{x_i x_{i-1}} (1 - \theta p)^{(1-x_i)x_{i-1}} \left[\frac{(1 - \theta p) p}{q} \right]^{x_i(1-x_{i-1})} \left[\frac{1 - 2p + \theta p^2}{q} \right]^{(1-x_i)(1-x_{i-1})},
$$
$$
(2.9) \quad\quad\quad\quad\quad P[X_1 = x_1] = p^{x_1} q^{1-x_1}.
$$

Substituting (2.8) and (2.9) into (2.7), the joint distribution becomes the product

$$
(2.10) \quad \left\{ \prod_{i=2}^{n} (\theta p)^{x_i x_{i-1}} (1 - \theta p)^{(1-x_i)x_{i-1}} \left[\frac{(1 - \theta p)p}{q} \right]^{x_i(1-x_{i-1})} \right.
$$
$$
\left. \left[\frac{1 - 2p + \theta p^2}{q} \right]^{(1-x_i)(1-x_{i-1})} \right\} p^{x_1} q^{1-x_1}
$$
$$
= \theta^{n_{11}} (1 - \theta p)^{(n_{01}+n_{10})} (1 - 2p + \theta p^2)^{n_{00}} p^{\sum_{i=1}^{n} x_i} q^{-\sum_{i=2}^{n-1} (1-x_i)},
$$

where

$$
n_{11} = \sum_{i=2}^{n} x_i x_{i-1} = \sum_{i=1}^{n-1} x_i x_{i+1},
$$
$$
n_{01} = \sum_{i=1}^{n-1} (1 - x_i) x_{i+1},
$$
$$
(2.11)
$$
$$
n_{10} = \sum_{i=1}^{n-1} x_i (1 - x_{i+1}),
$$
$$
n_{00} = \sum_{i=1}^{n-1} (1 - x_i)(1 - x_{i+1}),
$$

so that $n_{11} + n_{01} + n_{10} + n_{00} = n - 1$.

In this paper attention is restricted to inference on θ and it is assumed that p is known. The case where p is an unknown nuisance parameter is of interest but somewhat more complicated and will not be considered here.

3. Large sample theory

The model (2.10) is a particular case of the general Markov processes discussed by Billingsley [1], and the large sample theory developed there can be applied directly. Expression (2.8) corresponds to the notation $f(X_{i-1}, X_i; \theta)$ in [1]. If terms not depending on θ are neglected, the log likelihood (the log of (2.10)) can be written

$$(3.1) \quad L_n(\theta) = n_{11} \log \theta + (n_{01} + n_{10}) \log (1 - \theta p) + n_{00} \log (1 - 2p + \theta p^2).$$

The term $f(X_1, \theta)$ of [1] corresponds to (2.9) for the model and does not depend on θ. Thus, the exact likelihood (3.1) and the large sample approximate likelihood used by Billingsley are equivalent. Theorems (2.1) and (2.2) of [1] give the following.

THEOREM 1. *If θ is restricted to an open interval, there exists a sequence of estimators $\hat{\theta}(X_1, X_2, \cdots, X_n)$ which converge in probability to θ. The sequence $\hat{\theta}(X_1, X_2, \cdots, X_n)$ is a solution of*

$$(3.2) \quad \frac{dL_n(\theta)}{d\theta} = \frac{n_{11}}{\theta} - \frac{(n_{01} + n_{10})p}{(1 - \theta p)} + \frac{n_{00}p^2}{(1 - 2p + \theta p^2)} = 0,$$

with probability going to one as $n \to \infty$. Further, the asymptotic distribution of $\sqrt{n}(\hat{\theta} - \theta)$ is normal $N(0, \tau^2(\theta))$, where

$$(3.3) \quad \tau^2(\theta) = \frac{\theta(1 - \theta p)(1 - 2p + \theta p^2)}{p^2(1 - 2p + \theta p)}.$$

For testing the hypothesis $H:\theta = \theta_0$ against the alternative $A:\theta \neq \theta_0$, the log likelihood ratio test statistic has an asymptotic chi square distribution (1 degree of freedom):

$$(3.4) \quad 2[L_n(\hat{\theta}) - L_n(\theta)] \xrightarrow{\mathcal{L}} \chi_1^2$$

as $n \to \infty$ under H.

A large sample confidence interval for θ can be obtained by using (3.4). If $\chi_{1,\alpha}^2$ is the upper 100α per cent critical value of the chi square distribution (1 degree of freedom), then the set of θ values which satisfy

$$(3.5) \quad 2[L_n(\hat{\theta}) - L_n(\theta)] \leq \chi_{1,\alpha}^2$$

is a confidence interval for θ with confidence coefficient approaching $1 - \alpha$ as $n \to \infty$. It is an interval since $L_n(\theta)$ is concave ($L_n''(\theta) < 0$).

4. The exact distribution of the sufficient statistics

The joint distribution (2.10) can be rewritten in the form

$$(4.1) \quad \frac{(1 - 2p + \theta p^2)^{n-1}}{q^{n-2}} \left[\frac{\theta(1 - 2p + \theta p^2)}{(1 - \theta p)^2} \right]^{\sum_{i=1}^{n-1} x_i x_{i+1}}$$

$$\left[\frac{pq(1 - \theta p)^2}{(1 - 2p + \theta p^2)^2} \right]^{\sum_{i=1}^{n} x_i} \left[\frac{1 - 2p + \theta p^2}{(1 - \theta p)q} \right]^{x_1 + x_n}.$$

Denote $R = \sum_{i=1}^{n-1} X_i X_{i+1}$, $S = \sum_{i=1}^{n} X_i$, and $T = X_1 + X_n$. By the factorization theorem they are sufficient although not minimal since $N_{11} = R$ and

$$(4.2) \quad (N_{01} + N_{10}) = \sum_{i=1}^{n-1} X_{i+1}(1 - X_i) + X_i(1 - X_{i+1}) = 2(S - R) - T$$

are also sufficient, which can be seen from the likelihood expression (2.10) using $N_{00} = (n - 1) - N_{11} - (N_{01} + N_{10})$. However, the joint distribution of (R, S, T) seems easier to derive than that of $(N_{11}, N_{01} + N_{10})$.

Since the joint distribution (4.1) of $X_1, X_2, \cdots, X_n$ is constant for fixed values of R, S, and T, using (4.1), it follows that

$$(4.3) \qquad P[R = r, S = s, T = t] = M_n(r, s, t) C_{1n} \eta_1^r \eta_2^s \eta_3^t,$$

where

$$(4.4) \qquad C_{1n} = \frac{(1 - 2p + \theta p^2)^{n-1}}{q^{n-2}}, \qquad \eta_1 = \frac{\theta(1 - 2p + \theta p^2)}{(1 - \theta p)^2},$$

$$\eta_2 = \frac{pq(1 - \theta p)^2}{(1 - 2p + \theta p^2)^2}, \qquad \eta_3 = \frac{(1 - 2p + \theta p^2)}{(1 - \theta p)q},$$

and $M_n(r, s, t)$ is the number of sequences $(x_1, x_2, \cdots, x_n)$ of zeros and ones which have $\sum_{i=1}^{n-1} x_i x_{i+1} = r$, $\sum_{i=1}^{n} x_i = s$, and $x_1 + x_n = t$.

To count the number of such sequences for given (r, s, t), first note that there are $\binom{2}{t}$ different ways of getting a sum of t from $x_1 + x_n$. Next, since $\sum_{i=1}^{n} x_i = s$, there are a total of s ones in the sequence. If we count the number z of zero runs between the first and the last of these ones in the sequence, we have the relationship

$$(4.5) \qquad\qquad r = s - 1 - z.$$

The reason for this is that every time a run of zeros is inserted between consecutive ones, the value of R is decreased by one. The number of ways of putting $n - s$ zeros into $z + (2 - t)$ cells of zero runs where $z = s - 1 - r$ (from 4.5) and no cell is empty is given by

$$(4.6) \qquad\qquad \binom{n - s - 1}{z + (2 - t) - 1} = \binom{n - s - 1}{s - r - t}$$

(see, for example, Feller [5], p. 37). We define throughout $\binom{-1}{-1} = 1$, as is required for the special case $s = n$. Finally, the number of ways of inserting s ones into $z + 1$ cells of ones (where the cells of ones are separated by the z zero runs between the first and last ones) with no cell empty is given by

$$(4.7) \qquad\qquad \binom{s - 1}{z + 1 - 1} = \binom{s - 1}{s - 1 - r} = \binom{s - 1}{r},$$

again using Feller [5], p. 37, and (4.5). Thus, the total number of ways that these three conditions can hold (and which must hold so that $R = r$, $S = s$, and

$T = t$) is the product of

(4.8)
$$M_n(r, s, t) = \binom{2}{t}\binom{n - s - 1}{s - r - t}\binom{s - 1}{r}.$$

Summarizing, we have proved the following.

THEOREM 2. *If* $X_1, X_2, \cdots, X_n$ *is a Markov chain satisfying* (2.2) *through* (2.6), *then the sufficient statistics* $R, S,$ *and* T *have joint distribution given by*

(4.9)
$$P[R = r, S = s, T = t] = \binom{2}{t}\binom{n - s - 1}{s - r - t}\binom{s - 1}{r} C_{1n}\eta_1^r\eta_2^s\eta_3^t,$$

where $C_{1n}, \eta_1, \eta_2,$ *and* η_3 *are given by* (4.4).

Using (4.9), the joint distribution of $N_{11} = R$ and $N_{01} + N_{10} = 2(S - R) - T$ can be derived since

(4.10)
$$P[N_{11} = r, (N_{01} + N_{10}) = w] = \sum_t P[R = r, 2(S - R) - T = w, T = t]$$
$$= \sum_t P[R = r, S = r + \tfrac{1}{2}(w + t), T = t].$$

For even values $w = 2u,$

(4.11) $P[N_{11} = r, (N_{01} + N_{10}) = 2u]$
$$= P[R = r, S = r + u, T = 0] + P[R = r, S = r + u + 1, T = 2]$$
$$= \binom{r + u - 1}{r}\binom{n - r - u - 1}{u} C_{1n}\eta_1^r\eta_2^{r+u}$$
$$+ \binom{r + u}{r}\binom{n - r - u - 2}{u - 1} C_{1n}\eta_1^r\eta_2^{r+u+1}\eta_3^2$$
$$= C_{1n}(\eta_1\eta_2)^r\eta_2^u\left[\binom{r + u - 1}{r}\binom{n - r - u - 1}{u}\right.$$
$$\left. + \binom{r + u}{u}\binom{n - r - u - 2}{u - 1}\frac{p}{q}\right].$$

For odd values $w = 2u + 1,$ similarly,

(4.12) $P[N_{11} = r, N_{01} + N_{10} = 2u + 1]$
$$= P[R = r, S = r + u + 1, T = 1]$$
$$= 2\binom{r + u}{r}\binom{n - r - u - 2}{u} C_{1n}(\eta_1\eta_2)^r\eta_2^u\eta_2\eta_3.$$

5. The exact maximum of the likelihood

For maximizing the likelihood, consider the derivative equation $L_n'(\theta) = 0$ given by (3.2). This equation leads to a quadratic equation and we prove that the solution with the positive square root term maximizes the likelihood in all cases.

THEOREM 3. *The maximum likelihood estimator of θ is given by*

$$(5.1) \quad \hat{\theta}_+(n_{11}, (n_{01} + n_{10})) = \frac{1}{2}\left[\left\{\frac{2n_{11} + (n_{01} + n_{10}) + m}{mp} - \frac{(n_{11} + n_{10} + n_{01})}{mp^2}\right\}\right.$$

$$\left. + \left(\left\{\frac{2n_{11} + (n_{01} + n_{10}) + m}{mp} - \frac{(n_{11} + n_{01} + n_{10})}{mp^2}\right\}^2 + \frac{4n_{11}(1 - 2p)}{mp^3}\right)^{1/2}\right],$$

where $m = n - 1$.

PROOF. See the Appendix.

For the special case of $p = \frac{1}{2}$, (5.1) reduces to $\hat{\theta}_+ = 2[1 - ((n_{01} + n_{10})/m)]$.

6. Large sample distributions and small sample comparisons

Using (4.9) and writing $X = (R - (n - 1)\theta p^2)/\sqrt{n}$, $Y = (S - np)/\sqrt{n}$, it can be shown that the limiting distribution of (X, Y) and T is that of a bivariate normal $N((0, 0), \Sigma)$ and an independent binomial $B(2, p)$, where the asymptotic variance covariance matrix of X and Y is

$$(6.1) \quad \Sigma = \begin{pmatrix} 4\theta p^3 q + \dfrac{\theta p^2(1 - 2p + \theta p)(1 - 2p + \theta p^2)}{1 - \theta p} & \dfrac{2\theta p^2 q^2}{1 - \theta p} \\ \dfrac{2\theta p^2 q^2}{1 - \theta p} & \dfrac{pq(1 - 2p + \theta p)}{1 - \theta p} \end{pmatrix}.$$

This result, which should take no longer than a day to verify, was obtained by writing out the factorials in the binomial coefficients in (4.9), using Stirling's approximation and a log expansion, and taking the limit as $n \to \infty$.

Because of its greater simplicity, one is tempted to use the estimator of θ given by $R/[(n - 1)p^2]$, which is unbiased. However, from the asymptotic variance of X, we note for max $\{0, (2p - 1)/p^2\} < \theta < 1/p, 0 < p < 1$,

$$(6.2) \quad \lim_{n \to \infty} n \operatorname{Var}\left[\frac{R}{(n - 1)p^2}\right]$$

$$= \frac{1}{p^4}\left[4\theta p^2 q + \frac{\theta p^2(1 - 2p + \theta p)(1 - 2p + \theta p^2)}{1 - \theta p}\right]$$

$$> \frac{\theta(1 - \theta p)(1 - 2p + \theta p^2)}{p^2(1 - 2p + \theta p)} = \tau^2(\theta) = \lim_{n \to \infty} nE(\hat{\theta}_+ - \theta)^2.$$

For small sample comparisons, because of the complexity of $\hat{\theta}_+$ and the distribution (4.9), it seems unlikely that there exists a computationally convenient closed form expression for its mean and variance except for $p = \frac{1}{2}, \theta = 1$. In this exceptional case, $\hat{\theta}_+ = 2[1 - ((N_{01} + N_{10})/(n - 1))]$ and it can be shown, summing (4.11) and (4.12), that

$$(6.3) \qquad\qquad P[(N_{01} + N_{10}) = w] = \binom{n - 1}{w}\frac{1}{2^{n-1}},$$

so that $E\theta_+ = 1$, $\text{Var } \theta_+ = 1/(n - 1)$, and $n \text{ Var } \theta_+/\tau^2 = n/(n - 1)$. Also for $\theta = 1$ but $0 < p < 1$, we can calculate

$$(6.4) \qquad \frac{1}{n} \text{Var } R < p^2 q(1 + 3p)\left[1 - \frac{(1 + 5p)}{n(1 + 3p)}\right],$$

which has the extra factor $[1 - (1 + 5p)/(n(1 + 3p))]$ compared with the asymptotic value $p^2 q(1 + 3p)$ obtained from Σ. Although the maximum likelihood estimator is still preferred, the finite sample ratio of its variance or mean squared error to that of the unbiased is smaller than the asymptotic ratio for these cases.

For the general case, expectations and variances were numerically computed, in a metallurgical application of the model [8], by Dr. Charles A. Johnson at Argonne Laboratories and are reproduced in Table I. The computations were performed using (4.9) and so forth. For example,

$$(6.5) \qquad E\hat{\theta}_+ = \sum_r \sum_w \hat{\theta}_+(r, w)p[N_{11} = r, (N_{01} + N_{10}) = w],$$

with similar expressions for the variances. Table I gives $E\hat{\theta}_+$ and $\text{Var } \hat{\theta}_+$ for selected combinations of n, θ, p, and compares them with the asymptotic values θ and $\tau^2(\theta)$. It is interesting to note the oscillatory behavior of both $E\hat{\theta}_+$ and $\text{Var } \hat{\theta}_+$ and the size of the samples for good asymptotic approximation.

TABLE I

FINITE SAMPLE MEANS AND VARIANCES OF $\hat{\theta}_+$ AND COMPARISON
WITH THE ASYMPTOTIC APPROXIMATIONS θ, $\tau^2(\theta)$

p	θ	$\tau^2(\theta)$	n	$E\hat{\theta}_+$	$100(E\hat{\theta}_+ - \theta)/\theta$	$n \text{ Var } \hat{\theta}_+$	$100[n \text{ Var } \hat{\theta}_+ - \tau^2]/n \text{ Var } \hat{\theta}_+$
0.5	1.0	1.0	10	1.000	0.0%	1.111	10.0%
			40	1.000	0.0	1.026	2.5
			100	1.000	0.0	1.010	1.0
0.1	5.0	163.5	10	1.221	−75.6	197.1	17.1
			40	4.173	−16.5	252.6	35.3
			100	4.995	−0.1	205.5	20.5
			200	5.007	0.1	181.5	9.9
			500	4.999	0.0	169.8	3.8
			1000	4.996	−0.1	166.5	1.8
0.06	2.0	433.7	10	.360	−87.0	1230.0	64.7
			40	1.861	−7.0	1082.0	59.9
			100	2.192	9.6	736.3	41.1
			200	2.019	1.0	591.6	26.7
			500	1.997	−0.1	493.4	12.1
			1000	1.999	0.0	458.7	5.5
0.06	10.0	687.7	10	1.363	−86.4	4513.	84.8
			40	5.002	−50.0	1140.	39.6
			100	8.961	−10.4	1008.	31.8
			200	9.964	−0.4	843.	18.4
			500	10.008	0.0	741.	7.2
			1000	10.000	0.0	713.	3.5

7. Distribution theory for independent samples

When several independent, identically distributed samples are combined, the distribution theory is modified slightly. Denote each sample size by N_k, the corresponding individual sufficient statistics by (R_k, S_k, T_k) or N_{11k} and so forth, for $k = 1, 2, \cdots, K$, where K is the total number of samples to be combined. Using the factorization theorem on the combined joint distribution of (R_k, S_k, T_k), $k = 1, 2, \cdots, K$, or on N_{11k}, $(N_{01k} + N_{10k})$, $k = 1, 2, \cdots, K$, we have $R = \sum_{k=1}^{K} R_k$, $S = \sum_{k=1}^{K} S_k$, $T = \sum_{k=1}^{K} T_k$, are sufficient or, more minimally $N_{11} = \sum_k N_{11k} = R$, $(N_{01} + N_{10}) = \sum_k (N_{01k} + N_{10k}) = 2(S - R) - T$ are sufficient. We have the following.

THEOREM 4. *If (R_k, S_k, T_k) are independent for $k = 1, 2, \cdots, K$, then the joint distribution of R, S, T is given by*

$$(7.1) \quad P[R = r, S = s, T = t] = \binom{2K}{t}\binom{n - s - K}{s - r - t}\binom{s - K}{r} C_{Kn}\eta_1^r\eta_2^s\eta_3^t,$$

where $C_{Kn} = (1 - 2p + \theta p^2)^{n-K}/q^{n-2K}$, $n = \sum_k n_k$, and η_1, η_2, η_3 are given by (4.4).

PROOF. We can prove (7.1) by induction on K. For $K = 1$, (7.1) reduces to (4.9). For $K + 1$, we compute the joint distribution by convoluting (7.1) and (4.9):

$$(7.2) \quad \sum_{r_{K+1}=0}^{r} \sum_{s_{K+1}=0}^{s} \sum_{t_{K+1}=0}^{t}$$

$$\binom{2K}{t - t_{K+1}}\binom{n - n_{K+1} - (s - s_{K+1}) - K}{s - s_{K+1} - (r - r_{K+1}) - (t - t_{K+1})}\binom{s - s_{K+1} - K}{r - r_{K+1}}$$

$$\times \eta_1^{r-r_{K+1}}\eta_2^{s-s_{K+1}}\eta_3^{t-t_{K+1}}C_{Kn-n_{K+1}}$$

$$\times \binom{2}{t_{K+1}}\binom{n_{K+1} - s_{K+1} - 1}{s_{K+1} - r_{K+1} - t_{K+1}}\binom{s_{K+1} - 1}{r_{K+1}} \eta_1^{r_{K+1}}\eta_2^{s_{K+1}}\eta_3^{t_{K+1}}C_{1n_{K+1}}$$

$$= \binom{2(K + 1)}{t}\binom{n - s - (K + 1)}{s - r - t}\binom{s - (K + 1)}{r} C_{K+1n}\eta_1^r\eta_2^s\eta_3^t,$$

provided the combinatorial identity can be shown for the sums of the products of the binomial coefficients. To do this use the following three identities:

$$(7.3) \quad \sum_{t_{K+1}=0}^{t} \binom{2K}{t - t_{K+1}}\binom{2}{t_K} = \binom{2(K + 1)}{t},$$

$$(7.4) \quad \sum_{r_{K+1}=0}^{r} \binom{s - s_{K+1} - K}{r - r_{K+1}}\binom{s_{K+1} - 1}{r_{K+1}} = \binom{s - (K + 1)}{r},$$

$$(7.5) \quad \sum_{s_{K+1}=0}^{s} \binom{n - n_{K+1} - (s - s_{K+1}) - K}{s - s_{K+1} - (r - r_{K+1}) - (t - t_{K+1})}\binom{n_{K+1} - s_{K+1} - 1}{s_{K+1} - r_{K+1} - t_{K+1}}$$

$$= \binom{n - s - (K + 1)}{s - r - t}.$$

Both (7.3) and (7.4) hold since the hypergeometric distribution sums to one and (7.5) can be proved by induction on s. Note that (7.4) holds for any s_{K+1} and

(7.5) holds for any r_{K+1}, t_{K+1}. Taking the products of (7.3), (7.4), and (7.5) and using the above remark for appropriate orders of summation gives the required result.

The distribution of the more minimal sufficient statistics N_{11}, $(N_{01} + N_{10})$ can be obtained using (4.10) and (7.1).

The maximum likelihood estimate $\hat{\theta}_+$ is similarly given by (5.1) except that $m = n - K$ in the formula, since now $N_{00} + N_{01} + N_{10} + N_{11} = n - K$.

For independent samples, Theorem 1 is modified slightly to read:

$$(7.6) \qquad \sqrt{n}(\hat{\theta} - \theta) \xrightarrow{\mathcal{L}} N(0, \gamma\tau^2(\theta))$$

as $n \to \infty$, where $\gamma = \lim [n/(n - K)]$. The proof follows Billingsley [1] (p. 14) with $r = 1$ and g replaced by a $g^{(k)}$, which is the sum of the log of (2.8) over the kth sample sequence. A law of large numbers for independent nonidentical random variables and a similar central limit theorem is combined with the martingale argument there.

8. An application to birth order data

To apply the model and investigate possible Markov dependence of sex between successive births, appropriate family data was sought. Data was required from families not practicing family limitation by sex so that the fixed sample analysis of the model would be appropriate instead of complicated mixtures of inverse sampling schemes. Family limitation is a common difficulty in sex ratio studies [10] (p. 175), [3], [7].

A geneology of Amish families [6] appears to provide appropriate data. Birth control was considered sinful and the prescript "be fruitful and multiply" was followed [4]. The only type of limitation that might have been practiced was that of limiting the total number once the family size was considered enough. The data also support these considerations since, according to Edwards [3] (p. 343), families practicing limitation by sex composition would have an increased number of girl-boy or boy-girl outcomes in the last two children and the count of such sequences is 86 out of the 195 families in the sample.

Table II gives the coded sex composition in order of birth for selected Amish families. Families were chosen from Old Order Amish or Amish Mennonite parents born before or up to 1900–1910 and who were mostly farmers or carpenters. Families with multiple births were eliminated. To conserve space in the table, the girl and boy family sequence is considered as a binary number with girls corresponding to ones and boys to zeros, a leading one is placed at the front of the sequence and then the resulting sequence converted to the corresponding octal number code. Thus, for example, ggb, gbg, bbg, ggg, bbg is coded 165171. The leading one is used to denote the start of the sequence so that zero sequences of different length are not confused.

In the application of the model, we assume that data from different families are independent and identically distributed and that p and θ do not differ be-

TABLE II

OCTAL CODED BIRTH ORDER DATA FOR 195 AMISH FAMILIES
Convert the octal number to binary, drop the leading one, and associate
girls with ones and boys with zeros in the resulting sequence.

17	336	7443	106	240	42
167	235	264	63	6	4
203	17	16	75	24	1137
24	115	54	13726	2153	3004
21	11117	1670	760	35	237
342	17760	306	434	2636	130
1275	367	24	576	254	3200
63	1350	471	115	460	136
1703	503	211	13403	43677	24220
304	156	6	1402	25175	367
267	37	1575	5621	33	7702
4676	23241	56	234	56	4
206	12	120	1413	237	41
32	1556	37	70	13	1675
144654	2410	6211	353436	1100	7
4456	165171	16	640	5377	73
1205	4	4233	302	32	223
15020	110	171	100564	4602	4320
143	4	20	55	27431	33
713	103	46	7	161	147
1550	43	23	70	3054	267
10372	606	217	237	45207	70
7552	4350	2462	27	115	130
64	763	334	225	317	773
744	1175	11222	46240	61	561
131	3015	1135	1363	7450	2177
1254	47	14261	71	13	53
312134	13357	4	445	14	37
510	37	627	1112	127	652
70	11001	62	731	125	650
14	15533	41	57	52	1066
130	765	14	16240	144062	6370
47	3056	134137			

tween trials or families. Although there is some evidence that p can vary between families [11] (p. 645) and between trials [9] (p. 447), other evidence [2] (p. 249) suggests that this is a not unrealistic assumption for the overall model since the variation is slight. Applying model (7.1) with $K = 195$ families, we compute from Table II, $n = \Sigma n_k = 1466$, $R = \Sigma R_k = 337$, $S = \Sigma S_k = 723$, and $T = \Sigma T_k = 184$. Using either $p = 0.48$ or $p = 0.49$ for the probability of a female birth, we estimate $\hat{\theta}_+ \doteq 1.08$ applying (5.1) with $m = n - K = 1271$. Using (3.4) and $p = 0.49$, we reject the hypothesis that $\theta = 1$ in favor of $\theta \neq 1$ at the 0.01 level of significance, since $2[L_n(\hat{\theta}) - L_n(1)] \doteq 7.10 > 6.6 \doteq \chi^2_{1,.01}$. The 95 per cent confidence interval for θ, using (3.5), is $1.02 \leq \theta \leq 1.13$ to two decimals. Although the model is different, the finding of an increase in the con-

ditional probability of a girl given a previous girl is in agreement with Edwards
[3] (p. 343) and Renkonen [9].

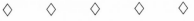

APPENDIX

PROOF OF THEOREM 3. To show that (5.1) maximizes the likelihood, we
consider two cases: $(n_{01} + n_{10}) > 0$, and $= 0$.

Case 1: $n_{01} + n_{10} > 0$. If we examine the derivative equation (3.2), we note
$L'_n(1/p) = -\infty$ and $L''_n(\theta) < 0$. Assume first that $L'_n(\max\{0, (2p - 1)/p^2\}) \leqq 0$.
Then $L_n(\theta)$ is decreasing and the maximum occurs on the boundary

(A.1) $$\theta = \max\{0, (2p - 1)/p^2\};$$

we must show $\hat{\theta}_+$ gives this value. If $p \leqq \frac{1}{2}$, the assumption reduces to $L'_n(0) \leqq 0$
so that from (3.2), $n_{11} = 0$ and $-(n_{01} + n_{10})p + [n_{00}p^2/(1 - 2p)] \leqq 0$. Using
$n_{11} = 0$, $n_{11} + n_{01} + n_{10} + n_{00} = m$, this condition becomes

(A.2) $$(mp - (n_{01} + n_{10})q) \leqq 0.$$

Consequently, evaluating (5.1),

(A.3)
$$\hat{\theta}_+ = \frac{1}{2}\left[\left\{\frac{n_{01} + n_{10} + m}{mp} - \frac{n_{01} + n_{10}}{mp^2}\right\} + \left(\left\{\frac{n_{01} + n_{10} + m}{mp} - \frac{(n_{01} + n_{10})}{mp^2}\right\}^2\right)^{\frac{1}{2}}\right]$$
$$= \frac{1}{2}\left[\frac{mp - (n_{01} + n_{10})q}{mp^2} - \frac{mp - (n_{01} + n_{10})q}{mp^2}\right] = 0.$$

If $p > \frac{1}{2}$, the assumption becomes $L'_n((2p - 1)/p^2) \leqq 0$ so that $n_{00} = 0$ and
$n_{11}p - (2p - 1)m \leqq 0$. Evaluating (5.1),

(A.4)
$$\hat{\theta}_+ = \frac{1}{2}\left[\left\{\frac{n_{11} + 2m}{mp} - \frac{m}{mp^2}\right\} + \left(\left\{\frac{n_{11}p}{mp^2} + \frac{2p - 1}{p^2}\right\}^2 - \frac{4n_{11}pm(2p - 1)}{m^2p^4}\right)^{\frac{1}{2}}\right]$$
$$= \frac{1}{2}\left[\frac{2p - 1}{p^2} + \frac{n_{11}p}{mp^2} + \left|\frac{n_{11}p}{mp^2} - \frac{2p - 1}{p^2}\right|\right] = \frac{2p - 1}{p^2}.$$

Thus, under the assumption $\hat{\theta}_+ = \max\{0, (2p - 1)/p^2\}$. Next assume
$L'_n(\max\{0, (2p - 1)/p^2\}) > 0$. Under this assumption there will be a root
which maximizes $L_n(\theta)$ in the open interval $(\max\{0, (qp - 1)/p^2\}, 1/p)$ since
$L''_n(\theta) < 0$ and $L'_n(1/p) = -\infty$. This root will be one of the two roots of the
quadratic equation

(A.5) $$\theta(1 - \theta p)(1 - 2p + \theta p^2)\left(\frac{n_{11}}{\theta} - \frac{(n_{01} + n_{10})p}{1 - \theta p} + \frac{n_{00}p^2}{1 - 2p + \theta p^2}\right) = 0$$

or

(A.6) $$\theta^2 - \theta\left\{\frac{2n_{11} + n_{01} + n_{10} + m}{mp} - \frac{(n_{11} + n_{01} + n_{10})}{mp^2}\right\} - \frac{n_{11}(1 - 2p)}{mp^3} = 0.$$

Since $\hat\theta_+$ is one of the roots of this equation, it remains to rule out the other root

$$(A.7) \quad \hat\theta_- = \frac{1}{2}\left[\left\{\frac{2n_{11}+n_{01}+n_{10}}{mp} - \frac{(n_{11}+n_{01}+n_{10})}{mp^2}\right\}\right.$$
$$\left. - \left(\left\{\frac{2n_{11}+n_{01}+n_{10}+m}{mp} - \frac{(n_{11}+n_{01}+n_{10})}{mp^2}\right\}^2 + \frac{4n_{11}(1-2p)}{mp^3}\right)^{\frac12}\right],$$

by showing $\hat\theta_- \leq \max\{0, (2p-1)/p^2\}$. Substituting $n_{01}+n_{10} = m - n_{11} - n_{00}$, we can rewrite

$$(A.8) \quad \hat\theta_- = \frac{1}{2}\left[\left\{\frac{2p-1}{p^2} + \frac{n_{11}p+n_{00}q}{mp^2}\right\}\right.$$
$$\left. - \left(\left\{\frac{2p-1}{p^2} + \frac{n_{11}p+n_{00}q}{mp^2}\right\}^2 + \frac{4n_{11}(1-2p)}{mp^3}\right)^{\frac12}\right].$$

For $p \leq \frac12$, if we replace the second term in the radical by zero, we obtain

$$(A.9) \quad \hat\theta_- \leq \frac{1}{2}\left[\left\{\frac{2p-1}{p^2} + \frac{n_{11}p+n_{00}q}{mp^2}\right\} - \left|\frac{2p-1}{p^2} + \frac{n_{11}p+n_{00}q}{mp^2}\right|\right] \leq 0.$$

For $p > \frac12$, rewrite $\hat\theta_-$ in the form

$$(A.10) \quad \hat\theta_- = \frac{1}{2}\left[\left\{\frac{2p-1}{p^2} + \frac{n_{11}p+n_{00}q}{mp^2}\right\}\right.$$
$$\left. - \left(\frac{2p-1}{p^2} + \frac{2(p-1)(-n_{11}p+n_{00}q)}{mp^2} + \left\{\frac{n_{11}p+n_{00}q}{mp^2}\right\}^2\right)^{\frac12}\right].$$

Replacing the $+n_{00}q$ term in the center of the radical by $-n_{00}q$, we obtain

$$(A.11) \quad \hat\theta_- \leq \frac{1}{2}\left[\left\{\frac{2p-1}{p^2} + \frac{n_{11}p+n_{00}q}{mp^2}\right\}\right.$$
$$\left. - \left(\left\{\frac{2p-1}{p^2} + \frac{(n_{11}p-n_{00}q)}{mp^2}\right\}^2\right)^{\frac12}\right] \leq \frac{2p-1}{p^2},$$

so that $\hat\theta_- \leq \max\{0, (2p-1)/p^2\}$.

Case 2: $n_{01}+n_{10} = 0$. If $n_{01}+n_{10} = 0$, then $L_n'(\theta) > 0$ so that $L_n(\theta)$ is increasing and maximized at the end point $\theta = 1/p$. Substituting in $\hat\theta_+$ with $n_{01}+n_{10} = 0$ gives

$$(A.12)$$
$$\hat\theta_+ = \frac{1}{2}\left[\left\{\frac{mp - n_{11}(1-2p)}{mp^2}\right\} + \left(\left\{\frac{mp-n_{11}(1-2p)}{mp^2}\right\}^2 + \frac{4n_{11}(1-2p)}{mp^3}\right)^{\frac12}\right]$$
$$= \frac{1}{2}\left[\left\{\frac{mp - n_{11}(1-2p)}{mp^2}\right\} + \left|\frac{mp+n_{11}(1-2p)}{mp^2}\right|\right] = \frac{1}{p}.$$

Q.E.D.

Note, $mp + n_{11}(1-2p) = (n_{11}+n_{01}+n_{10}+n_{00})p + n_{11}(1-2p) \geq 0$. Methods similar to those used to rule out $\hat\theta_-$ can be used to verify $\max\{0, (2p-1)/p^2\} \leq \hat\theta_+ \leq 1/p$.

◇   ◇   ◇   ◇   ◇

The model was first considered in a metallurgical application with the late Charles Johnson. Conversations with John McDonald, Nathan Keyfitz, and Tom Espenshade (who provided the data) were most helpful.

REFERENCES

[1] P. BILLINGSLEY, *Statistical Inference for Markov Processes*, Chicago, University of Chicago Press, 1961.
[2] A. W. F. EDWARDS and M. FRACCARO, "Distribution and sequences of sexes in a selected sample of Swedish families," *Ann. Hum. Genet.*, Vol. 24 (1960), pp. 245–252.
[3] A. W. F. EDWARDS, "Sex-ratio data analysed independently of family limitation," *Ann. Hum. Genet.*, Vol. 29 (1966), pp. 337–346.
[4] T. J. ESPENSHADE, "A new method for estimating the level of natural fertility in populations practicing birth control," *Demography*, Vol. 8 (1971), pp. 525–536.
[5] W. FELLER, *An Introduction to Probability Theory and Its Applications*, Vol. I, New York, Wiley, 1957 (2nd ed.).
[6] J. M. FISHER, *Descendants and History of the Christian Fisher Family*, published by Amos L. Fisher, Rt. 1, Ranks, Pa., 1957.
[7] L. A. GOODMAN, "Some possible effects of birth control on the human sex ratio," *Ann. Hum. Genet.*, Vol. 25 (1961), pp. 75–81.
[8] C. A. JOHNSON and J. H. KLOTZ, "The atom probe and Markov chain statistics of clustering," University of Wisconsin Statistics Department Technical Report No. 267, 1971.
[9] K. O. RENKONEN, "Is the sex ratio between boys and girls correlated to the sex of precedent children?" *Ann. Med. Exp. Biol. Fenn.*, Vol. 34 (1956), pp. 447–451.
[10] K. O. RENKONEN, O. MÄKELÄ, and R. LEHTOVAARA, "Factors affecting the human sex ratio," *Ann. Med. Exp. Biol. Fenn.*, Vol. 39 (1961), pp. 173–184.
[11] L. B. SHETTLES, "Factors influencing sex ratios," *Int. J. Gynaecol. Obstet.*, Vol. 8 (1970), pp. 643–647.

AN EQUALITY IN STOCHASTIC PROCESSES

CHIN LONG CHIANG
UNIVERSITY OF CALIFORNIA, BERKELEY

1. Introduction

The equality presented in this paper is extremely simple, but has proven useful on a number of occasions in deriving certain transition probabilities where other approaches such as the Laplace transform or the generating function become untidy (see, for example, [7]). The equality is not completely unknown; it has appeared, in a slightly different form, in a two dimensional process ([2], p. 102); and it is obvious for the simple Poisson process. The purpose of this paper is to state it in a general form and to demonstrate its validity and usefulness with a number of examples.

2. The equality

Let $\{X(t); t \in T\}$ be a time dependent Markov process defined over the interval $T: [0, \infty)$. For each $t \in T$, the random variable $X(t)$ assumes nonnegative integer values with the transition probability

$$(1) \qquad P_{ik}(t_0, t) = Pr\{X(t) = k | X(t_0) = i\},$$
$$0 \le t_0 \le t < \infty, \ i \le k; \ i, k = 0, 1, \cdots.$$

Our discussion is related only to nondecreasing processes where the value of $X(t)$ is increased by the occurrence of an event (for example, the pure birth process), or the nonincreasing processes (for example, the pure death process). The equality will be presented only for the former cases. However, an example of the pure death process will be given in Section 3.

For each i, we assume the existence of a continuous function $\lambda_i(\tau)$ such that

$$(2) \qquad \frac{\partial}{\partial t} P_{ij}(\tau, t) \bigg|_{t=\tau} = \begin{cases} \lambda_i(\tau) & \text{for } j = i+1, \\ -\lambda_i(\tau) & \text{for } j = i, \\ 0 & \text{otherwise.} \end{cases}$$

It follows that the transition probabilities in (1) satisfy the forward differential equations

$$(3) \qquad \frac{d}{dt} P_{ii}(t_0, t) = -\lambda_i(t)P_{ii}(t_0, t),$$

$$\frac{d}{dt} P_{ik}(t_0, t) = -\lambda_k(t)P_{ik}(t_0, t) + \lambda_{k-1}(t)P_{i,k-1}(t_0, t),$$
$$i \le k; \ i, k = 0, 1, \cdots.$$

187

The first equation in (3) has the solution

$$(4) \qquad P_{ii}(t_0, t) = g_i(t_0, t)$$

where $g_i(t_0, t)$ denotes $\exp\left\{-\int_{t_0}^{t} \lambda_i(\xi)\, d\xi\right\}$, while the second equations give the recursive relationship

$$(5) \qquad P_{ik}(t_0, t) = \int_{t_0}^{t} P_{i,k-1}(t_0, t_{k-1})\lambda_{k-1}(t_{k-1})P_{kk}(t_{k-1}, t)\, dt_{k-1}.$$

The probability $P_{i,k-1}(t_0, t_{k-1})$ may be written in the form of (5):

$$(6) \qquad P_{i,k-1}(t_0, t_{k-1}) = \int_{t_0}^{t_{k-1}} P_{i,k-2}(t_0, t_{k-2})\lambda_{k-2}(t_{k-2})P_{k-1,k-1}(t_{k-2}, t_{k-1})\, dt_{k-2}.$$

Substituting (6) in (5) yields

$$(7) \qquad P_{i,k}(t_0, t) = \int_{t_0}^{t} \int_{t_0}^{t_{k-1}} P_{i,k-2}(t, t_{k-2}) \prod_{\ell=k-2}^{k-1} \lambda_\ell(t_\ell)P_{\ell+1,\ell+1}(t_\ell, t_{\ell+1})\, dt_\ell,$$

or, upon integration with respect to t_{k-1},

$$(8) \qquad P_{i,k}(t_0, t) = \int_{0}^{t} P_{i,k-2}(t_0, t_{k-2})\lambda_{k-2}(t_{k-2})P_{k-1,k}(t_{k-2}, t)\, dt_{k-2}.$$

Equation (8) indicates a sequence of transitions taking place in the interval $(t_0, t): i \to k - 2$ in (t_0, t_{k-2}), $k - 2 \to k - 1$ in $(t_{k-2}, t_{k-2} + dt_{k-2})$, and $k - 1 \to k$ in $(t_{k-2} + dt_{k-2}, t)$, for $t_0 \leq t_{k-2} \leq t$.

Equation (7) can be extended by repeated substitutions of (5) in (7) beginning with $k = k - 2$. Consequently, we arrive at a formula,

$$(9) \qquad P_{ik}(t_0, t) = \int_{t_0}^{t} \int_{t_0}^{t_{k-1}} \cdots \int_{t_0}^{t_{k-i+1}} P_{ii}(t_0, t_i) \prod_{\ell=i}^{k-1} \lambda_\ell(t_\ell)P_{\ell+1,\ell+1}(t_\ell, t_{\ell+1})\, dt_\ell,$$

which shows the occurrence of each transition from ℓ to $\ell + 1$ in $(t_\ell, t_\ell + dt_\ell)$. Now the transitions can be regrouped in any meaningful way one wishes by integrating the right side of (9). When a particular transition, $j \to j + 1$, is of concern, we integrate the right side of (9) with respect to t_ℓ, for $i \leq \ell < j$ and $j < \ell \leq k$ to obtain *the equality. Let j be an arbitrary but fixed integer, for $i \leq j < k$, then*

$$(10) \qquad P_{ik}(t_0, t) = \int_{t_0}^{t} P_{ij}(t_0, \tau)\lambda_j(\tau)P_{j+1,k}(\tau, t)\, d\tau.$$

Clearly, (5) is a special case of the equality (10).

An equality for the continuous case also can be derived, where we will be dealing with the density function $f_{xz}(t_0, t)$ instead of the probability $P_{ik}(t_0, t)$.

A similarity between the present equality and the Chapman-Kolmogorov equation should be noted. The transition probability in (1) involves the parameter t and the values of the random variable $X(t)$ (or the states of the system). The Chapman-Kolmogorov equation,

$$(11) \qquad P_{ik}(t_0, t) = \sum_{j} P_{ij}(t_0, \tau)P_{jk}(\tau, t),$$

is related to a fixed but arbitrary time τ and varying states j at τ; whereas in equality (10) a state j is fixed and the integral is taken over the values of τ. This, however, is the extent of the similarity. In equality (10), we *require* a transition from j to $j + 1$ to take place in $(\tau, \tau + d\tau)$ for which a probability $\lambda_j(\tau)\, d\tau$ is included, while in the Chapman-Kolmogorov equation there is no such requirement. This additional factor nullifies a complete analogy between the two equalities.

3. Examples

3.1. *The Poisson process.* In the nonhomogeneous case, the intensity $\lambda_i(\tau) = \lambda(\tau)$ is a function of time; the transition probability is given by

$$
(12) \qquad P_{ik}(t_0, t) = \frac{\exp\left\{-\int_{t_0}^{t} \lambda(\xi)\, d\xi\right\}\left[\int_{t_0}^{t} \lambda(\xi)\, d\xi\right]^{k-i}}{(k - i)!}, \qquad i \leqq k.
$$

According to equality (10), we should have

$$
(13) \quad \frac{g(t_0, t)}{(k - i)!}\left(\int_{t_0}^{t} \lambda(\xi)\, d\xi\right)^{k-i}
$$

$$
= \int_{t_0}^{t}\left[\frac{g(t_0, \tau)}{(j - i)!}\left(\int_{t_0}^{\tau} \lambda(\xi)\, d\xi\right)^{j-i}\right]\lambda(\tau)\left[\frac{g(\tau, t)}{(k - j - 1)!}\left(\int_{\tau}^{t} \lambda(\xi)\, d\xi\right)^{k-j-1}\right] d\tau.
$$

where $g(t_0, t)$ denotes $\exp\left\{-\int_{t_0}^{t} \lambda(\xi)\, d\xi\right\}$ and $g(\tau, t)$ denotes $\exp\left\{-\int_{\tau}^{t} \lambda(\xi)\, d\xi\right\}$. To verify (13), we introduce a function

$$
(14) \qquad \theta(\tau) = \frac{\int_{t_0}^{\tau} \lambda(\xi)\, d\xi}{\int_{t_0}^{t} \lambda(\xi)\, d\xi}, \qquad d\theta(\tau) = \frac{\lambda(\tau)\, d\tau}{\int_{t_0}^{t} \lambda(\xi)\, d\xi},
$$

and rewrite the right side of (13) as

$$
(15) \quad \frac{g(t_0, t)}{(j - i)!(k - j - 1)!}\left(\int_{t_0}^{t} \lambda(\xi)\, d\xi\right)^{k-i}\int_{0}^{1}[\theta(\tau)]^{j-i}[1 - \theta(\tau)]^{k-j-1}\, d\theta(\tau)
$$

$$
= \frac{g(t_0, t)}{(k - i)!}\left(\int_{t_0}^{t} \lambda(\xi)\, d\xi\right)^{k-i},
$$

and recover the left side of (13).

When $\lambda(\tau) = \lambda$, and $t_0 = 0$, (13) becomes

$$
(16) \qquad \frac{e^{-\lambda t}(\lambda t)^{k-i}}{(k - i)!} = \int_{0}^{t}\frac{e^{-\lambda \tau}(\lambda \tau)^{i-i}}{(j - i)!}\lambda\,\frac{e^{-\lambda(t-\tau)}[\lambda(t - \tau)]^{k-j-1}}{(k - j - 1)!}\, d\tau.
$$

3.2. *The Yule process.* When the intensity $\lambda_i(\tau) = i\lambda(\tau)$, the differential equations in (3) define the Yule process,

$$
(17) \qquad P_{ik}(t_0, t) = \frac{(k - 1)!}{(k - i)!(i - 1)!}\, (g(t_0, t))^i(1 - g(t_0, t))^{k-i}.
$$

To verify equality (10), we need to show that

(18) $\quad \dfrac{(k-1)!}{(k-i)!(i-1)!} (g(t_0, t))^i (1 - g(t_0, t))^{k-i}$

$$= \int_{t_0}^{t} \frac{(j-1)!}{(j-i)!(i-1)!} (g(t_0, \tau))^i (1 - g(t_0, \tau))^{i-i} j \lambda(\tau)$$

$$\frac{(k-1)!}{(k-j-1)!j!} (g(\tau, t))^{j+1} (1 - g(\tau, t))^{k-j-1} d\tau,$$

where $g(t_0, \tau)$ denotes $\exp\left\{-\int_{t_0}^{\tau} \lambda(\xi)\, d\xi\right\}$. Let

(19) $$\theta(\tau) = \frac{1 - g(\tau, t)}{1 - g(t_0, t)},$$

so that

(20) $\quad d\theta(\tau) = \dfrac{-g(\tau, t)\lambda(\tau)\, d\tau}{1 - g(t_0, t)}$ and $\quad 1 - \theta(\tau) = \dfrac{g(\tau, t) - g(t_0, t)}{1 - g(t_0, t)}.$

Substituting (19) and (20) in the right side of (18) and simplifying yields

(21) $\quad \dfrac{(k-1)!}{(j-i)!(i-1)!(k-j-1)!} (g(t_0, t))^i (1 - g(t_0, t))^{k-i}$

$$\int_{0}^{1} [1 - \theta(\tau)]^{j-i} [\theta(\tau)]^{k-j-1}\, d\theta(\tau)$$

$$= \frac{(k-1)!}{(k-i)!(i-1)!} (g(t_0, t))^i (1 - g(t_0, t))^{k-i},$$

which is equal to the left side of (18), proving (18).

3.3. *The pure birth process.* To verify equality (10) for the present case, we need the following lemma.

LEMMA 1. *Whatever may be distinct real numbers,* $\lambda_1, \lambda_2, \cdots, \lambda_n$,

(22) $$\frac{1}{\prod\limits_{\gamma=2}^{n} (\lambda_1 - \lambda_\gamma)} + \cdots + \frac{1}{\prod\limits_{\gamma=1}^{n-1} (\lambda_n - \lambda_\gamma)} = 0.$$

Several proofs of the lemma are given in Chiang [2], p. 126; we do not present the details here.

The pure birth process is a different form from the Yule process in that the intensity function $\lambda_i(\tau) = \lambda_i$ is a function of i, but is assumed to be independent of time τ. When λ_i are distinct for different i, then the differential equation (3) has the solution (see Feller [5], p. 449, and [2], p. 51),

(23) $$P_{ik}(t_0, t) = (-1)^{k-i} \lambda_i \lambda_{i+1} \cdots \lambda_{k-1} \sum_{\alpha=i}^{k} \frac{\exp\{-\lambda_\alpha(t - t_0)\}}{\prod\limits_{\gamma=i, \gamma \neq \alpha}^{k} (\lambda_\alpha - \lambda_\gamma)}.$$

Similarly,

(24) $$P_{ij}(t_0, \tau) = (-1)^{j-i} \lambda_i \lambda_{i+1} \cdots \lambda_{j-1} \sum_{\alpha=i}^{j} \frac{\exp\{-\lambda_\alpha(\tau - t_0)\}}{\prod\limits_{\gamma=i, \gamma \neq \alpha}^{j} (\lambda_\alpha - \lambda_\gamma)}$$

and

$$(25) \quad P_{j+1,k}(\tau, t) = (-1)^{k-j-1} \lambda_{j+1} \lambda_{j+2} \cdots \lambda_{k-1} \sum_{\beta=j+1}^{k} \frac{\exp\{-\lambda_\beta(t-\tau)\}}{\displaystyle\prod_{\delta=j+1,\delta\neq\beta}^{k} (\lambda_\beta - \lambda_\delta)}.$$

When (24) and (25) are substituted in (10), we find on the right side of (10),

$$(26) \quad \int_{t_0}^{t} P_{ij}(t_0, \tau) \lambda_j P_{j+1,k}(\tau, t)\, d\tau$$

$$= (-1)^{k-i-1} \lambda_i \lambda_{i+1} \cdots \lambda_{k-1} \sum_{\alpha=i}^{j} \sum_{\beta=j+1}^{k} \frac{\displaystyle\int_{t_0}^{t} \exp\{-\lambda_\alpha(\tau - t_0)\} \exp\{-\lambda_\beta(t - \tau)\}\, d\tau}{\displaystyle\prod_{\gamma=i,\gamma\neq\alpha}^{j} (\lambda_\alpha - \lambda_\gamma) \prod_{\delta=j+1,\delta\neq\beta}^{k} (\lambda_\beta - \lambda_\delta)},$$

where

$$(27) \quad \int_{t_0}^{t} \exp\{-\lambda_\alpha(\tau - t_0)\} \exp\{-\lambda_\beta(t - \tau)\}\, d\tau$$

$$= -\left[\frac{\exp\{-\lambda_\alpha(t - t_0)\}}{\lambda_\alpha - \lambda_\beta} + \frac{\exp\{-\lambda_\beta(t - t_0)\}}{\lambda_\beta - \lambda_\alpha} \right].$$

Therefore, (26) may be rewritten

$$(28)$$

$$(-1)^{k-i} \lambda_i \lambda_{i+1} \cdots \lambda_{k-1} \left[\sum_{\alpha=i}^{j} \sum_{\beta=j+1}^{k} \frac{\exp\{-\lambda_\alpha(t - t_0)\}}{(\lambda_\alpha - \lambda_\beta) \displaystyle\prod_{\gamma=i,\gamma\neq\alpha}^{j} (\lambda_\alpha - \lambda_\gamma) \prod_{\delta=j+1,\delta\neq\beta}^{k} (\lambda_\beta - \lambda_\delta)} \right.$$

$$\left. + \sum_{\alpha=i}^{j} \sum_{\beta=j+1}^{k} \frac{\exp\{-\lambda_\beta(t - t_0)\}}{(\lambda_\beta - \lambda_\alpha) \displaystyle\prod_{\gamma=i,\gamma\neq\alpha}^{j} (\lambda_\alpha - \lambda_\gamma) \prod_{\delta=j+1,\delta\neq\beta}^{k} (\lambda_\beta - \lambda_\delta)} \right].$$

In the first term inside the brackets, for each α, we compute the sum

$$(29) \quad \left\{ \sum_{\beta=j+1}^{k} \frac{1}{(\lambda_\alpha - \lambda_\beta) \displaystyle\prod_{\delta=j+1,\delta\neq\beta}^{k} (\lambda_\beta - \lambda_\delta)} \right\} \frac{\exp\{-\lambda_\alpha(t - t_0)\}}{\displaystyle\prod_{\gamma=i,\gamma\neq\alpha}^{j} (\lambda_\alpha - \lambda_\gamma)}$$

$$= \left\{ \frac{1}{\displaystyle\prod_{\delta=j+1}^{k} (\lambda_\alpha - \lambda_\delta)} \right\} \frac{\exp\{-\lambda_\alpha(t - t_0)\}}{\displaystyle\prod_{\gamma=i,\gamma\neq\alpha}^{j} (\lambda_\alpha - \lambda_\gamma)} = \frac{\exp\{-\lambda_\alpha(t - t_0)\}}{\displaystyle\prod_{\gamma=i,\gamma\neq\alpha}^{k} (\lambda_\alpha - \lambda_\gamma)},$$

since, according to Lemma 1, for any distinct numbers λ_α, λ_{j+1}, λ_{j+2}, $\cdots$, λ_k,

$$(30) \quad \frac{1}{(\lambda_\alpha - \lambda_{j+1}) \displaystyle\prod_{\gamma=j+2}^{k} (\lambda_{j+1} - \lambda_\gamma)} + \cdots + \frac{1}{(\lambda_\alpha - \lambda_k) \displaystyle\prod_{\gamma=j+1}^{k-1} (\lambda_k - \lambda_\gamma)}$$

$$= \frac{1}{\displaystyle\prod_{\gamma=j+1}^{k} (\lambda_\alpha - \lambda_\gamma)}.$$

Similarly, in the second term inside the brackets of (28) we find for each β,

(31)

$$\left[\sum_{\alpha=i}^{j} \frac{1}{(\lambda_\beta - \lambda_\alpha) \prod\limits_{\gamma=i, \gamma \neq \alpha}^{j} (\lambda_\alpha - \lambda_\gamma)}\right] \frac{\exp\{-\lambda_\beta(t - t_0)\}}{\prod\limits_{\delta=j+1, \delta \neq \beta}^{k} (\lambda_\beta - \lambda_\delta)} = \frac{\exp\{-\lambda_\beta(t - t_0)\}}{\prod\limits_{\delta=i, \delta \neq \beta}^{k} (\lambda_\beta - \lambda_\delta)}.$$

Substituting (29) and (31) in (28) yields

(32)
$$(-1)^{k-i} \lambda_i \lambda_{i+1} \cdots \lambda_{k-1} \sum_{\alpha=i}^{k} \frac{\exp\{-\lambda_\alpha(t - t_0)\}}{\prod\limits_{\gamma=i, \gamma \neq \alpha}^{k} (\lambda_\alpha - \lambda_\gamma)},$$

which is equal to (23), as was to be shown.

3.4. *The Pólya process.* The Pólya process is determined by the differential equation (3) with the intensity function

(33)
$$\lambda_k(t) = \frac{\lambda + \lambda a k}{1 + \lambda a t},$$

where both λ and a are nonnegative constants. Solving (3) for $P_{ik}(t_0, t)$, we have

(34)
$$P_{ik}(t_0, t) = \frac{\Gamma(k + 1/a)}{(k - i)!\Gamma(i + 1/a)} \left(\frac{1 + \lambda a t_0}{1 + \lambda a t}\right)^{i+1/a} \left(1 - \frac{1 + \lambda a t_0}{1 + \lambda a t}\right)^{k-i}.$$

Using this general formula for the probabilities $P_{ij}(t_0, \tau)$ and $P_{j+1,k}(\tau, t)$ in (10), we obtain

(35)
$$\int_{t_0}^{t} P_{ij}(t_0, \tau) \lambda_j(\tau) P_{j+1,k}(\tau, t) \, d\tau$$

$$= \frac{\Gamma(j + 1/a)}{(j - i)!\Gamma(i + 1/a)} \frac{\Gamma(k + 1/a)}{(k - j - 1)!\Gamma(j + 1 + 1/a)} \int_{t_0}^{t} \left(\frac{1 + \lambda a t_0}{1 + \lambda a \tau}\right)^{i+1/a}$$

$$\left(1 - \frac{1 + \lambda a t_0}{1 + \lambda a \tau}\right)^{j-i} \left(\frac{\lambda + \lambda a j}{1 + \lambda a \tau}\right) \left(\frac{1 + \lambda a \tau}{1 + \lambda a t}\right)^{j+1+1/a} \left(1 - \frac{1 + \lambda a \tau}{1 + \lambda a t}\right)^{k-j-1} d\tau,$$

where the integral is simply

(36)

$$(1 + \lambda a t_0)^{i+1/a}(1 + \lambda a t)^{-(k+1/a)}(\lambda a)^{k-i-1}(\lambda + \lambda a j) \int_{t_0}^{t} (\tau - t_0)^{i-i}(t - \tau)^{k-j-1} \, d\tau$$

$$= (1 + \lambda a t_0)^{i+1/a}(1 + \lambda a t)^{-(k+1/a)}(\lambda a)^{k-i-1}$$

$$(\lambda + \lambda a j)(t - t_0)^{k-i} \frac{(j - i)!(k - j - 1)!}{(k - i)!}$$

$$= \left(\frac{1 + \lambda a t_0}{1 + \lambda a t}\right)^{i+1/a} \left(1 - \frac{\lambda a t_0}{1 + \lambda a t}\right)^{k-i} \left(j + \frac{1}{a}\right) \frac{(j - i)!(k - j - 1)!}{(k - i)!}.$$

When the last expression in (36) is substituted for the integral in (35), the right side member of (35) becomes identical to that in (34), proving equality (10) for the Pólya process.

3.5. *The pure death process.* The pure death process is different from all the preceding processes; in this case the population size is decreasing instead of increasing with time t. The transition probability $P_{ik}(t_0, t)$ holds for $k \leqq i$ and satisfies the differential equation

$$(37) \qquad \frac{d}{dt} P_{ik}(t_0, t) = -k\mu(t)P_{ik}(t_0, t) + (k+1)\mu(t)P_{i,k+1}(t_0, t),$$

$$k = 0, 1, \cdots, i,$$

where the intensity function $\mu(t)$ is also known as the force of mortality. The solution of (37) is

$$(38) \qquad P_{ik}(t_0, t) = \frac{i!}{k!(i-k)!} (h(t_0, t))^k (1 - h(t_0, t))^{i-k},$$

where $h(t_0, t)$ denotes $\exp\left\{-\int_{t_0}^{t} \mu(\xi)\, d\xi\right\}$. The equality for the death process assumes a form slightly different from (10);

$$(39) \qquad P_{ik}(t_0, t) = \int_{t_0}^{t} P_{ij}(t_0, \tau)j\mu(\tau)P_{j-1,k}(\tau, t)\, d\tau, \qquad 0 \leqq k < j \leqq i.$$

Verification of (39) is straightforward. Using (37) we can write

$$(40) \quad \int_{t_0}^{t} P_{ij}(t_0, \tau)j\mu(\tau)P_{j-1,k}(\tau, t)\, d\tau$$

$$= \int_{t_0}^{t} \frac{i!}{j!(i-j)!} (h(t_0, \tau))^i (1 - h(t_0, \tau))^{i-j}j\mu(\tau)$$

$$\frac{(j-1)!}{k!(j-1-k)!} (h(\tau, t))^k (1 - h(\tau, t))^{i-1-k}\, d\tau,$$

where $h(\tau, t)$ denotes $\exp\left\{-\int_{\tau}^{t} \mu(\xi)\, d\xi\right\}$ and $h(t_0, \tau)$ denotes $\exp\left\{-\int_{t_0}^{\tau} \mu(\xi)\, d\xi\right\}$.

Now let

$$(41) \qquad \theta(\tau) = \frac{1 - h(t_0, \tau)}{1 - h(t_0, t)}, \qquad d\theta(\tau) = \frac{h(t_0, \tau)\mu(\tau)\, d\tau}{1 - h(t_0, t)}.$$

Then (40) may be rewritten as

(42)

$$\frac{i!}{(i-j)!k!(j-1-k)!} (h(t_0, t))^k (1 - h(t_0, t))^{i-k} \int_{0}^{1} (\theta(\tau))^{i-i}(1 - \theta(\tau))^{j-1-k}\, d\theta(\tau)$$

$$= \frac{i!}{k!(i-k)!} (h(t_0, t))^k (1 - h(t_0, t))^{i-k}$$

$$= P_{ik}(t_0, t),$$

which proves the equality in (39).

4. An application

Theoretical significance of equality (10) is yet to be assessed, depending to a great extent on its relevance in developing stochastic processes. The following example illustrates its usefulness as a means of deriving certain transition probabilities.

The example in question is the so-called "simple stochastic epidemic," which has been extensively studied by N. T. J. Bailey [1]. According to this model, a population consists of two groups of individuals: infectives and susceptibles. At the initial time t_0, there are one infective and N susceptibles. For each t, for $t \in [t_0, \infty)$, there are $X(t)$ infectives and $N + 1 - X(t)$ susceptibles. The probability distribution of the random variable $X(t)$ satisfies the system of differential equations

$$(43) \qquad \frac{d}{dt} P_{1k}(t_0, t) = -a_k \beta(t) P_{1k}(t_0, t) + a_{k-1} \beta(t) P_{1,k-1}(t_0, t),$$

$$k = 1, \cdots, N + 1,$$

where

$$(44) \qquad a_k = k(N + 1 - k) \qquad k = 1, \cdots, N; a_0 = a_{N+1} = 0,$$

with the initial condition $P_{11}(t_0, t_0) = 1$, and the constant $\beta(t)$ is known as the infection rate. The Laplace transform and the probability generating function have been used to solve the differential equations (43). Because the coefficient a_k is a quadratic function of k, for each k, the computations involved are quite complex. The partial differential equation for the probability generating function, for example, is of the second order. However, when equality (10) is used, one can write down the solution almost immediately. The complete solution and the detailed discussion on related points have been given in [7], and will not be repeated here.

5. The equalities in a two dimensional process

Equality (10) can be extended to multidimensional processes, where the random variables concerned are the number of transitions rather than population sizes. To be specific, we use a two dimensional process for illustration. In the birth, death and other processes discussed in Section 3, there is only one transient state for each individual: the state of "living." In a two dimensional process, each individual may be in either one of two transient states, S_1 and S_2. State S_1 may be interpreted as the healthy state, and S_2 the illness state. In addition, there is an absorbing state R, the death state. A person is in state S_1 if he is well, in S_2 if he is ill. A transition from S_1 to S_2 means the occurrence of an illness or a relapse, while a transition from S_2 to S_1 means recovery. When a person dies, he enters the death state R from either S_1 or S_2 depending upon whether he is in state S_1 or S_2 at the time of death. Fix and Neyman have discussed extensively this model in their study of the probabilities of relapse, recovery, and death for cancer patients [6] (see also Du Pasquier [4]).

During a time interval (t_0, t) an individual may leave one transient state for another. We are interested in the number of transitions that he makes between the two transient states and the corresponding probabilities, which are defined as follows:

(45) $\begin{aligned} P_{\alpha\beta}^{(m)}(t_0, t) &= Pr \text{ \{an individual in state } S_\alpha \text{ at time } t_0 \text{ will leave } S_\alpha \, m \text{ times} \\ &\qquad \text{during } (t_0, t) \text{ and will be in } S_\beta \text{ at time } t\} \\ &= Pr\{M_{\alpha\beta}(t_0, t) = m\}, \qquad\qquad \alpha, \beta = 1, 2; m = 0, 1, \cdots. \end{aligned}$

The random variable $M_{\alpha\beta}(t_0, t)$, corresponding to the probability $P_{\alpha\beta}^{(m)}(t_0, t)$, is thus the number of times the individual leaves S_α for S_β before he reaches S_β at time t. The sums

(46)
$$\sum_{m=0}^{\infty} P_{\alpha\alpha}^{(m)}(t_0, t) = P_{\alpha\alpha}(t_0, t),$$
$$\sum_{m=1}^{\infty} P_{\alpha\beta}^{(m)}(t_0, t) = P_{\alpha\beta}(t_0, t), \qquad \alpha \neq \beta; \alpha, \beta = 1, 2,$$

are the probabilities that the individual will be at time t in S_α and S_β, respectively, regardless of the number of transitions he makes between t_0 and t. We assume that, for each τ, for $t_0 \leq \tau \leq t$, the derivatives

(47) $\left.\dfrac{\partial}{\partial t} P_{\alpha\alpha}(\tau, t)\right|_{t=\tau} = \nu_{\alpha\alpha}, \qquad \left.\dfrac{\partial}{\partial t} P_{\alpha\beta}(\tau, t)\right|_{t=\tau} = \nu_{\alpha\beta}$

exist and are independent of time τ, so that $\nu_{\alpha\alpha}$ is a negative constant and $\nu_{\alpha\beta}$ a positive constant. Explicit formulas of the probabilities $P_{\alpha\beta}^{(m)}(t_0, t)$ have been derived in terms of $\nu_{\alpha\alpha}$ and $\nu_{\alpha\beta}$ (see [2], Chapter 5).

Corresponding to equality (10) there are four equalities in the two dimensional process. They are

(48) $P_{\alpha\beta}^{(m)}(t_0, t) = \displaystyle\int_{t_0} P_{\alpha\alpha}^{(j)}(t_0, \tau)\nu_{\alpha\beta}P_{\beta\beta}^{(m-j-1)}(\tau, t)\, d\tau,$

(49) $P_{\alpha\beta}^{(m)}(t_0, t) = \displaystyle\int_{t_0}^{t} P_{\alpha\beta}^{(j)}(t_0, \tau)\nu_{\beta\alpha}P_{\alpha\beta}^{(m-j)}(\tau, t)\, d\tau,$

(50) $P_{\alpha\alpha}^{(m)}(t_0, t) = \displaystyle\int_{t_0}^{t} P_{\alpha\beta}^{(j)}(t_0, \tau)\nu_{\beta\alpha}P_{\alpha\alpha}^{(m-j)}(\tau, t)\, d\tau,$

and

(51) $P_{\alpha\alpha}^{(m)}(t_0, t) = \displaystyle\int_{t_0}^{t} P_{\alpha\alpha}^{(j)}(t_0, \tau)\nu_{\alpha\beta}P_{\beta\alpha}^{(m-j)}(\tau, t)\, d\tau,$

for any fixed but arbitrary j, for j between 0 and m. Equality (48), for example, holds for $j = 0, \cdots, m - 1$; while (49) holds for $j = 1, \cdots, m - 1$. These four equalities can be verified in a similar manner as equality (10). For the verification of the equality in (48), consider that an individual in state S_α at time t_0 will leave S_α m times and be in S_β at time t, and let j be a fixed number with $0 \leq j < m$. Let the $(j + 1)$th exit transition from S_α to S_β take place in

$(\tau, \tau + d\tau)$, so that at τ he is in state S_α, the remaining $m - j - 1$ transitions from S_β occurring during (τ, t); the probability of this sequence of events is

$$(52) \qquad P_{\alpha\alpha}^{(j)}(t_0, \tau)[\nu_{\alpha\beta}\, d\tau]P_{\beta\beta}^{(m-j-1)}(\tau, t).$$

Integrating (52) from $\tau = t_0$ to $\tau = t$ gives the equality in (48).

It has been shown in [2], pp. 102 to 104, that the multiple transition probabilities $P_{\alpha\beta}^{(m)}(t_0, t)$ and $P_{\alpha\alpha}^{(m)}(t_0, t)$ satisfy the equalities (48) through (51) for every m. Two simple cases are given below.

It is obvious that for $m = 0$,

$$(53) \qquad P_{\alpha\alpha}^{(0)}(t_0, t) = \exp\{\nu_{\alpha\alpha}(t - t_0)\}, \qquad P_{\beta\beta}^{(0)}(t_0, t) = \exp\{\nu_{\beta\beta}(t - t_0)\}.$$

For $m = 1$, $P_{\alpha\beta}^{(1)}(t_0, t)$ is the probability that exactly one transition from S_α to S_β occurs in (t_0, t), and $P_{\alpha\alpha}^{(1)}(t_0, t)$ is the first return probability to the original state S_α at t after having left S_α once. The first passage probability is given by

$$(54) \qquad P_{\alpha\beta}^{(1)}(t_0, t) = \frac{\nu_{\alpha\beta}}{\nu_{\alpha\alpha} - \nu_{\beta\beta}} (\exp\{\nu_{\alpha\alpha}(t - t_0)\} - \exp\{\nu_{\beta\beta}(t - t_0)\}), \qquad \alpha \neq \beta.$$

According to equality (48), we have

$$(55) \qquad P_{\alpha\beta}^{(1)}(t_0, t) = \int_{t_0}^{t} P_{\alpha\alpha}^{(0)}(t_0, \tau)\nu_{\alpha\beta}P_{\beta\beta}^{(0)}(\tau, t)\, d\tau,$$

or, substituting (53) and (54) in (55),

$$(56) \qquad \frac{\nu_{\alpha\beta}}{\nu_{\alpha\alpha} - \nu_{\beta\beta}} (\exp\{\nu_{\alpha\alpha}(t - t_0)\} - \exp\{\nu_{\beta\beta}(t - t_0)\})$$
$$= \int_{t_0}^{t} \exp\{\nu_{\alpha\alpha}(\tau - t_0)\}\nu_{\alpha\beta}\exp\{\nu_{\beta\beta}(t - \tau)\}\, d\tau,$$

which is easily shown to be true.

Equalities (48) and (50) (or (49) and (51)) can also be used to derive the general formulas for the probabilities $P_{\alpha\alpha}^{(m)}(t_0, t)$ and $P_{\alpha\beta}^{(m)}(t_0, t)$. The probability $P_{\alpha\beta}^{(1)}(t_0, t)$, if it is unknown, can be obtained from (55). Using the known probability $P_{\alpha\beta}^{(1)}(t_0, t)$, we can derive the first return probability $P_{\alpha\alpha}^{(1)}(t_0, t)$ from equality (50) for $m = 1$, $j = 1$,

$$(57) \qquad P_{\alpha\alpha}^{(1)}(t_0, t) = \int_{t_0}^{t} P_{\alpha\beta}^{(1)}(t_0, \tau)\nu_{\beta\alpha}P_{\alpha\alpha}^{(0)}(\tau, t)\, d\tau.$$

Substituting (56) for $P_{\alpha\beta}^{(1)}(t_0, \tau)$ and (53) for $P_{\alpha\alpha}^{(0)}(\tau, t)$ in (57) and integrating the resulting expression yields

$$(58) \quad P_{\alpha\alpha}^{(1)}(t_0, t) = \frac{\nu_{\alpha\beta}\nu_{\beta\alpha}}{(\nu_{\alpha\alpha} - \nu_{\beta\beta})^2} [(\nu_{\alpha\alpha} - \nu_{\beta\beta})(t - t_0)\exp\{\nu_{\alpha\alpha}(t - t_0)\}$$
$$- (\exp\{\nu_{\alpha\alpha}(t - t_0)\} - \exp\{\nu_{\beta\beta}(t - t_0)\})].$$

Now using equalities (48) and (50) successively for $m = 2$, we obtain the second passage probability

(59)

$$P_{\alpha\beta}^{(2)}(t_0, t) = \frac{\nu_{\alpha\beta}^2\nu_{\beta\alpha}}{(\nu_{\alpha\alpha} - \nu_{\beta\beta})^3} \left[(\nu_{\alpha\alpha} - \nu_{\beta\beta})(t - t_0)(\exp\{\nu_{\alpha\alpha}(t - t_0)\} + \exp\{\nu_{\beta\beta}(t - t_0)\}) \\ - 2(\exp\{\nu_{\alpha\alpha}(t - t_0)\} - \exp\{\nu_{\beta\beta}(t - t_0)\}) \right]$$

and the second return probability

$$(60) \quad P_{\alpha\alpha}^{(2)}(t_0, t) = \frac{\nu_{\alpha\beta}^2\nu_{\beta\alpha}^2}{(\nu_{\alpha\alpha} - \nu_{\beta\beta})^4} \left[\tfrac{1}{2}(\nu_{\alpha\alpha} - \nu_{\beta\beta})^2(t - t_0)^2 \exp\{\nu_{\alpha\alpha}(t - t_0)\} \right.$$

$$- (\nu_{\alpha\alpha} - \nu_{\beta\beta})(t - t_0)(2 \exp\{\nu_{\alpha\alpha}(t - t_0)\} + \exp\{\nu_{\beta\beta}(t - t_0)\})$$

$$\left. + 3(\exp\{\nu_{\alpha\alpha}(t - t_0)\} - \exp\{\nu_{\beta\beta}(t - t_0)\}) \right].$$

The probabilities $P_{\alpha\beta}^{(m)}(t_0, t)$ and $P_{\alpha\alpha}^{(m)}(t_0, t)$ can all be successively derived in the same manner beginning with $m = 3$. It is interesting to note that, using this approach, the multiple transition probabilities can be derived even when the intensity functions $\nu_{\alpha\alpha}(t)$ and $\nu_{\alpha\beta}(t)$ are functions of time.

REFERENCES

[1] N. T. J. BAILEY, "The simple stochastic epidemic: a complete solution in terms of known functions," *Biometrika*, Vol. 50 (1963), pp. 235–240.
[2] C. L. CHIANG, *Introduction to Stochastic Processes in Biostatistics*, New York, Wiley, 1968.
[3] K. L. CHUNG, *Markov Chains with Stationary Transition Probabilities*, New York, Springer-Verlag, 1967.
[4] L. G. DU PASQUIER, "Mathematische Theorie du Invaliditätsversicherung," *Mitt. Verein. Schweiz. Versich.-Math.*, Vol. 8 (1913), pp. 1–153.
[5] W. FELLER, *An Introduction to Probability Theory and Its Applications*, Vol. 1, New York, Wiley, 1968 (3rd ed.).
[6] E. FIX and J. NEYMAN, "A simple stochastic model for recovery, relapse, death and loss of patients," *Hum. Biol.*, Vol. 23 (1951), pp. 205–241.
[7] G. L. YANG and C. L. CHIANG, "A time dependent simple stochastic epidemic," *Proceedings of the Sixth Berkeley Symposium on Mathematical Statistics and Probability*, Berkeley and Los Angeles, University of California Press, 1972, Vol. 4, pp. 147–158.

A SYSTEMATIC APPROACH TO GRAPHICAL METHODS IN BIOMETRY

M. TARTER and S. RAMAN
UNIVERSITY OF CALIFORNIA, BERKELEY

1. Introduction

This paper deals with certain new graphical techniques which may be of value in exploratory biometry. In two senses, emphasis is placed upon the systematization of graphical procedures. One, a new theoretical result is obtained which gives conditions under which nonparametric histogram procedures of Parzen [11], Rosenblatt [13], Watson and Leadbetter [25], as well as others, can be treated as a special case of Fourier series methods of Cencov [2], Tarter and Kronmal [8], [19], [22], and Watson [24]. Two, by utilizing alternative weighted Fourier series, most hitherto considered graphical procedures such as the histogram, scatter diagram, and cumulative polygon are placed within a single computational framework. This systematization is shown to provide a researcher with both a comprehensive as well as a statistically and computationally efficient approach to graphical data analysis.

In Section 6 of this paper, an example of the graphical display of biomedical data is presented. The bivariate case, for example, generalizations of the scatter diagram, is considered in detail and the biomedical variable pair, bone age and chronological age, is used to demonstrate the application of this new graphical procedure.

Before proceeding to the sections of this paper that deal with the systematization and exemplification of graphical methods in biometry, it may be worthwhile to offer a brief explanation concerning what we consider to be the particular relevance of the *new* graphical procedures to biometry. By way of contrast, the following quotation ([1], p. 1), provides a clear exposition of the purpose underlying what might be called the *old* graphical procedures:

"Time after time it happens that some ignorant or presumptuous member of a committee or a board of directors will upset the carefully-thought-out plan of a man who knows the facts, simply because the man with the facts cannot present his facts readily enough to overcome the opposition. It is often with impotent exasperation that a person having the knowledge sees some fallacious

Research supported in part by small grant to faculty—Dr. M. Tarter General Research Support Grant 5 S01 RR5441-10.

199

conclusion accepted, or some wrong policy adopted, just because known facts cannot be marshalled and presented in such manner as to be effective."

This quotation clearly indicates that the primary function the older graphical methods were usually designed to fulfill was the summarization of information once this information had been obtained.

It is the contention of the authors that while the older methods emphasized the *expository*, the newer graphical methods place an emphasis on the *exploratory*. While it is certainly important for the biometrician or biostatistician to be able to *present* his "conclusions," the process of *reaching* these conclusions would now seem to be an equally important application of graphics.

Unquestionably, the major impetus leading to exploratory graphics has been the availability of high speed digital computation. In particular, recent developments involving the transmission of digitized graphical information over voice grade phone lines may substantially increase the potential for graphical presentation. Unlike the now fairly common IBM 2250 graphics configuration, which usually requires cathode ray tube (CRT) display units to be located within one hundred feet of a large central computer, the new IMLAC and other terminals will make interactive graphics economical for those with access only to a small computer or to a distant time shared computer system.

Before providing details of several new biostatistical graphic methods, one additional comment should be made. In a context where a new and substantially more powerful means of implementation becomes available, it may be of value to thoroughly reconsider traditional methods and the modes of thinking which engendered them and were engendered by them. The histogram, fractile diagram, scatter diagram, and other graphical tools were devised to meet certain specific goals and to cope with a narrow range of practical limitations. Today it is rarely necessary to group continuous data as a preliminary to the computation of sample moments (and then apply Sheppard's corrections). The construction of the traditional histogram based on the division of the range of the random variable into class intervals may be similarly reconsidered.

In the next section, the recent evolution of the histogram will be described. Fortunately, in this situation the methods which in our opinion are the most suitable for biostatistical graphics will be shown to include histogram procedures as a special case. However, it may not always be true that an elaboration of a conventional procedure is the most suitable alternative when matched with new means of implementation. For example, in Section 4, where an alternative to the fractile diagram is considered briefly, and in Section 6 which primarily concerns alternatives to the scatter diagram, it appears that the traditional graphical methods may be supplanted or at least supplemented by substantially different procedures.

2. Nonparametric and series graphical procedures

In this section, the symbolic or mathematical substructure of certain new graphical procedures will be presented. Following an heuristic introduction to the generalized histogram, a nonparametric procedure, introduced in [13] and investigated in [11], [25], [22], and others, it will be shown that for most practical purposes generalized histogram type nonparametric procedures can be treated as special cases of the series procedures, investigated in [2], [8], [22], and [24], as well as Schwartz [14]. Although this identity between nonparametric and series procedures was previously mentioned in [8], it was not explicitly presented, primarily because of the lack of a practical method for implementing this result. However, new procedures devised by Tarter and Fellner [18] have recently been found to make it practical and desirable to consider nonparametric procedures from a series point of view.

The process of constructing a typical "old style" histogram can be considered as consisting of two separate steps. In Step 1 (see Figure 1), the domain of

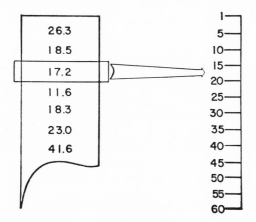

FIGURE 1

Step 1.

interest is divided into equally spaced class intervals and it is ascertained into which interval each data point is to be allocated. In Step 2 (see Figure 2), for each data point X_j, $j = 1, \cdots, n$, a *rectangular* block, with width equal to the class interval length h and with height equal to $(nh)^{-1}$ is added to the pile of blocks already piled within the class interval which contains X_j. It is apparent that Step 1, which is the geometrical analog of moment computation using a frequency table of grouped data, is necessary only if hand rather than machine calculation is used. It is more sensible and efficient to center the jth data point at the exact value assumed by X_j. The resulting irregularly packed pile of blocks can be easily "compressed" numerically by even the smallest digital computer (see Figure 3).

Once one revises Step 1, it is a simple matter to generalize Step 2 and consider alternatives to the rectangular shape of the blocks or counters that compile the contribution of the individual data points to the final graph of the density estimator $\hat{f}$ (see Figure 4).

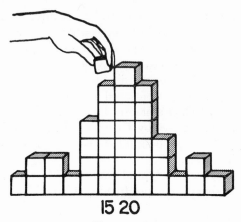

I5 20

FIGURE 2

Step 2.

At this point, it is advisable to switch from graphical to symbolic expression. Let $f(x)$ represent the joint probability density function of the p dimensional random variate column vectors $\{X_j\}, j = 1, \cdots, n$, where the X_j will be assumed to be independent and identically distributed. Let k represent an arbitrary column vector of integers or p-tuples and let N represent the set of all k. For a fixed sample size n, a generalized histogram $\hat{f}$, that is, nonparametric estimator of f [13], can be expressed as

$$(1) \qquad \hat{f}(x) = \frac{1}{n} \sum_{j=1}^{n} \delta_n(x - X_j).$$

If Step 1 but not Step 2 is revised so that the rectangular shape of each counter is retained but the jth counter is centered at X_j, then

$$(2) \qquad \delta_n(z) = \frac{I_H(z)}{h^p},$$

Contribution Centered at the Data Point

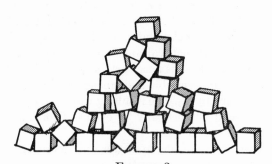

FIGURE 3

Improving Step 1.

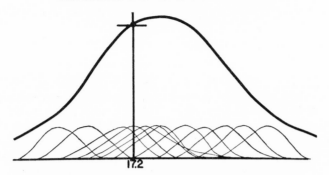

Contribution Distributed Over the Entire Range

FIGURE 4

Improving Step 2.

where H is a p dimensional rectangular parallelopiped within space E^p with diagonal corners $\pm(\tilde{x}_1, \tilde{x}_2, \cdots, \tilde{x}_p)$, where $\tilde{x}_k = h/2$ for all k and I_H represents the indicator function of H.

We will now show that a broad class of nonparametric estimators can be expressed as series estimators. The latter were introduced independently in [2], [8], [22], as well as [24]. This result is somewhat surprising since at least two authors, Schwartz [14] and Wegman [26], have stressed comparisons between nonparametric and series estimators and, hence, given the impression that there are fundamental mathematical and statistical differences between them. Theorem 1 tends to indicate that for almost all purposes, nonparametric and series estimators can be treated as being different forms of the same estimator. Thus, in our opinion, the choice between the two alternatives should be made solely on the basis of computational criteria.

THEOREM 1. *Assume that we are interested in the estimation of the multivariate density f over a finite subregion of the p dimensional Euclidean space. (Without loss of generality we will define the support of f to be the hypercube*

$$(3) \qquad U \equiv \{X: -\tfrac{1}{4} < X_s \leq \tfrac{1}{4}, s = 1, \cdots, p\},$$

where X_s is the sth component of X.) Assume that the p dimensional nonparametric kernel, as defined in expression (1) has a uniformly convergent Fourier expansion on the hypercube

$$(4) \qquad V = \{X: -\tfrac{1}{2} < X_s < \tfrac{1}{2}, s = 1, \cdots, p\}$$

of the form

$$(5) \qquad \delta_n(X) \equiv \sum_{k \in N} b_k \exp\{2\pi i k'(X - R)\},$$

where $R' = (-\tfrac{1}{2}, \cdots, -\tfrac{1}{2})$. Then at every point X of the support region of f, the "nonparametric" estimator $\hat{f}$ defined by expression (1) is identical to the "series" estimator

(6) $$\sum_{k \in N} \hat{B}_k b_k \exp \{2\pi i k'(X - R)\},$$

where

(7) $$\hat{B}_k = n^{-1} \sum_{j=1}^{n} \exp \{-2\pi i k'(X_j - R)\}.$$

The proof of Theorem 1 is obtained through simple algebraic substitution and interchange of the order of summation. It is, of course, not necessary to expand δ about the point R. However, expansion about R helps to establish the identity between expression (7) and the definition of $\hat{B}_k$ given in [22]. (In the remaining sections of this paper we will use the earlier definition, that is, omit R and assume V to be the usual unit hypercube.) It might also be noted that if the function $\tilde{f}$ is defined as

(8) $$\tilde{f}(X) = \begin{cases} 1/n & \text{if } X = X_j, \ j = 1, \cdots, n, \\ 0 & \text{otherwise,} \end{cases}$$

then the Fourier series associated with $\tilde{f}$ is

(9) $$\tilde{f}(X) \sim \sum_{k \in N} \hat{B}_k \exp \{2\pi i k'(X - R)\}$$

and

(10) $$\hat{f}(X) = \int_V \tilde{f}(Z) \, \delta_n(X - Z) \, dZ,$$

where the integral is taken in the Lebesgue-Stieltjes sense. Hence, $\hat{f}$ can be considered to be the convolution of $\tilde{f}$ with δ_n.

Now define the Fourier coefficient of the density f as

(11) $$B_k = \int_V \exp \{-2\pi i k'(X - R)\} f(X) \, dX$$

and the usual goodness of fit criterion [22], [25], mean integrated square error (MISE), as

(12) $$J = E \int_V |f(X) - \hat{f}(X)|^2 \, dX.$$

By simple algebraic manipulation as in [24] and [18], one finds that the MISE of nonparametric-series estimator $\hat{f}$ equals

(13) $$J(f, \hat{f}) = \sum_{k \in N} \{n^{-1}|b_k|^2(1 - |B_k|^2) + |1 - b_k|^2|B_k|^2\}.$$

Consequently, for f and δ as defined in the statement of Theorem 1, the problem of optimal choice of the "best" kernel δ is identical to the problem of choice of "best" weights, $b_k = b_k^{\text{opt}}$, in expression (6). This problem has been considered in [24] as well as [18] with the result that

(14) $$b_k^{\text{opt}} = \frac{n|B_k|^2}{1 + (n - 1)|B_k|^2}.$$

The estimation of b_k^{opt} is considered separately by Fellner and Tarter in [18], where an estimator

(15) $$\hat{b}_k^{\text{opt}} = \frac{n}{n - 1} - \frac{1}{(n - 1)|\hat{B}_k|^2}$$

is derived as an analog to the inclusion rule for the choice of $b_k = 0$ or 1 investigated in [22].

3. Computational considerations

It is not usually feasible to directly apply the series estimator derived in Theorem 1. For biomedical and other applications, graphical procedures must be considered from computational as well as statistical points of view. While optimum weights (14) are estimable from given data, it is impractical to compute more than a moderate number of these coefficients. On the other hand, the estimators considered in [22] result in a very simple inclusion rule, namely, include the coefficient B_k if and only if

$$(16) \qquad |B_k|^2 > \frac{1}{n+1},$$

which is the dichotomous analog of weight (14) or, in the usual situation where B_k is unknown, use

$$(17) \qquad |\hat{B}_k|^2 > \frac{2}{n+1},$$

which is the dichotomous analog of weight (15).

Furthermore, since the asymptotically optimal kernel is the Dirac δ function (see [24]), the above procedure approaches optimality, that is, the MISE approaches zero as n approaches infinity. Investigations with real data by Raman [12] indicate that satisfactory results may be obtained by using the above technique with sample size as low as 45 pairs of observations to estimate certain bivariate distributions.

In contradistinction to series methods, the use of nonparametric estimates of form (1) for graphical purposes requires that the entire file of data points be either stored or reentered into the computer in order to graph $\hat{f}$ at each specific value of x. Since the estimator $\hat{B}_k$ and the inclusion rule (17) are symmetric functions of the observations, there is no need to allocate memory space in the computer for the storage of data. On heuristic considerations, we propose as a stopping rule the termination of the search for a subsequence of coefficients (in the bivariate case) as soon as two consecutive coefficients become negligible in a horizontal and vertical scan of the array of coefficients.

Since the inclusion rule is the same for B_k and B_{-k}, it becomes necessary to compute and store the real and imaginary parts of only half the total number of coefficients. This again results in saving of computer memory and time.

To further optimize the running time, we test the coefficients by the inclusion and stopping rule after reading each set of 100 data points. Since the observations are assumed independent, these intermediate estimates are unbiased. However, to be conservative we perform the test with the final sample size substituted for n in the right side of inequality (17).

In a typical example with 1000 pairs of observations from a 50 per cent mixture of Gaussian distributions, the computation of the Fourier coefficients took about nine minutes on an IBM 1130. The computational advantage of the method will be evident by noting that in the above situation, the first 100 observations took three minutes, the second 100 took one and a half minutes, the third 100 took one minute, the fourth and the rest took half a minute each. Moreover, the economy of summarizing the characteristic density by the series technique can be appreciated by noting that the number of coefficients needed in the above situation was only 23. Studies performed by Kronmal and Tarter [8] have shown that the number of parameters required in the univariate case is less than fifteen for most distributions, sample sizes, and intervals of estimation.

Besides the advantage of series forms that is related to the condensation of statistical information into a relatively few estimators, one might note a second closely related computational property possessed by most series procedures and, in particular, by expression (6). The statistics $\hat{B}_k$ are symmetric functions of the observations and, hence, can be computed iteratively.

The utility of the iterative computation of $\hat{B}_k$ is best illustrated by the application of univariate modifications of expression (6) to the problem of estimating a cumulative distribution function. Consider that the process of graphing the sample cumulative is almost identical to the process of ranking the data points. This has led to investigations [8] and [21] which deal with the use of series estimators as replacements for the sample cumulative.

In the next section, a general result is derived for which a special case, related to estimation of the cumulative distribution function, has been considered by Kronmal and Tarter [8]. It has been shown ([8], Section 7) that the same subset of indices M, minimizes the MISE of estimator $\hat{F}_M$ that minimizes the MISE of density estimator $\hat{f}_M$. Specifically, in the notation of this paper, letting $p = 1$, and $\bar{x}$ represent the sample mean, and defining density estimator $\hat{f}_M$ and cumulative estimator $\hat{F}_M$, respectively, as

$$(18) \qquad \hat{f}_M(x) = 1 + \sum_{k \in M} \hat{B}_k \exp\{2\pi ikx\}$$

and

$$(19) \qquad \hat{F}_{M'}(x) = (\tfrac{1}{2} + x - \bar{x}) + \sum_{k \in M'} (2\pi ik)^{-1} \hat{B}_k \exp\{2\pi ikx\},$$

where $0 \notin M$ or M', then if goodness of fit is measured in terms of MISE, the set M should equal the set M'. Note that one can treat the term

$$(20) \qquad \sum_{k \in M'} (2\pi ik)^{-1} \hat{B}_k \exp\{2\pi ikx\}$$

of expression (19) as a special case of the general series estimator defined by expression (6), where

$$(21) \qquad b_k = \begin{cases} (2\pi ik)^{-1} & \text{if} \quad k \in M', \\ 0 & \text{otherwise.} \end{cases}$$

4. Weighted series estimators of functions derived from the density

In Sections 4 and 5, the choice of specific predetermined sequences of b_k will be considered from the following two points of view. One, the researcher may wish to obtain an estimate of a distribution *density* which possesses certain desirable mathematical or statistical properties. (Weights chosen for this purpose will be considered in Section 5.) For example, one may wish to constrain a density estimator to be nonnegative. Two, the target of the estimation process, rather than the density itself, may be a function derived from the density. For example, as previously discussed, one may wish to estimate and graph the cumulative distribution function. In this section, we will consider approaches to the latter class of problems which may be desirable from both a computational and statistical point of view.

It may be of value to distinguish between the previously described two classes of problems by examining the MISE criteria associated with estimates of the *density* as opposed to the MISE between a statistical construct *derived* from a density and alternative estimates of this construct. If this latter construct can be expressed as a weighted sum of the coefficients of the Fourier series expansion of the density, then the following result applies.

THEOREM 2. *Define*

$$(22) \qquad g(x) \equiv \sum_{k \in N} b_k B_k \exp \{2\pi i k' x\}$$

and

$$(23) \qquad \hat{g}(x) \equiv \sum_{k \in M} b_k \hat{B}_k \exp \{2\pi i k' x\},$$

where $\{b_k\}$, $k \in N$, is a preselected sequence of complex valued constants, N, B_k and $\hat{B}_k$ are as defined in Section 2, and $M \subseteq N$. Then the same set M minimizes the MISE $J(g, \hat{g})$ for all sequences $\{b_k\}$.

PROOF. From Theorem 1 of [22], one finds that

$$(24) \qquad J(g, \hat{g}) = \sum_{k \in M} \text{Var} \, (b_k \hat{B}_k) + \sum_{k \in (N \cap \overline{M})} b_k^2 |B_k|^2.$$

Therefore, the error increment ΔJ_{k_0} due to adding a term $k_0 \in M$ (as defined in Corollary 2 [22]) equals

$$(25) \qquad b_k^2 ((\text{Var} \, \hat{B}_k) - |B_k|^2).$$

Theorem 2 follows from the observation that for all nonzero b_k, the sign of expression (25) is identical to the sign of

$$(26) \qquad (\text{Var} \, \hat{B}_k) - |B_k|^2.$$

It is easily seen that estimates of density derivatives can be obtained, for which Theorem 2 applies. Also, consider the problem of estimating the function

$$(27) \qquad g(x) = f(x) + C \frac{\partial f(x)}{\partial x_s},$$

which may (at least in the univariate case) be of value in empirical Bayes investigations (here x_s is the sth component of the vector x). To estimate $g(x)$, one might choose estimator $\hat{g}(x)$ of expression (23) with

$$(28) \qquad\qquad b_k = 1 + 2\pi i C k_s,$$

where k_s is the sth component of p-tuple k. If MISE is chosen as the measure of fit of $\hat{g}$ to g, then Theorem 2 implies that M can be determined by means of inclusion rule (17). Naturally, it is also possible to modify "Fellner weights" (15) to obtain a more statistically efficient estimator of expression (27). The decision of whether to use an inclusion rule or a weighting procedure should, of course, take into account computational as well as statistical properties of the alternative procedures.

A function derived from the density, which differs substantially from the integrals or derivatives of f, will be considered in the remainder of this section. Define $g^{(\lambda)}(x)$ as a univariate special case of expression (22) with

$$(29) \qquad\qquad b_k = \exp\{2(\pi k\lambda)^2\}.$$

Consider the following special case of the Fourier coefficients B_k of density f,

$$(30) \qquad\qquad B_k = \sum_{s=1}^{c} p_s \exp\{2\pi k\mu_s - 2(\pi k\sigma_s)^2\}.$$

If all values of μ_s and σ_s are sufficiently small, then f closely approximates a superposition of c Gaussian densities with component means equal to $\{\mu_s\}$, $s = 1, \cdots, c$, component standard deviations equal to $\{\sigma_s\}$, $s = 1, \cdots, c$, and mixing parameters $\{p_s\}$, $s = 1, \cdots, c$. Moreover, assuming $\lambda < \sigma_s$ for all s, the function $g^{(\lambda)}(x)$ closely approximates a superposition of Gaussian densities which differs from $f(x)$ only in that the set of component variances equals

$$(31) \qquad\qquad \{(\sigma_s^2 - \lambda^2)\}, \qquad\qquad s = 1, \cdots, c.$$

Thus, if $\hat{B}_k$ is obtained from independent and identically distributed data arising from a superposition of c Gaussian densities, one can estimate $g^{(\lambda)}(x)$ by substituting the special case of b_k given by expression (29) into expression (23) and then determining the set M by means of inclusion rule (17).

It may be of interest to mention that a very slight modification of the method of decomposing superpositions described above can be shown to be identical to a particular form of nonparametric density estimation procedure considered in [11] (see p. 1068) and elsewhere. From expression (5), one finds that

$$(32) \qquad\qquad b_k = \int_V \delta(x) \exp\{-2\pi i k'(x - R)\}\, dx.$$

If one considers the univariate Gaussian kernel δ (see [11], p. 1068), one finds that b_k of expression (32), that is, a constant times the Gaussian characteristic function evaluated at $t = -2\pi k$, is identical to expression (29) with $\lambda = \sigma i$ (where σ is the standard deviation of the Gaussian kernel). Hence, the method for decomposing superpositions of distribution functions described in this section and considered from other points of view in [3], [4], [7], [9], [10], and [15] is closely connected to the nonparametric method for estimating densities based upon Gaussian kernels. In fact, as M approaches N the specific series estimator $\hat{g}$ with b_k given in expression (29), which is used to decompose superpositions of Gaussian densities, approaches the specific nonparametric estimator (1) with δ_n set equal to a complex Gaussian function with $\mu = 0$ and $\sigma = \lambda i$. Interestingly, this particular choice of δ *reduces* the variances of superimposed Gaussian components while a choice of δ with a real positive variance can be shown from expression (10) to cause the variance of the density estimate to be greater than that of the density which is estimated.

Although functions of form g of expression (22) are of interest and of practical value in biomedical investigations, the display of composite functions, especially transgenerations of f and F are probably of primary biomedical utility (at least in the univariate case). Consider, for example, the ratio of $f(x)$ to the survival curve $1 - F(x)$, that is, the hazard function or, in some applications, the age specific death rate.

It would not be appropriate to give an extensive survey of composite graphical functions here, and hence, the remaining sections of the paper will deal with a discussion and examples of the use of $\hat{g}$ with various choices of b_k for the purpose of estimating a multivariate *density*. However, before leaving the topic of composite functions and statistical constructs derived from the density, two general comments seem appropriate.

One, the inclusion rule given by Theorem 2 applies to derived functions g of expression (20). Composite functions such as the hazard, fractile [6], confidence band [16], transformation selection [20], [17] functions may make use of combinations of derived functions $\hat{g}$. However, there is no guarantee that the particular choices of $\hat{g}$ which are optimal (even in the weak sense of inclusion rule (16)) for the purpose of estimating various choices of g *singly* will, when combined to form a composite estimate, be optimal.

Two, the computational convenience of the various estimators, which can be put into form $\hat{g}$, makes it feasible to try new and more complex composite functions. For example, Tarter and Kowalski [20] have found graphs of the function

$$(33) \qquad \frac{\phi \Phi^{-1} \hat{F}(x)}{\hat{f}(x)}$$

(where ϕ and Φ represent the standard Gaussian and $\hat{f}$ and $\hat{F}$ the estimated unknown density and cumulative) to be superior in many instances to the usual fractile diagram for the purpose of selecting a transformation of data to normality.

5. Series density estimators utilizing a predetermined sequence of weights

In this section a hybrid form of density estimator will be taken up. Consider the case where one is interested in density estimates that are constrained to satisfy certain mathematical properties, for example, be nonnegative. Alter-

natively, suppose that one wishes to find a computationally convenient estimator that corresponds as closely as possible to a conventional statistical form,
for example, a histogram that utilizes rectangular blocks. We will consider in
this section a hybrid or compromise technique that tends to retain certain
of the above prespecified mathematical properties while it approaches the statistical and computational efficiency of the series estimators introduced in Section 2.

Consider a specific nonparametric estimator, or equivalently, a series estimator
$\hat{g}$ with coefficients b_k chosen to satisfy some mathematical constraint. For example, let $\hat{f}$ be defined by expression (1) with δ_n given by expression (2). Here

$$(34) \qquad\qquad b_k = \frac{\sin \pi k' h}{\pi k' h}.$$

Alternatively, if one wishes to estimate a density f with an estimator $\hat{f}$ that is
constrained to be nonnegative one might, in the univariate case, choose coefficients b_k to be the Fejer weights

$$(35) \qquad\qquad b_k = \begin{cases} \left(1 - \dfrac{k}{m+1}\right) & \text{if } |k| \leq m, \\ 0 & \text{elsewhere,} \end{cases}$$

where m is some predetermined constant. Fejer forms of series estimators are
considered in the univariate case in [8] and in the multivariate case in [16].

This section deals with density estimators $\hat{g}$ of form (23) with predetermined
sequences of weights b_k, for example, as given in expressions (34) or (35). Theorem 3 concerns the choice of an appropriate inclusion rule (choice of set M)
for such density estimators.

THEOREM 3. *Let δ be any prespecified kernel whose Fourier expansion (assumed, as in Theorem 1, to converge in V) generates the weight sequence $\{b_k\}$.
Then the weighted series estimator $\hat{g}$ of form (21), chosen so that an index $k_0 \in M$
if and only if*

$$(36) \qquad n^{-1}|b_{k_0}|^2 < |B_{k_0}|^2(1 + n^{-1}|b_{k_0}|^2 - |1 - b_{k_0}|^2),$$

*has at least as small a MISE as the nonparametric estimator obtained by substituting
δ into expression (1).*

The proof of Theorem 3 follows directly from MISE expression (13). Note
that if we assume that δ is a symmetric kernel, then the b_k are all real and the
above inequality reduces to

$$(37) \qquad\qquad b_k < \frac{2n|B_k|^2}{1 + (n-1)|B_k|^2},$$

which is equivalent to

$$(38) \qquad\qquad b_k < 2b_k^{\text{opt}}$$

(see expression (14)).

An alternative interpretation of inclusion rule (37) can be obtained as follows.
Define $\delta^{\text{opt}}(z)$ by using the values of b_k^{opt} given in expression (14) as the coefficients of the Fourier expansion of $\delta^{\text{opt}}(z)$ (see expression (5)). Consider that by

Parseval's theorem the integrated square error ISE between δ and δ^{opt}, that is, $\int (\delta(z) - \delta^{\mathrm{opt}}(z))^2 \, dz$, equals $\sum_{k \in N} (b_k - b_k^{\mathrm{opt}})^2$. Hence, to minimize the ISE one should include index k in the set M if and only if $(b_k - b_k^{\mathrm{opt}})^2 < (b_k^{\mathrm{opt}})^2$, that is, if $b_k < 2b_k^{\mathrm{opt}}$, which is identical to inequality (38).

It is, of course, necessary to check whether estimate $\hat{g}$, to which the above inclusion rule is applied, retains the mathematical properties of the nonparametric estimators based upon δ. However, empirical studies with prespecified sequences of b_k, for example, Fejer weights (35), have tended to show that guaranteed possession of "mathematical" property, for example, nonnegativity, can usually be purchased only with an unacceptable increase in MISE. Thus, the hybrid procedures considered in this section may offer a reasonable compromise in certain applications.

While the choice of prespecified Fejer weight sequence (35) in conjunction with inclusion rule (38) appears to be a useful graphical method, we are not at all certain of the value of prespecified sequences of b_k, as given by expressions (34) and (29), for the purpose of density estimation. Like most procedures which arise from nonparametric estimator (1), the effective use of weights (34) and (29) depends on the estimation of at least one parameter, for weight (34) the class interval length h and for weight (29) the kernel standard deviation λ. Although it is, of course, possible to estimate the parameters of "prespecified" b_k by fitting b_k, considered as a function of h or λ, to b_k^{opt}, this seems to be a roundabout way of handling the estimation problem. Hence, in the example which will be considered in the next section, estimation is implemented from the series point of view, using the computational procedures described in Section 3.

6. Biomedical application

In this section, we consider a specific application of the computational methods outlined in Section 3, for estimating a bivariate density.

The basic data used in these calculations were measurements of chronological age and bone age of children included in the Child Development Studies (Kaiser Foundation, Oakland, California). The children included were a 10 per cent sample, stratified by sex, race, and height (classified as tall, medium, short). For purposes of illustration, we have included here the data for white males of medium height. The particular bone selected is hamate and the bone ages are determined by matching the X-ray picture of the child with the standard radiological atlas prepared by Gruelich and Pyle [5]. The values read in are close to within three months of the actual bone age since the graduation of the atlas is in intervals of three months.

The program computes the bivariate probability density nonparametrically from the data, using the technique of Fourier approximation of multivariate densities (see [22]). The x variable is the chronological age in months and the y variable is the bone age in months. The lower and upper limits are obtained by calculating the maximum and minimum values and choosing the closest number in tenths. Table I gives the Fourier coefficients calculated from the data for the upper half plane. The values for the lower half plane can be obtained as conjugates of the values on the upper half plane.

TABLE I

HAMATE BONE AGE STUDY, GROUP II: WHITE MALES, MEDIUM HEIGHT
X lower = 30.0, X upper = 130.0, Y lower = 20.0,
Y upper = 130.0. Number of observations = 98.

X coord	Y coord	Fourier coefficients (upper half plane) Real	Imaginary
−3	1	−0.16353922E−04	0.79695746E−05
−3	2	−0.11921363E−04	−0.73126666E−05
−2	0	−0.26822795E−04	0.13461094E−04
−2	1	−0.16394707E−04	−0.22885004E−04
−2	2	0.40507031E−04	−0.24095239E−04
−1	0	−0.17124028E−04	−0.31696021E−04
−1	1	0.75077390E−04	−0.18168164E−04
−1	2	−0.22633103E−05	0.23782737E−04
0	0	0.90909103E−04	0.00000000E 00
0	1	−0.12383168E−04	0.32439042E−04
0	2	−0.18815233E−04	−0.34065936E−06
0	3	−0.13230197E−04	−0.13690030E−04
1	0	−0.17124028E−04	0.31696021E−04
1	1	−0.27838021E−04	−0.83455852E−05
1	2	−0.52113328E−05	−0.19308896E−04
2	0	−0.26822795E−04	−0.13461094E−04
2	1	0.41055191E−05	−0.16014244E−04

Table II shows the bivariate probability density calculated from the Fourier coefficients for the grid of points within the specified limits. The corresponding scatter diagram for these limits are shown in Table III. The limits chosen for the display of scatter diagram and bivariate density are not the same as the ones used for the calculation of the Fourier coefficients, which accounts for the discrepancy in the number of observations shown on the scatter diagram. Since total probability density is always unity, the appropriate actual density height in Table II can be obtained by dividing the number shown by the scale factor given in the title.

For ease of visualization, the table was converted to a contour diagram which is shown in Table IV. In the preparation of this table, numbers to be displayed were truncated to tenths. The table displays only those numbers starting with even second digits which are greater than or equal to 20.

By abstracting the essential features of the scatter diagram, the contour chart clearly exhibits distributional features of the data. For example, Table IV indicates the possible decomposition of the data into a bivariate normal distribution and a degenerate uniform distribution.

TABLE II

BIVARIATE PROBABILITY DENSITY (TIMES 110,000)

HAMATE BONE AGE STUDY, GROUP II: WHITE MALES, MEDIUM HEIGHT

Number of observations = 98.

Bone age in months	Age in months 35	52	69	86	103	120
130						9 12
126						11 18
123						14 25
119						18 32
115						21 37
112					8	22 40
108					8 20 15	21 40
104				9	25 35 32	17 35
101				11 25	45 51 45	12 27
97				16 24 37	65 68 59	5 17
93			6	20 38 47	82 82 74	0 7
90			9 5	24 41 54	89 93 84	0 0
86			14 11 9	27 42 57	90 97 88	0 0
82			20 18 18	31 41 57	82 93 85	0 0
79		5	25 25 26	33 39 54	69 82 76	0 0
75		8 5	30 28 31	36 36 49	52 66 64	0 0
71		14 9 5	31 30 31	35 31 42	41 49 50	5 5
68		18 13 7	31 31 31	31 26 35	31 32 36	5 5
64		18 15 9	28 30 30	26 21 26	21 17 24	0 0
60	5	18 16 10	25 28 25	23 13 18	11 7 13	0 0
57	6	16 16 11	24 25 17	20 10	5 5	0 0
53	9	14 17 13	22 18 8	15 7	6 5	0 0
49	8 13	12 18 16	18 12 5	7 0	0 5	0 0
46	13 16	11 20 17	16 9	8	0 6	0 0
42	17 19	11 22 22	14 7	10 5	0 8	0 0
38	19 21	9 22 21	12 6	9 6	7 9	5 0
35	17 21	7 22 18	11	9 8	8 9	7 0
31	12 16	0 21 13	9	9 9	9 6	7 7
27	6 10	0 18 7	6	7 5	5	8 7
24	0 0	0 13 0		6 6	6	0
20	0 0	0 7 0		6	6	0

TABLE III

SCATTER DIAGRAM

HAMATE BONE AGE STUDY, GROUP II: WHITE MALES, MEDIUM HEIGHT

Number of observations = 96.

Bone age in months	____ Age in months ____					
	35	52	69	86	103	120
130						
126					1	
123					2	
119					1	2
115					1 3	
112				4 1	1	
108				2 3		
104				1 1	2 3	
101				2 1 1 4	1 1	
97				1 2		
93				1 1 2 1	2 1	
90				1 1 1		
86			1 1 1 1			
82			1 1 1 1			
79			2 1 1 2			
75			1 1 1			
71	1		1 1			
68		1 1 1				
64		1 1 2 1				
60		1				
57		1 1				
53		1				
49	1	1				
46						
42	1	1				
38	2	1				
35	1	1				
31	1 1					
27						
24		1				
20						

TABLE IV

CONTOURS OF PROBABILITY DENSITY (TIMES 110,000)

HAMATE BONE AGE STUDY, GROUP II: WHITE MALES, MEDIUM HEIGHT

Number of observations = 98. Values below 20 have been suppressed.

Bone age in months	\	\	Age in months	\	\	\
	35	52	69	86	103	120
130						
126						20
123					20	20
119					40	40
115					60	40
112				20	80	60
108				40	80	40
104				60	80	40
101				80	60	40
97				80	40	20
93			20	80	20	
90			20	60		
86			40	40		
82			40	40		
79			40	20		
75			20	20		
71		20	20			
68		20	20			
64		20	20			
60		20	20			
57		20	20			
53		20	20			
49		20	20			
46	20	20				
42	20	20				
38	20	20				
35	20	20				
31	20	20				
27	20					
24	20					
20	20					

TABLE V

Conditional Probability Density
Hamate Bone Age Study, Group II: White Males, Medium Height
Number of observations = 98.

Age in months

Bone age in months	35	52	69	86	103	120
130						4
126					1	6
123					3	7
119				2	5	9
115				4	8	10
112				6	10	11
108				7	12	9
104				8	12	6
101				9	12	2
97				9	10	
93				9	8	
90				8	6	
86			2	8	4	
82			4	6	2	
79			6	5		
75			8	3		
71			11	1		
68		3	14			
64		5	15			
60		7	14			
57		8	12			
53		8	9			
49	8	8	6			
46	14	7	3			
42	18	7				
38	20	7				
35	18	7				
31	13	6				
27	6	6				
24		5				
20		3				

Table V shows the empirical conditional probability distribution $\hat{f}(Y|X)$ (obtained by dividing the bivariate probability density by the marginal density).

Also shown, in Table VI, are the estimated regression $E(Y|X)$, the standard deviation, mode, median, and the two quartiles of $\hat{f}(Y|X)$.

TABLE VI

ESTIMATED MODE, QUARTILES, MEDIAN, REGRESSION, CONDITIONAL STANDARD
DEVIATION, VARIANCE, AND CORRECTION

X	Mode	$Q(1)$	$Q(3)$	Median	$E(Y|X)$	S.D.	$V(Y|X)$	Correction
35.0	34.6	31.7	36.8	34.3	35.0	6.1	38.20	0
38.4	34.6	31.6	42.9	33.6	35.7	6.9	47.79	2
41.8	34.6	31.5	42.2	33.3	36.1	7.2	52.19	5
45.2	34.5	30.0	44.2	37.8	43.4	20.7	432.55	1
48.6	38.3	34.7	55.1	47.4	49.3	21.7	473.22	0
52.0	38.3	39.6	59.0	50.6	49.3	14.8	220.58	2
55.4	64.0	41.9	62.2	51.2	53.9	14.2	202.41	1
58.8	63.9	49.3	66.2	60.2	58.8	13.0	171.01	0
62.2	67.7	56.5	71.1	63.4	63.8	9.9	99.70	−1
65.6	67.6	60.3	69.7	68.5	66.5	8.3	69.52	0
69.0	67.5	65.4	75.8	66.9	68.2	7.6	58.18	0
72.4	71.4	63.3	73.9	72.2	70.4	7.4	55.68	1
75.8	71.2	68.7	79.1	70.3	72.3	7.5	57.16	3
79.2	75.0	66.7	81.5	74.3	74.2	14.2	203.40	4
82.6	78.6	70.7	88.1	83.3	78.9	18.4	339.89	3
86.0	89.6	73.2	96.8	84.7	84.3	18.6	346.65	1
89.4	97.0	82.7	100.1	94.5	89.4	17.3	301.94	0
92.8	96.9	85.2	104.2	97.9	94.1	15.1	230.55	−1
96.2	100.6	89.2	109.1	102.4	97.4	13.8	190.81	−1
99.6	104.4	93.2	106.7	99.7	101.1	10.6	114.47	−1
103.0	104.3	98.0	111.9	104.8	103.5	10.4	109.38	0
106.4	104.2	95.7	110.1	102.8	105.6	10.1	102.50	0
109.8	108.0	100.8	115.3	108.1	107.8	9.9	99.85	1
113.2	107.9	105.9	113.6	106.2	109.9	9.6	93.53	3
116.6	111.7	104.9	119.6	112.3	108.7	17.5	307.17	7
120.0	111.6	101.4	119.7	113.3	98.2	32.1	1032.62	21

Biologically, for the average normal child the bone age should be the same as the chronological age. In practice, however, there are sources of error due to observer bias. Further, the atlas on which the assessments are based was calibrated 40 years ago and, hence, the possibility of a secular trend on the osteological maturation of California's children cannot be ruled out. Consequently, a correction at each age to within three months can be obtained from the difference of the chronological age and the regression estimate shown in the last column of Table VI. After applying the correction to the original data, we then recomputed the bivariate distribution. The corresponding results are shown in Tables VII, VIII, and IX. It can be seen from Table X that the second order corrections are now negligible, at least at those levels where there are observations. Further, the contour chart after the correction shows a sharper segregation of the com-

TABLE VII

BIVARIATE PROBABILITY DENSITY (TIMES 110,000)
HAMATE BONE AGE STUDY, GROUP II: WHITE MALES, MEDIUM HEIGHT
Number of observations = 98.

Age in months

Bone age in months	35			52			69			86			103			120
130													8	10	10	6
126												17	21	20	16	9
123											10	34	36	32	24	13
119										18	28	54	52	45	32	17
115										37	48	71	67	55	38	21
112									8	58	68	85	76	61	42	23
108								11	24	76	85	92	79	61	41	19
104								26	43	89	95	91	76	56	36	13
101								42	60	95	98	82	65	46	27	6
97								55	75	94	92	68	51	33	17	
93								65	84	85	80	50	34	19	7	
90								70	86	72	64	32	19	7		
86							9	66	82	56	46	17	6			
82						6	18	59	73	40	29	5				
79					7	11	27	50	61	26	15					
75				6	13	16	32	41	48	14	5					
71				11	18	21	35	32	35	5						
68			7	15	22	25	33	22	23							
64		8	13	18	25	28	30	14	14							
60	5	14	17	21	25	30	24	6	6							
57	9	20	21	22	23	29	18									
53	14	24	24	22	20	26	11									
49	18	25	25	20	16	21	7									
46	19	23	23	17	13	16										
42	17	18	18	14	10	11										
38	12	15	13	11	7	6										
35	9	8	9	9	5											
31	5	5														
27																
24																
20																

TABLE VIII

SCATTER DIAGRAM

HAMATE BONE AGE STUDY, GROUP II: WHITE MALES, MEDIUM HEIGHT

Number of observations = 96.

TABLE IX

Contours of Probability Density (Times 110,000)

Hamate Bone Age Study, Group II: White Males, Medium Height

Number of observations = 98. Values below 20 have been suppressed.

Age in months

Bone age in months	35	52	69	86	103	120
130					20	20
126					20	20
123					40	20
119					60	40
115					60	40
112				80	80	60
108				80	80	60
104				60	80	
101				60	80	40
97				80	60	40
93				80	60	20
90			20	60	40	
86			20	40	40	
82			20	40	20	
79		20	20	20	20	
75		20	20	20		
71		20	20			
68		20	20	20		
64		20	20	20		
60		20	20	20		
57		20	20			
53		20	20			
49		20				
46		20				
42	20	20				
38	20	20				
35	20	20				
31	20	20				
27						
24						
20						

TABLE X

ESTIMATED MODE, QUARTILES, MEDIAN, REGRESSION, CONDITIONAL STANDARD
DEVIATION, VARIANCE, AND CORRECTION

X	Mode	$Q(1)$	$Q(3)$	Median	$E(Y|X)$	S.D.	$V(Y|X)$	Correction
35.0	34.6	31.4	36.6	34.0	35.2	6.1	37.78	0
38.4	34.6	31.6	42.9	33.6	35.7	6.9	47.71	2
41.8	34.6	31.5	41.8	33.2	39.2	18.9	359.02	2
45.2	34.6	31.2	40.2	39.6	40.8	20.3	414.60	4
48.6	34.5	36.1	58.1	42.3	46.6	20.3	415.92	1
52.0	38.3	33.7	65.7	44.9	48.7	15.6	244.81	3
55.4	67.7	36.5	67.9	51.2	53.8	15.9	253.14	1
58.8	67.6	49.3	72.3	59.0	59.4	13.7	187.86	0
62.2	67.6	55.3	70.3	62.3	64.7	9.9	98.65	−2
65.6	67.6	59.6	76.7	68.0	67.0	8.2	67.57	−1
69.0	67.5	65.3	75.8	66.9	68.3	7.5	57.15	0
72.4	71.4	63.7	74.7	72.9	69.6	7.0	49.84	2
75.8	71.3	62.1	80.1	71.2	71.4	7.5	56.62	4
79.2	75.0	68.1	77.3	76.4	72.1	12.4	154.25	7
82.6	74.9	72.7	84.8	79.1	76.7	16.4	271.27	5
86.0	82.3	75.2	98.4	86.9	82.9	18.2	334.86	3
89.4	93.3	76.9	100.4	88.1	88.6	17.4	304.33	0
92.8	96.9	85.9	104.0	98.0	93.9	15.4	237.68	−1
96.2	100.6	88.7	108.5	101.9	98.2	13.2	175.87	−2
99.6	104.3	92.6	106.2	99.2	101.6	10.7	114.89	−2
103.0	104.3	97.4	111.4	104.2	104.1	10.4	108.39	−1
106.4	108.0	102.4	117.0	109.6	106.1	10.0	100.14	0
109.8	107.9	100.3	115.1	107.7	108.2	9.8	97.14	1
113.2	107.9	105.7	113.6	113.4	109.9	9.5	90.45	3
116.6	111.7	105.3	120.2	112.7	108.3	16.7	280.88	8
120.0	111.7	100.6	120.7	106.3	101.0	27.3	748.79	18

ponents. Also, it will be noted that the quartiles after correction give a more reasonable range between the $P_{0.25}$ and $P_{0.75}$ quartiles.

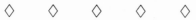

The authors would like to thank Professor J. Yerushalmy for making available the data utilized in Section 6 and Dr. W. Fellner and Dr. R. Brand for suggestions concerning statistical aspects of this paper.

REFERENCES

[1] W. C. BRINTON, *Graphic Methods for Presenting Facts*, New York, The Engineering Magazine Company, 1917.
[2] N. N. CENCOV, "Evaluation of an unknown distribution density from observations," *Soviet Math. Dokl.*, Vol. 3 (1962), pp. 1559–1562.
[3] G. DOETSCH, "Zerlegung einer Function in Gauss'sche Fehlerkurven," *Math. Z.*, Vol. 41 (1936), pp. 283–318.
[4] J. GREGOR, "An algorithm for the decomposition of a distribution into Gaussian components," *Biometrics*, Vol. 25 (1969), pp. 79–93.

[5] W. W. Gruelich and S. I. Pyle, *Radiographic Atlas of Skeletal Development of the Hand and Wrist*, Stanford, Stanford University Press, 1966 (2nd ed.).

[6] A. Hald, *Statistical Theory with Engineering Applications*, New York, Wiley, 1952.

[7] R. A. Kronmal, "The estimation of probability densities," unpublished Ph.D. thesis, Division of Biostatistics, University of California, Los Angeles, 1964.

[8] R. A. Kronmal and M. Tarter, "The estimation of probability densities and cumulatives by Fourier series methods," *J. Amer. Statist. Assoc.*, Vol. 63 (1968), pp. 925–952.

[9] P. Medgyessy, "The decomposition of compound probability distributions," *Hungar. Acad. Sci. Inst. Appl. Math.*, Vol. 2 (1953), pp. 165–177. (In Hungarian.)

[10] ———, *Decomposition of Superpositions of Distribution Functions*, Budapest, Pub. House of the Hungarian Academy of Sciences, 1961.

[11] E. Parzen, "On estimation of a probability density function and mode," *Ann. Math. Statist.*, Vol. 33 (1962), pp. 1065–1076.

[12] S. Raman, "Contribution to the theory of Fourier estimation of multivariate probability density functions with application to data on bone age determinations," unpublished Ph.D. thesis, Department of Biostatistics, University of California, Berkeley, 1971.

[13] M. Rosenblatt, "Remarks on some nonparametric estimates of a density function," *Ann. Math. Statist.*, Vol. 27 (1956), pp. 832–837.

[14] S. C. Schwartz, "Estimation of probability density by an orthogonal series," *Ann. Math. Statist.*, Vol. 38 (1967), pp. 1961–1965.

[15] D. F. Stanat, "Nonsupervised pattern recognition through the decomposition of probability functions," Technical Report, University of Michigan, Sensory Intelligence Laboratory, 1966.

[16] M. Tarter, "Variance and covariance formulas for evaluations of estimated orthogonal expansions," to appear.

[17] ———, "Inverse cumulative approximation and applications," *Biometrika*, Vol. 55 (1968), pp. 29–42.

[18] M. Tarter and W. Fellner, "Some new results concerning density estimates based on Fourier series," *Proceedings of the Fifth Conference on the Interface Between Statistics and Computation*, North Hollywood, Western Periodicals, 1972.

[19] M. Tarter, R. Holcomb, and R. A. Kronmal, "A description of new computer methods for estimating the population density," *Proc. Assoc. for Computing Machinery*, Vol. 22 (1967), pp. 511–519.

[20] M. Tarter and C. J. Kowalski, "A new test for, and class of transformations to, normality," *Technometrics*, Vol. 50 (1972), in press.

[21] M. Tarter and R. A. Kronmal, "Estimation of the cumulative by Fourier series methods and application to the insertion problem," *Proc. Assoc. for Computing Machinery*, Vol. 23 (1968), pp. 491–497.

[22] ———, "On multivariate density estimates based on orthogonal expansions," *Ann. Math. Statist.*, Vol. 41 (1970), pp. 718–722.

[23] J. Van Ryzin, "Bayes risk consistency of classification procedures using density estimation," *Sankhyā Ser. A*, Vol. 28 (1966), pp. 261–270.

[24] G. S. Watson, "Density estimation by orthogonal series," *Ann. Math. Statist.*, Vol. 40 (1969), pp. 1496–1498.

[25] G. S. Watson and M. R. Leadbetter, "On the estimation of the probability density, I," *Ann. Math. Statist.*, Vol. 34 (1963), pp. 480–491.

[26] E. J. Wegman, "Nonparametric probability density estimation," University of North Carolina at Chapel Hill, Institute of Statistics Mimeo Series, No. 638, 1969.

APPLICATIONS OF NEYMAN'S $C(\alpha)$ TECHNIQUE

F. N. DAVID

UNIVERSITY OF CALIFORNIA, RIVERSIDE

1. Introduction

The χ^2 techniques are possibly the most widely used in statistical methods in that they are simple in application and interpretation. This very generality, however, leads to a lack of sensitivity of the test criterion since the hypotheses alternate to that under test are commonly only vaguely specified. During the past few years there have been procedures put forward which enable more sensitive tests to be made. We give here a series of models for the alternative hypothesis under χ^2 type situations and the appropriate test criteria. The technique used to derive the test criteria is that put forward by Neyman [1] and loosely referred to by us as the $C(\alpha)$ procedure. The power functions of these tests may be calculated, and in such cases as we have investigated, they show the chosen criteria to be comparable in sensitivity to others which may be proposed.

2. Models reflecting a change in the location parameter

Suppose two groups of individuals with n in the first group (A) and N in the second group (B). On each individual the same characteristic X is measured. These measurements are used to divide the groups into $s + 1$ categories, so that we have Table I.

TABLE I

| | \multicolumn{4}{c}{Categories of measurement} | |
	1	2	$\cdots$	$s + 1$	Total
A	n_1	n_2	$\cdots$	n_{s+1}	n
B	N_1	N_2	$\cdots$	N_{s+1}	N
Totals	M_1	M_2	$\cdots$	M_{s+1}	M

It is apparent that if the measurements of the characteristic X are accurate and there are no "tied" values, a rank sum criterion is the appropriate quantity

This investigation was partially supported by USPHS Research Grant No. GM-10525-08, National Institutes of Health, Public Health Service.

to test for possible differences in the location parameters of the populations generating groups A and B. There are, however, many situations in experimental data where ties are abundant, particularly in the first (or last) categories where often all that is recorded is that the measurement was less (or greater) than a given value. The χ^2 criterion will test the null hypothesis that there is no difference between the population location parameters, but it will be sensitive to all alternative hypotheses instead of just that of a possible difference. A model set up by J. Neyman [2] would appear to be appropriate for this situation.

Let the hypothesis alternative to the null be that the location parameter of the population generating group B is greater than that of the population generating group A. Accordingly, we postulate the setup in Table II with $\xi = 0$ for the null hypothesis, and the obvious restraints on ξ for the alternate hypothesis.

TABLE II

| | Categories of measurement | | | | | | |
	1	2	3	$\cdots$	s	$s+1$	Total
A	p_1	p_2	p_3	$\cdots$	p_s	p_{s+1}	1
B	$p_1(1-\xi)$	$p_2 + \xi(p_1 - p_2)$	$p_3 + \xi(p_2 - p_3)$	$\cdots$	$p_s + \xi(p_{s-1} - p_s)$	$p_{s+1} + \xi p_s$	1

Using Neyman's procedure we have, conditional on n and N, that the test criterion T is

$$(1) \quad T = \sum_{j=1}^{s} (p_{j-1} - p_j)\left[\frac{N_j}{p_j} - \frac{N_{s+1}}{p_{s+1}}\right] - \frac{N}{M} \sum_{j=1}^{s} (p_{j-1} - p_j)\left[\frac{M_j}{p_j} - \frac{M_{s+1}}{p_{s+1}}\right]$$

with $p_0 = 0$. Writing

$$(2) \qquad A_r = \sum_j \frac{(p_{j-1} - p_j)^{r+1}}{p_j^r} + \frac{p_s^{r+1}}{p_{s+1}^r},$$

we have, under H_0,

$$(3) \qquad \mu_1'(T) = 0, \qquad\qquad \mu_2(T) = \frac{nN}{M} A_1,$$

$$\mu_3(T) = \frac{nN}{M}\left(\frac{n^2 - N^2}{M^2}\right) A_2, \qquad \kappa_4(T) = \frac{nN}{M}\left(\frac{n^3 + N^3}{M^3}\right)[A_3 - 3A_1^2],$$

indicating that for reasonable sized M the approximation to normality is satisfactory.

3. Power function of the test

Conditional on n and N as before, we have under H_1 ($\xi > 0$) that

$$(4) \qquad\qquad \mu_1'(T) = \frac{nN}{M}[A_1\xi]$$

and

$$(5) \qquad\qquad \mu_2(T) = \frac{nN}{M}\left[A_1 + \xi A_2 \frac{n}{M} - \xi^2 A_1^2 \frac{n}{M}\right].$$

Consequently, following the usual procedure and assuming that T is normally distributed, the power of the test may be computed.

4. Approximations involved in the test

The criterion T may be written as

$$(6) \qquad T = \frac{1}{M} \left[\sum_{j=1}^{s} (nN_j - Nn_j)\left(\frac{p_{j-1} - p_j}{p_j}\right) + (nN_{s+1} - Nn_{s+1})\frac{p_s}{p_{s+1}} \right]$$

with $p_0 = 0$. The parameters p will not generally be known and estimates of them will usually be substituted. Since $\xi = 0$ under the null hypothesis, we put $p_j = M_j/M$ obtaining

$$(7) \qquad \hat{T} = \frac{1}{M} \left[\sum_{j=1}^{s} (nN_j - Nn_j)\left(\frac{M_{j-1} - M_j}{M_j}\right) + (nN_{s+1} - Nn_{s+1})\frac{M_s}{M_{s+1}} \right].$$

It is easy to show that $\mathcal{E}\hat{T} = 0$ under the null hypothesis. Further, if we write for the denominator

$$(8) \qquad \frac{nN}{M^2}\left(\sum \frac{(M_{j-1} - M_j)^2}{M_j} + \frac{M_s^2}{M_{s+1}}\right),$$

it has expected value

$$(9) \qquad \frac{nN}{M}\left[\left(\sum_{j=1}^{s} \frac{(p_{j-1} - p_j)^2}{p_j} + \frac{p_s^2}{p_{s+1}}\right) + \frac{1}{M}\sum_{j=1}^{s+1}\left(\frac{p_{j-1}^2}{p_j^2} + \frac{p_{j-1}}{p_j}\right)\right]$$

if we exclude terms of higher order than $1/M$. This indicates that substituting the estimates of the p will tend to make the denominator too large, on the average, and the nominal significance levels will, accordingly, underestimate significance, a fault on the right side. To order $1/M$ the covariance between the numerator and the denominator is zero.

5. Neyman's randomization approach

Neyman [2] put forward the model given above but with an essential difference. He assumed that a total of M elements was given, but that the dichotomy of the M into the two samples A and B was achieved as the result of a random experiment. Once the dichotomy is made the n and N elements were each subjected to measurement and categorization as described above. The test criterion

$$(10) \qquad T_R = \sum_{j=1}^{s} (p_{j-1} - p_j)\left(\frac{N_j}{p_j} - \frac{N_{s+1}}{p_{s+1}}\right) - \Pi \sum_{j=1}^{s} (p_{j-1} - p_j)\left(\frac{M_j}{p_j} - \frac{M_{s+1}}{p_{s+1}}\right),$$

where Π is the probability that one of the M elements is assigned to the sample, is the same as in the conditional case if we put $\Pi = N/M$. The variance of T_R is

$$(11) \qquad \sigma_{T_R}^2 = \Pi(1 - \Pi)\sum_{j=1}^{s}\frac{(p_{j-1} - p_j)^2}{p_j} + \frac{p_s^2}{p_{s+1}}$$

and as before, the assumption is made that (T_R/σ_{T_R}) is a unit normal variable. The expectation of T_R is zero under H_0. Clearly, Π is determined by the initial random experiment.

Under the alternate hypothesis

$$(12) \qquad \mathcal{E}(T_R|\xi) = \xi\Pi(1 - \Pi)\left(\sum_{j=1}^{s} \frac{(p_{j-1} - p_j)^2}{p_j} + \frac{p_s^2}{p_{s+1}}\right)$$

and

$$(13) \quad \mathrm{Var}\,(T_R|\xi) = \mathrm{Var}\,(T_R|\xi = 0) + \xi\Pi(1 - \Pi)^2\left[\sum_{j=1}^{s} \frac{(p_{j-1} - p_j)^3}{p_j^2} + \frac{p_s^3}{p_{s+1}^2}\right]$$

$$- \xi^2[\mathrm{Var}\,(T_R|\xi = 0)]^2.$$

6. Example (Neyman's random experiment)

In an experiment to determine whether the larvae of *Lema triliveata daturaphila* (a kind of potato beetle) have a sense of smell, a target was made with an attractant at the "bull's eye." Twenty larvae were released individually 13 mm from the target center and the performance of each was classified as being nondirectional, intermediate, and directional, the dichotomy into classes being made on the basis of the distance traveled and the time taken. Twenty more larvae were released individually from a target distance of 23 mm and the same classification of performance made. The results of the experiments were as shown in Table III.

TABLE III

PERCEPTION TESTS FOR LARVAE

Distance from target center (mm)	Categories Nondirectional	Intermediate	Directional	Total
13	2 (N_1)	5 (N_2)	13 (N_3)	20
23	4 (n_1)	7 (n_2)	9 (n_3)	20
Totals	6 (M_1)	12 (M_2)	22 (M_3)	40

Under the null hypothesis of no difference of sense of smell with distance there should be no real difference between the performances at the two distances. Under the alternate hypothesis the larvae should perform better at 13 mm than they do at 23 mm. Here we have $s = 2$, $N = n = 20$, and the test criterion is

$$(14) \qquad -(N_1 - \Pi M_1) - (N_2 - \Pi M_2)\left(1 - \frac{p_1}{p_2}\right) + \frac{p_2}{p_3}(N_3 - \Pi M_3)$$

or, taking $\Pi = \frac{1}{2}$ and substituting estimates for the p,

$$(15) \qquad \frac{1}{2}\left[-(N_1 - n_1) + \left(\frac{M_1 - M_2}{M_2}\right)(N_2 - n_2) + \frac{M_2}{M_3}(N_3 - n_3)\right].$$

Calculations give an equivalent normal deviate of less than unity indicating that there is no significance.

7. Example (conditional test)

Fisher [3] gives data concerning the infestation of sheep by ticks for two different distributions. We adapt his data by dividing the distributions into four categories, namely, light infestation, medium, fairly heavy, and very heavy, as given in Table IV. The conditional criterion based on the $C(\alpha)$ technique will be appropriate here. Either the $C(\alpha)$ criterion or the χ^2 criterion is very significant indicating that the population of which II is a sample is probably more heavily infested than that of I.

TABLE IV

Sets of sheep	Infestation				Total
	Light	Medium	Fairly heavy	Very heavy	
I	24	21	12	3	60
II	20	19	19	24	82
Totals	44	40	31	27	142

8. Differences in dispersion parameters

It is clear from the setup of Table II that the alternative to the hypothesis under test is equivalent to that of a difference in the location parameters of the two populations generating the samples. This indicates the possibility of writing variants on the setup which will allow the alternative to the hypothesis under test to be equivalent to a difference in the dispersion parameters of the two populations. Such a situation frequently arises in experimental work when two treatments designed to have the same average effect are being compared and it is desired to know whether one treatment is more variable than the other.

Under the alternate hypothesis there will be (possibly) a diminution of probabilities at the tails when one population is compared with the other, and a heaping up at the center. Assume that there is an even number of categories. (This is not an important restriction and the result for an odd number of categories can easily be obtained.) We write, for $\xi > 0$, the setup in Table V.

TABLE V

Population	Categories							Total
	1	2	$\cdots$	s	$s+1$	$\cdots$	$2s$	
A	p_1	p_2	$\cdots$	p_s	p_{s+1}	$\cdots$	p_{2s}	1
B	$p_1 - \xi p_1$	$p_2 + \xi(p_1 - p_2)$	$\cdots$	$p_s + \xi p_{s-1}$	$p_{s+1} + \xi p_{s+2}$	$\cdots$	$p_{2s}(1 - \xi)$	1

If the sample values are

$$\text{(16)} \qquad \sum_{j=1}^{2s} n_j = n, \qquad \sum_{j=1}^{2s} N_j = N, \qquad\qquad n + N = M,$$

we have conditionally that, assuming $M_0 = 0 = M_{2s+1}$,

$$\text{(17)} \quad T = \sum_{j=1}^{s-1} \left(\frac{M_{j-1} - M_j}{M_j} \right) \left[N_j - \frac{NM_j}{M} \right] + \frac{M_{s-1}}{M_s} \left(N_s - \frac{N}{M} M_s \right)$$
$$+ \frac{M_{s+2}}{M_{s+1}} \left(N_{s+1} - \frac{N}{M} M_{s+1} \right) + \sum_{\ell=s+2}^{2s} \frac{(M_{\ell+1} - M_\ell)}{M_\ell} \left(N_\ell - \frac{N}{M} M_\ell \right)$$

and

$$\text{(18)} \quad \text{Var } T = \frac{Nn}{M} \left(\sum_{j=1}^{s} \frac{(M_{j-1} - M_j)^2}{M_j} + \frac{M_{s-1}^2}{M_s} + \frac{M_{s+2}^2}{M_{s+1}} + \sum_{\ell=s+2}^{2s} \frac{(M_{\ell+1} - M_\ell)^2}{M_\ell} \right).$$

Since the expected value of T is zero under H_0, the test criterion is $T/(\text{Var } T)^{1/2}$, significance being judged from normal tables.

Under H_1 we have

$$\text{(19)} \quad T = \frac{nN\xi}{M} \left[\sum_{j=1}^{s-1} \frac{(p_{j-1} - p_j)^2}{p_j} + \sum_{\ell=s+2}^{2s} \frac{(p_{\ell+1} - p_\ell)^2}{p_\ell} + \frac{p_{s-1}^2}{p_s} + \frac{p_{s+2}^2}{p_{s+1}} \right]$$

and

$$\text{(20)} \quad \text{Var } T = \frac{nN}{M} \left[\sum_{j=1}^{s-1} \frac{(p_{j-1} - p_j)^2}{p_j} + \sum_{\ell=s+2}^{2s} \frac{(p_{\ell+1} - p_\ell)^2}{p_\ell} + \frac{p_{s-1}^2}{p_s} + \frac{p_{s+2}^2}{p_{s+1}} \right]$$
$$+ \frac{n^2 N}{M^2} \xi \left[\sum_{j=1}^{s-1} \frac{(p_{j-1} - p_j)^3}{p_j^2} + \sum_{\ell=s+2}^{2s} \frac{(p_{\ell+1} - p_\ell)^3}{p_\ell^2} + \frac{p_{s-1}^3}{p_s^2} + \frac{p_{s+2}^3}{p_{s+1}^2} \right]$$
$$- N[\mathcal{E}(T)]^2,$$

so that the power of the test to detect a positive value of ξ may be computed. It will be recognized that the choice of a central dichotomy—in this case I have made a dichotomy between the sth and the $(s + 1)$st categories—is an arbitrary one. Further, if there is a change in the location parameter at the same time as the change in the dispersion parameter, the first change will tend to mask the second. This is, however, a situation which is always present in "nonparametric" tests for dispersion.

9. Number of groups

Commonly in the use of χ^2 and allied tests, the number of groups used for calculating the test criterion is fixed by the conditions under which the data are gathered. It is, therefore, useful to look at such $C(\alpha)$ tests as may be regarded as competitors of χ^2 with the purpose of determining the number of groups which will give optimum power. Calculations were carried out regarding the power, assuming equal probabilities for each group under H_0, and letting $n = N = M/2$. Under these assumptions, the conclusions reached were that the smallest number of groups consistent with the H_1 model should be aimed for. Thus, we have the following.

(i) *Change in location.*
  Models:

$$H_0 \quad \begin{array}{cc} p_1 & 1 - p_1 \\ p_1 & 1 - p_1 \end{array} \; \begin{array}{c} 1 \\ 1 \end{array} \qquad H_1 \quad \begin{array}{cc} p_1(1 - \xi) & 1 - p_1(1 - \xi) \\ p_1 & 1 - p_1 \end{array} \; \begin{array}{c} 1 \\ 1 \end{array}$$

Sample setup:

$$\begin{array}{cc|c} N_1 & N_2 & N \\ n_1 & n_2 & n \\ \hline M_1 & M_2 & M \end{array}$$

The test criterion is

(21) $$T = \frac{Nn_1 - nN_1}{M_2} = \frac{M_1N_2 - N_1M_2}{M_2}$$

and

(22) $$\operatorname{Var} T = \frac{nN}{M} \frac{M_1}{M_2}.$$

(ii) *Change in dispersion.*
  Models:

$$H_0 \quad \begin{array}{ccc} p_1 & p_2 & p_3 \\ p_1 & p_2 & p_3 \end{array} \; \begin{array}{c} 1 \\ 1 \end{array} \qquad H_1 \quad \begin{array}{ccc} p_1 & p_2 & p_3 \\ p_1(1 - \xi) & p_2 + \xi(p_1 + p_2) & p_3(1 - \xi) \end{array} \; \begin{array}{c} 1 \\ 1 \end{array}$$

Sample setup:

$$\begin{array}{ccc|c} n_1 & n_2 & n_3 & n \\ N_1 & N_2 & N_3 & N \\ \hline M_1 & M_2 & M_3 & M \end{array}$$

The test criterion is

(23) $$T = \frac{nN_2 - Nn_2}{M_2}$$

and

(24) $$\operatorname{Var} T = \frac{nN(M_1 + M_3)}{MM_2}.$$

10. Model for fatal road accidents

It is clear that the alternative hypothesis H_1 can be built suitable to the conditions of any particular problem provided that this building is done before any set of data is scrutinized. For example, suppose we remember that the age and sex of pedestrians killed by moving vehicles are both recorded and published. It may be desired to test whether the age distribution for males is the same as the age distribution for females. An opinion is expressed that more little boys would tend to be killed than little girls because they are more active and, therefore, have more exposure to risk and similarly that more of the aged killed would be men. The Ministry of Transport's (U.K.) Report on Fatal Road Accidents (1922) gives the information in Table VI.

TABLE VI

AGE AND SEX OF PEDESTRIANS KILLED

Sex	Years of age					Totals
	0 to 10	10 to 20	20 to 40	40 to 60	60+	
Male	304	68	73	162	366	973
Female	187	37	47	116	221	608
Totals	491	105	120	278	587	1581

Assuming the model

$$p_1 \quad p_2 \quad p_3 \quad p_4 \quad p_5 \quad 1$$
$$p_1 \quad p_2 \quad p_3 \quad p_4 \quad p_5 \quad 1,$$

we have χ_4^2 equals 1.93, or nonsignificance. The opinion expressed as to what may be found in the data suggests that for an application of Neyman's $C(\alpha)$ technique we might choose for our alternate setup

$$p_1 + p_2\xi \quad p_2 + (p_3 - p_2)\xi \quad p_3(1 - \xi) \quad p_4(1 - \xi) \quad p_5 + p_4\xi \quad 1$$
$$p_1 \qquad\qquad p_2 \qquad\qquad p_3 \qquad\qquad p_4 \qquad\qquad p_5 \qquad 1$$

The test criterion is

$$(25) \quad T = \left(N_1 - \frac{NM_1}{M}\right)\frac{M_2}{M_1} + \left(N_2 - \frac{NM_2}{M}\right)\left(\frac{M_3 - M_2}{M_2}\right) - \left(N_3 - \frac{NM_3}{M}\right)$$
$$- \left(N_4 - \frac{NM_4}{M}\right) + \frac{M_4}{M_5}\left(N_5 - \frac{NM_5}{M}\right).$$

Under H_0 the expected value of T is zero and

$$(26) \qquad \operatorname{Var} T = \frac{nN}{M^2}\left[\frac{M_2^2}{M_1} + \frac{(M_3 - M_2)^2}{M_2} + M_3 + M_4 + \frac{M_4^2}{M_5}\right].$$

From the table above, using $N = 973$, $n = 608$, we have

$$(27) \qquad\qquad T = 13.06, \quad \operatorname{Var} T = 131.18, \quad \frac{T}{\sigma_T} = 1.14.$$

This is still not significant, so we would not reject the null hypothesis of no difference in the proportions.

REFERENCES

[1] J. NEYMAN, *Probability and Statistics; The Harald Cramér Volume*, New York, Wiley, 1959, pp. 213–234.
[2] ———, "Statistical problems in science. The symmetric test of a composite hypothesis," *J. Amer. Statist. Assoc.*, Vol. 64 (1969), pp. 1154–1171.
[3] R. A. FISHER, "The negative binomial distribution," *Ann. Eugenics*, Vol. 11 (1941), pp. 182–187.

ON A MATHEMATICAL THEORY
OF QUANTAL RESPONSE ASSAYS

PREM S. PURI and JEROME SENTURIA
PURDUE UNIVERSITY

1. Introduction

About seven years ago, one of the authors (Puri [16]) was confronted with the following biological phenomenon. At time $t = 0$, each member of a group of hosts such as animals is injected with a dose of a specified virulent organism such as viruses or bacteria, which elicit a characteristic response from the host during the course of time. This response may be death, development of a tumor, or some other detectable symptom. If $n(t)$ denotes the number of hosts not responding by time t, the plot against t of either $n(t)$ itself or of the proportion $n(t)/n(0)$ is known as the time dependent response curve. These response curves differ with the dose and with the type of the organism. However, generally speaking, the larger the injected dose, the sooner the host responds. The question was raised as to how one could explain these observed response curves through a suitable stochastic model. Upon a search of the existing literature at the time, it was found that most of the models considered until then, were based on the hypothesis of existence of a fixed threshold, namely, while the organisms are undergoing certain growth processes within the host, as soon as their number touches a fixed threshold N, the host responds. In [16], this hypothesis was abandoned; first, because this hypothesis is not strictly correct; second, it is not clear what value one ought to choose for N in a given situation, and third, because this hypothesis makes the algebra unnecessarily intractable due to the involvement of the first passage time problem. Instead an alternative hypothesis originally suggested by Professor Lucien LeCam was adopted. Here, unlike in the threshold hypothesis, the connection between the number $Z(t)$ of organisms in a host at time t and the host's response is indeterministic in character. More exactly, it is assumed that the value of $Z(t)$ (or possibly of a random variable whose distribution is dependent on the process $\{Z(t)\}$) determines not the presence or the absence of response, but only the probability of response of the host. Mathematically, this amounts to postulating the existence of a nonnegative risk function $f(x, t)$ such that

The work of Prem S. Puri was supported in part by the U.S. Public Health Service, N.I.H. Grant GM-10525, at the Statistical Laboratory, University of California, Berkeley. The work of Jerome Senturia was supported by the National Science Foundation Traineeship Grant 3392-80-1399 at Purdue University.

(1) $P\{$host responds during $(t, t + \tau)|$not responded until t and $Z(t) = x\}$
$$= \delta f(x, t)\tau + o(\tau),$$

where $\delta \geqq 0$ and f satisfies certain mild regularity conditions. Stochastic models based on this more appropriate alternative hypothesis have been explored with a reasonable amount of success in a paper which appeared in the last Berkeley Symposium [16] and again in a later paper connected with bacteriophage reproduction (Puri [17]). In fact, in [16] it is assumed that the risk function f depends not only on $Z(t)$ but also on the integral $\int_0^t Z(\tau) \, d\tau$, which is contemplated as a measure of the amount of toxin produced by the live bacteria during the interval $(0, t)$ assuming, of course, that the toxin excretion rate is constant per bacterium per unit time.

The above models (see [16], [17]) apply to the situations where the response causing agents are selfreproducing such as viruses, bacteria, and so on. A natural question arises as to how a similar model based on the alternative hypothesis would behave in situations where the agent is not selfreproducing. Such would be the case where, for instance, the agent is a chemical poison, insecticide, or a drug. This then brings up the typical phenomenon that one faces in what is commonly described as *quantal response assays*. The classical theory of quantal response assays can be found in books such as Finney [7], [8], Bliss [6], and others. One of the purposes of this theory has been to help to arrive at an estimate of the relative potency of one drug against another by using measures such as E.D. 50, the dose which is just about enough to cause response among, on the average, about 50 per cent of the subjects. Here, typically the experimenter chooses a set of doses of each drug and tests each dose on a batch of subjects. At the end of the test, the experimenter records how many of the subjects responded. In order to analyze the data so obtained, it has been customary to make the following assumptions.

(i) For each subject there exists a tolerance limit or a threshold level T. This limit for a subject is the dose which will be just sufficient to produce the response, so that the subject will respond if $z \geqq T$ and will not if $z < T$, where z is the dose injected.

(ii) The threshold level T is assumed to be a random variable varying over the population of subjects, with a common distribution. Thus, the probability that a randomly chosen subject responds after receiving a dose z, is given by

(2) $P(z) = P(T \leqq z).$

It is common practice for the experimenters to use log dose or $x = \log z$, known as the dose metameter of z. Now if $g(y)$ is a probability density function so that $\int_{-\infty}^{\infty} g(y) \, dy = 1$, the form of the distribution of $\log T$ typically can be represented by the density

(3) $dQ(x) = \eta g(\gamma + \eta x) \, dx,$

where γ and η are the usual location and scale parameters, respectively. With this, one easily obtains

(4) $$P(z) = \int_{-\infty}^{\gamma + \eta \log z} g(y) \, dy.$$

In practice, the choice of $g(y)$ and, hence, of the distribution of the tolerance limit T is rather arbitrary. Some of the typical choices of $g(y)$ that have been used in literature are given below:

(5) $$g(y) = (2\pi)^{-\frac{1}{2}} \exp\{-y^2/2\}, \qquad -\infty < y < \infty,$$

(6) $$g(y) = \begin{cases} \sin 2y, & 0 \leq y \leq \pi/2, \\ 0, & \text{otherwise,} \end{cases}$$

(7) $$g(y) = \tfrac{1}{2} \operatorname{sech}^2 y, \qquad -\infty < y < \infty.$$

The last one has been used by Berkson in his well-known work in this area (see [5]).

While the above classical theory has been found useful and is still being used, there are, however, certain unattractive features in it that make one feel like giving it another look. Some of these are as follows. First is the above mentioned objection of assuming the existence of a tolerance limit or a threshold level for each subject even though the random element is introduced only through allowing this limit to vary randomly from subject to subject. Second, the model as it stands does not lend itself to the consideration of any biological mechanism going on within the host leading to its response. And third, it does not allow the consideration of the time when the response actually occurs if it does; all it considers is whether the response does or does not occur within a fixed length of time. These same features also underlie the more recent work of Ashford [1], Ashford and Smith [2], and Plackett and Hewlett [13], [14], in the case of mixture of drugs.

It is the purpose of this paper to give the classical theory of quantal response assays a fresh look and to construct new stochastic models that attempt to eliminate the above objections. This has been achieved by adopting the alternative approach of the nonthreshold type as discussed above. For the biological phenomenon under consideration, a typical stochastic model of the present type would involve the consideration of the following three main components.

The input process. This describes the manner in which the drug is introduced into the subject. We call it the "input process." One could visualize, depending upon the situation in question, several possibilities of inputs such as a continuous time deterministic input, discrete time deterministic input, or a random input according to some random mechanism.

The release process. This describes the manner in which the subject attempts to reduce the level of the drug within its body. This may be carried out either through the process of direct elimination of the drug through natural means or by changing the composition of the drug itself through biochemical processes. We call this the "release process." In principle, this would involve the mechanism going on within the body of the subject that takes into account the manner in which the subject copes with the drug. In experimental situations, the input process is generally controlled by the experimenter. The release process, on the other hand, is much more involved. It requires a great deal of experience and knowledge of the biological system on the part of the experimenter. It involves, in general, a considerable amount of experimentation while probing into the nature of the release mechanism. There has been, in fact, much work done in the past in an attempt to describe this mechanism for certain situations. For instance, the compartment models of, among others, Sapirstein, Vidt, Mandel, and Hanusek [22], Bellman [3], [4], are attempts toward a better understanding of functioning of specific organs and of various biological systems. Unfortunately, not too many of these models are stochastic in nature. Again, the models in dam theory (see Moran [11], Gani [9], and Prabhu [15], to cite only three references from this vast literature) could be found suitable for combining the aspects of both the input and the release processes.

The risk function. The most important aspect that does not appear to have been considered before in the context of the classical quantal response assays is the consideration of a risk function that relates the input and the release processes of the drug to the causation of the subject's response. Whether, in any given situation, the risk function depends only on the level $Z(t)$ of the drug at time t, or on some other factors characterizing the biological mechanism going on within the body of the subject, would entail a considerable knowledge of the biological system.

In the next few sections, we shall attempt to incorporate the three aspects listed above into a stochastic model. Although, this has been done here under rather simplified assumptions, the results do indicate that there is something to be gained by approaching this problem from a structural point of view. In this context the reader may also find, among others, the work of Neyman and Scott [12] of great interest. Here the response causing agent is urethane, while the response is the appearance of tumors in mice.

2. A stochastic model based on a quantal response process

2.1. *Assumptions and notation.* As a first attempt, we consider here a simple stochastic model along the lines discussed above. More comprehensive models incorporating detailed mechanisms suitable for certain situations shall be reported elsewhere. Following the lines of classical quantal response assays, we assume that for each subject the experiment starts with the administration (input) of a single dose $Z(0) = z$ at time $t = 0$, with no other inputs thereafter. Thus, if $Z(t)$ denotes the amount of drug present at time t in the body of the subject, it is evident that with probability one $Z(t)$ is nonincreasing with t. The release process is assumed to have two components. The first one determines how often and at what times the releases occur, while the second one associates with each such occurrence a nonnegative random variable Y denoting the amount of the drug to be released if available. More specifically, if $N(t)$ denotes the number of releases occurring during $(0, t]$, we assume, for simplicity, that $N(t)$ is a Poisson process with parameter $\mu > 0$. Also, given $N(t)$, let $Y_1, Y_2, \cdots, Y_{N(t)}$ denote the random amounts to be released if available, at the release time points as determined by the Poisson process. In particular, it is assumed that conditionally given $N(t)$, the random variables $Y_1, Y_2, \cdots, Y_{N(t)}$ are independently distributed with a common distribution having the probability density function

(8)
$$h(y) = \begin{cases} \beta \exp\{-\beta y\}, & y > 0, \\ 0, & \text{elsewhere,} \end{cases}$$

where $\beta > 0$. Of course, if at any time the random amount Y_i is greater than the amount actually available, all the available amount is then released. From the above construction, it follows that

(9)
$$z(t) \equiv \max\left\{0, Z(0) - \sum_{j=0}^{N(t)} Y_j\right\}, \qquad t \geq 0,$$

where by convention $Y_0 = 0$. Under the Poisson process assumption, it is clear that how often and at what times the releases occur is not influenced by the changes over time in the amount of the drug actually present. This, however, may not be realistic in certain situations. In Section 5, we shall consider briefly a more general model incorporating this dependence in an appropriate manner. Finally, we introduce what we shall call a *quantal response process* $\chi(t)$ defined as

(10)
$$\chi(t) = \begin{cases} 1, & \text{if the subject does not respond until } t, \\ 0, & \text{otherwise,} \end{cases}$$

where $\chi(0) = 1$. Also it is assumed that

(11)
$$P\{\chi(t + \tau) = 0 | \chi(t) = 1, Z(t) = x\} = \delta f(x, t)\tau + o(\tau),$$

where $\delta > 0$, and $f(\cdot, \cdot)$ defined for $x \geq 0$ and $t \geq 0$, is a nonnegative bounded function, assumed to be continuous almost everywhere with respect to both of its arguments. Using a standard argument, it is easy to show that

(12)
$$P\{\chi(t) = 1 | \omega\} = \exp\left\{-\delta \int_0^t f(Z(\tau, \omega), \tau) \, d\tau\right\},$$

where $Z(\tau, \omega)$ denotes the state of the process $\{Z(t)\}$ at time τ for a given realization ω of this process. From (12), we easily obtain the transform

(13)
$$E[\chi(t) \exp\{-sZ(t)\}] = E\left[\exp\left\{-sZ(t) - \delta \int_0^t f(Z(\tau), \tau) \, d\tau\right\}\right],$$

where $\text{Re}(s) \geq 0$. In particular, this yields

(14)
$$P\{L > t\} = P\{\chi(t) = 1\} = E[\chi(t)] = E\left[\exp\left\{-\delta \int_0^t f(Z(\tau), \tau) \, d\tau\right\}\right],$$

where L is the length of time the subject takes to respond. Taking δ in (14) as a dummy variable, it follows that the response time distribution can be studied equivalently by obtaining the distribution of the integral $\int_0^t f[Z(\tau), \tau] \, d\tau$. The reader may find this particular connection explored in detail elsewhere (see Puri [18], [19], [20], [21]). Again, in general, the random variable L may not be a proper random variable, so that

(15) $P\{L = \infty\} = P\{\text{no response}\}$

$$= \lim_{t \to \infty} E[\chi(t)] = E\left[\exp\left\{-\delta \int_0^\infty f(Z(\tau), \tau)\, d\tau\right\}\right].$$

At this point, we introduce the following notation:

$$W_1(t, z, x) = P\{Z(t) \leq x, \chi(t) = 1 | Z(0) = z, \chi(0) = 1\},$$

$$W_1(t, z) = P\{\chi(t) = 1 | Z(0) = z, \chi(0) = 1\},$$

$$W(t, z, x) = P\{Z(t) \leq x | Z(0) = z\},$$

(16) $$\phi_1(\theta, z, x) = \int_0^\infty \exp\{-\theta t\}\, W_1(t, z, x)\, dt,$$

$$\phi_1(\theta, z) = \int_0^\infty \exp\{-\theta t\}\, W_1(t, z)\, dt,$$

$$\phi(\theta, z, x) = \int_0^\infty \exp\{-\theta t\}\, W(t, z, x)\, dt,$$

where $\mathrm{Re}(\theta) > 0$, $0 \leq x \leq z$, and

(17) $$\begin{aligned} W(t, 0, x) &= W(t, z, z) = 1, & x &\geq 0, \\ W(t, z, x) &= W_1(t, z, x) = 0, & x &< 0. \end{aligned}$$

Here the last line follows from the fact that zero is an absorption state for the process $Z(t)$.

In the next subsection, we shall attempt to obtain expressions for the quantities defined above, by setting up the usual Kolmogorov backward integral equations involving these quantities.

2.2. *Certain integral equations and their solutions.*   Unless stated to the contrary, we assume henceforth that the risk function f does not explicitly depend on time t and that it depends only on the level $Z(t)$. Moreover, it is assumed that $f(x)$ is differentiable for all $x \geq 0$.

By considering the moment of the first release during $(0, t)$ and the amount to be released, it is easy to establish the following Kolmogorov backward integral equation for the probability $W_1(t, z, x)$ for $x < z$,

(18) $W_1(t, z, x)$

$$= \mu\beta \int_0^t \exp\{-[\mu + \delta f(z)]u\} \left[\int_0^{z-x} W_1(t - u, z - y, x) \exp\{-\beta y\}\, dy\right.$$

$$+ \int_{z-x}^z W_1(t - u, z - y) \exp\{-\beta y\}\, dy$$

$$+ \left. \exp\{-\delta f(0)(t - u)\} \int_z^\infty \exp\{-\beta y\}\, dy\right]\, du.$$

Taking the Laplace transform of both sides of (18), we have for Re $\theta > 0$,

(19) $[\mu + \theta + \delta f(z)]\phi_1(\theta, z, x) = \mu\beta \int_0^{z-x} \phi_1(\theta, z - y, x) \exp \{-\beta y\} \, dy$

$$+ \mu\beta \int_{z-x}^z \phi_1(\theta, z - y) \exp \{-\beta y\} \, dy$$

$$+ \exp \{-\beta z\} [\mu/(\theta + \delta f(0))].$$

Similarly, we have the corresponding equation for $W_1(t, z)$ given by

(20)
$W_1(t, z) = \exp \{-[\mu + \delta f(z)]t\}$

$$+ \mu\beta \int_0^t \exp \{-[\mu + \delta f(z)]u\} \int_0^z W_1(t - u, z - y) \exp \{-\beta y\} \, dy \, du$$

$$+ \mu \exp \{-\beta z\} \int_0^t \exp \{-[\mu + \delta f(z)]u - \delta f(0)(t - u)\} \, du,$$

or equivalently in terms of its Laplace transform, by

(21) $[\mu + \theta + \delta f(z)]\phi_1(\theta, z) = 1 + \exp \{-\beta z\} [\mu[\theta + \delta f(0)]^{-1}]$

$$+ \mu\beta \exp \{-\beta z\} \int_0^z \exp \{\beta v\} \phi_1(\theta, v) \, dv.$$

Equation (21) can easily be converted into the differential equation

(22) $\phi_1' + \phi_1[\beta + (\delta f' - \mu\beta)(\mu + \theta + \delta f)^{-1}] = \beta(\mu + \theta + \delta f)^{-1},$

where ϕ_1' and f' are the corresponding derivatives with respect to z. Solving (22) subject to the initial condition

(23) $\phi_1(\theta, 0) = [\theta + \delta f(0)]^{-1},$

we obtain

(24) $\phi_1(\theta, z) = [\theta + \mu + \delta f(z)]^{-1} \exp \left\{- \beta \int_0^z A(u) \, du\right\}$

$$\left[(A(0))^{-1} + \beta \int_0^z \exp \left\{\beta \int_0^v A(u) \, du\right\} dv\right],$$

where

(25) $A(u) = [\theta + \delta f(u)][\theta + \mu + \delta f(u)]^{-1},$ $u \geqq 0.$

Substituting (24) in (19) and solving (19) in an analogous manner, we have the solution for (19) given by

(26) $\phi_1(\theta, z, x) = [\theta + \mu + \delta f(z)]^{-1} \exp \left\{-\beta \int_0^z A(u) \, du\right\}$

$$\left[(A(0))^{-1} - \exp \left\{\beta \int_0^x A(u) \, du\right\} + \beta \int_0^x \exp \left\{\beta \int_0^v A(u) \, du\right\} dv\right],$$

where $x < z$. As a check, letting $x \to z$ in (26) and subtracting the result from (24) we obtain, as expected,

$$(27) \qquad \int_0^\infty P\{Z(t) = z, \chi(t) = 1 | Z(0) = z, \chi(0) = 1\} \exp\{-\theta t\}\, dt$$
$$= \phi_1(\theta, z) - \phi_1(\theta, z, z-) = [\theta + \mu + \delta f(z)]^{-1}.$$

The expressions for the transforms given by (24) and (26), in principle, are sufficient for determining the joint distribution of $\chi(t)$ and $Z(t)$. Unfortunately, to carry out the inversion of these transforms in this generality is rather cumbersome. Later on, we shall carry out their inversion for a special case. Again, if $f(0) > 0$, using a Tauberian argument, it follows from (24) that

$$(28) \qquad \psi(z) \equiv P\{L = \infty | Z(0) = z\} = \lim_{\theta \to 0} \theta \phi_1(\theta, z) = 0,$$

so that L is a proper random variable. In fact, using the relation

$$(29) \qquad \phi_1(\theta, z) = \int_0^\infty \exp\{-\theta t\} P\{L > r\}\, dt = \theta^{-1}(1 - E[\exp\{-\theta L\}])$$

and (24), we have

$$(30) \qquad E[\exp\{-\theta L\}] = 1 - [\theta + \mu + \delta f(z)]^{-1} \exp\left\{-\beta \int_0^z A(u)\, du\right\}$$
$$\left[\theta(A(0))^{-1} + \beta\theta \int_0^z \exp\left\{\beta \int_0^v A(u)\, du\right\} dv\right].$$

Now one could easily obtain moments of L from (30). In particular, it follows from (29) that

$$(31) \qquad E(L) = \lim_{\theta \to 0} \phi_1(\theta, z) = \phi_1(0, z).$$

2.3. *Probability of no response for the case with $f(0) = 0$.* If $f(0) > 0$, this would mean that the response could be caused even without the presence of the drug. However, in most of the practical situations this appears unrealistic, except when the response is the death of the subject. Even in the latter case, one could define response as the death caused by the drug and not by other causes; or as an approximation to the actual situation one could ignore the other causes, in which case $f(0) = 0$ would be a reasonable requirement. A more realistic model of this latter situation would be the one which incorporates other causes besides the one due to the drug, since, in principle, all these causes simultaneously compete against each other for the life of the subject. However, at present we shall not venture into this refinement and instead assume $f(0) = 0$ in what follows. With this assumption, the random variable L is no longer a proper random variable, since the probability that the subject never responds will be positive. Again, in quantal response assays, where the actual response times are often not reported, one is typically interested only in the probability that the subject never responds. This is valid only as an approximation assuming, of course, that the subject has been under observation for a sufficient length of time. Using (24) with $f(0) = 0$, this probability, denoted by $\psi(z)$, is now given by

$$(32) \quad \psi(z) = P\{\text{subject never responds} | Z(0) = z\}$$
$$= \lim_{\theta \to 0} \theta \phi_1(\theta, z) = \mu[\mu + \delta f(z)]^{-1} \exp\left\{-\beta \delta \int_0^z f(u)[\mu + \delta f(u)]^{-1}\, du\right\}.$$

Alternatively, one could easily justify, either from (28) and (21) with $f(0) = 0$ or by a direct probabilistic argument, that $\psi(z)$ must satisfy the integral equation

$$(33) \qquad \psi(z) \exp \{\beta z\} [\mu + \delta f(z)] = \mu + \mu\beta \int_0^z \exp \{\beta v\} \, \psi(v) \, dv.$$

This, when solved subject to the boundary condition $\psi(0) = 1$, again yields the expression (32). In the next section, we exhibit a comparison of the quantal response model with the present one through the use of expression (32).

3. A comparison of the present model with the classical one

It appears rather natural at this stage to look for some kind of direct comparison between the present theory and the classical one. Unfortunately, there does not appear to be any simple way of making such a comparison, mainly because the two theories are based on entirely different points of view. However, if we insist on making one for the sake of amusement, the only way which appears reasonable is to equate the end result common to both the theories. More specifically, by equating the probability of no response under the classical theory, namely,

$$(34) \qquad 1 - P\{z\} = P\{T > z\} = \int_{\gamma + \eta \log z}^{\infty} g(y) \, dy,$$

to the probability of no response under the present model, namely $\psi(z)$, we ask what risk function $f(\cdot)$ of the present model would correspond to a given density function $g(y)$ used in the classical theory. To this end, one can easily solve (32) for $f(z)$ in terms of ψ yielding

$$(35)$$
$$\delta f(z) = [\psi(z)]^{-1} \exp \{-\beta z\} \left[\mu(1 - \psi(z) \exp \{\beta z\}) + \mu\beta \int_0^z \exp \{\beta v\} \psi(v) \, dv \right].$$

Now by replacing $\psi(z)$ with $1 - P(z)$, one obtains the desired risk function f corresponding to a given density g of the classical model. For instance, the risk function corresponding to the normal density (5) is given by

$$(36) \quad \delta f(z) = \mu \exp \{-\beta z\} [1 - H(\gamma + \eta \log z)]^{-1}$$

$$\left[1 - \exp \{\beta z\} (1 - H(\gamma + \eta \log z)) \right.$$

$$\left. + \beta \int_0^z \exp \{\beta v\} (1 - H(\gamma + \eta \log v)) \, dv \right];$$

where $H(x) = (2\pi)^{-\frac{1}{2}} \int_{-\infty}^{x} \exp \{-\tau^2/2\} \, d\tau$. Similarly, for the density function of (7) we have

$$(37) \quad \delta f(z) = \mu \exp \{-\beta z\} [1 + \exp \{2(\gamma + \eta \log z)\}]$$

$$\left(1 - \exp \{\beta z\} [1 + \exp \{2(\gamma + \eta \log z)\}]^{-1} \right.$$

$$\left. + \beta \int_0^z \exp \{\beta v\} [1 + \exp \{2(\gamma + \eta \log v)\}]^{-1} \, dv \right).$$

As expected, since $P(0) = 0$, we have $f(0) = 0$ in the above formulas. Similar expressions can be obtained for f that correspond to other densities often used in the classical theory. Unfortunately, as is evident, all such expressions will usually be complicated, so that there appears to be no rationale for choosing one or the other form of the risk function in practice. In the next section, we consider the simplest form of the risk function, namely the linear function $\delta f(x) = \delta x$, which appears reasonable at least as a first approximation. The results obtained by using this simple risk function are then applied to some observed data.

4. An application of the model to observed data

We shall now restrict ourselves to the case of a linear risk function with $\delta f(x) = \delta x$. For this, we have from (26),

$$(38) \quad \phi_1(\theta, z, x) = (\theta + \mu + \delta z)^{-1}[C(z)]^{-1} \exp \{-\beta z\}$$
$$\left[(1 + \mu\theta^{-1}) - C(x) \exp \{\beta x\} + \beta \int_0^x C(v) \exp \{\beta v\} \, dv\right],$$

where $x < z$ and

$$(39) \quad C(v) = [(\theta + \mu)(\theta + \mu + \delta v)^{-1}]^{\beta\mu/\delta}, \qquad v \geqq 0.$$

Also expression (24) now takes the form

$$(40) \quad \phi_1(\theta, z) = [(\theta + \mu)(\theta + \mu + \delta z)^{-1}][C(z)]^{-1} \exp \{-\beta z\}$$
$$\left[\theta^{-1} + (\beta(\mu + \theta)^{-1}) \int_0^z C(v) \exp \{\beta v\} \, dv\right].$$

The transforms (38) and (40) can be easily inverted to produce the expressions for $W_1(t, z, x)$ and $W_1(t, z)$, respectively; for instance, when $\beta\mu/\delta$ is not an integer,

$$(41) \quad W_1(t, z) = \sum_{k=0}^{\infty} \frac{1}{k!} \left[A_k \left(\frac{\beta\mu}{\delta} - 1\right) \left(\frac{\delta z}{\mu + \delta z}\right)^k \exp \{-\beta z\} I_{k, \mu+\delta z}(t)\right.$$
$$\left. + A_k \left(\frac{\beta\mu}{\delta}\right) \left(\frac{\delta}{\beta}\right)^k I_{k+1,\beta}(z)t^k \exp \{-(\mu + \delta z)t\}\right],$$

where

$$(42) \quad A_k(x) = x(x + 1)(x + 2) \cdots (x + k - 1), \qquad k \geqq 1; \qquad A_0(x) \equiv 1,$$

and for $\alpha > 0$,

$$(43) \quad I_{k,\alpha}(x) = \int_0^x \frac{\alpha^k y^{k-1}}{\Gamma(k)} \exp \{-\alpha y\} \, dy, \qquad k \geqq 1; \qquad I_{0,\alpha}(x) \equiv 1.$$

It is easy to verify that by letting δ tend to zero in (38), one obtains

$$(44) \quad \lim_{\delta \to 0} \phi_1(\theta, z, x) = \phi(\theta, z, x)$$
$$= \mu[\theta(\theta + \mu)]^{-1} \exp \{-\beta\theta(\theta + \mu)^{-1}(z - x)\}, \qquad x < z,$$

a result for the process $Z(t)$ alone without the consideration of the quantal response process $\chi(t)$. Again, for the present case with $f(x) = x$, we have from (32) the expression for the probability of no response, given by

$$(45) \qquad \psi(z) = \exp\left\{-\beta z\right\}\left(1 + \frac{\delta}{\mu}z\right)^{-1+\beta\mu/\delta}.$$

It is this probability which is relevant to the fitting of our model to appropriate data on quantal response assays. Expression (45) contains essentially two parameters, since μ and δ always appear as μ/δ. However, for fitting the above formula to suitable data, it was found convenient to introduce the reparameterization

$$(46) \qquad \rho = \frac{\delta}{\mu}, \qquad \lambda = \rho(\beta - \rho),$$

so that

$$(47) \qquad \psi(z) = (1 + \rho z)^{\lambda/\rho^2} \exp\left\{-\left(\rho + \frac{\lambda}{\rho}\right)z\right\}.$$

Let Z_0 (E.D. 50) denote the dose which will produce a response with probability one half. From (47), it follows that Z_0 satisfies the relation

$$(48) \qquad \log\frac{1}{2} = -\left(\rho + \frac{\lambda}{\rho}\right)Z_0 + \frac{\lambda}{\rho^2}\log\left(1 + \rho Z_0\right).$$

Formula (41) was fitted to the data based on a study of the toxicity of an insecticide known as Deguelin. The data are due to Martin [10] and have also been used by Berkson [5] in an attempt to fit the classical model of the quantal response assays. In the study proper, concentrations at different dose levels z_i of Deguelin were prepared in an alcohol medium. These were then sprayed on groups of respective sizes n_i of the test insects (adult apterousfe male) *Aphis rumicis*. These sprayings were performed in a carefully controlled way using a special atomizer. After spraying, without further handling the insects were placed in tubes with a small amount of bean foliage. They were checked after about 20 hours for the number r_i of deaths in the ith group. These data are given in Table I.

TABLE I

MARTIN'S DATA ON TOXIC EFFECT OF DEGUELIN

Concentration mg/litre z_i	10.1	20.2	30.3	40.4	50.5
Total number n_i	48	48	49	50	48
Number of deaths r_i	18	34	47	47	48

Formula (47) was fitted to the above data by using the standard method of minimum chi square. The fit appears quite satisfactory, since the observed value of the chi square is 3.69 (three degrees of freedom), which is not significant at the five per cent level, where the table value is 7.81. Also, the method of maximum likelihood led to the estimates for the parameters ρ and μ, along with their standard errors, as given in (49). Using these and the relation (48), an estimate

$\hat{Z}_0$ of E.D. 50 was obtained by using a computer search procedure for finding the appropriate root $\hat{Z}_0$ of (48). The various estimates of the standard errors, as given here, are based on the standard large sample formulas valid for the maximum likelihood estimates:

$$
\begin{array}{lll}
\hat{\lambda} = 0.00526, & \hat{\rho} = 0.02428, & \hat{Z}_0 = 13.117 \\
\text{S.E.}(\hat{\lambda}) = 0.00102, & \text{S.E.}(\hat{\rho}) = 0.0143, & \text{S.E.}(\hat{Z}_0) = 1.435.
\end{array}
$$
(49)

As a passing remark, it may be appropriate to mention here that we also fitted Formula (47) to data reported in [5] which pertain to responses to certain bacteria. Here, as expected, the fit was considerably worse. For the four degrees of freedom available in that case, the observed chi square was 12.9. This being significant indicates the sensitivity of the present model to situations where the response causing agent is selfreproducing. The models appropriate for such situations have already been dealt with elsewhere (see [16], [17]). The present model is, of course, not designed for such situations.

5. A model with a generalization of the release process

In the release process as adopted in the above model, how often and at what times the releases occur is not influenced by the changes over time in the amount of the drug actually present in the subject. When the above work was presented at this Symposium a question was raised from the audience inquiring whether it was possible to modify the release process of the model in order to take into account the possible effect of the changes over time in the level of the drug on the frequency of the releases. We attempt here to accomplish this through a generalization of the Poisson process of Section 2. Let $\mu(z)$ be a nonnegative bounded function, which may be called the risk function for the release, such that

$$
\begin{aligned}
&P\{\text{a release occurs during } (t, t + \tau)|Z(t) = z\} = \mu(z)\tau + o(\tau), \\
&P\{\text{more than one release occurs during } (t, t + \tau)|Z(t) = z\} = o(\tau).
\end{aligned}
$$
(50)

The random variables $Y_1, Y_2, \cdots$, denoting the amounts to be released, if available, at the release points governed by (50), are as before independently distributed with the common distribution given by (8). Clearly, when $\mu(z)$ is a positive constant, we are back to the case of the Poisson release process. All the other assumptions of the model as outlined in Section 2 remain the same with the exception of (50); we assume that $f(0) = 0$. It may be remarked here that there is no loss in generality so far as the distribution of the quantal response process $\chi(t)$ is concerned, if we allow $\mu(0)$ to be positive. In the latter case we can still talk fictitiously of the releases, even though the level of the drug may be zero. Thus, we assume that $\mu(0) > 0$, for convenience. Let $N(t)$ denote the number of releases occurring during $(0, t]$. Also we introduce the following notation:

$$
\begin{aligned}
V_1(k, t, z) &= P\{\chi(t) = 1, N(t) = k|Z(0) = z, \chi(0) = 1\}, & k \geq 0, \\
V_1(t, z) &= P\{\chi(t) = 1|Z(0) = z, \chi(0) = 1\}, \\
V(k, t, z) &= P\{N(t) = k|Z(0) = z\}, & k \geq 0.
\end{aligned}
$$
(51)

It is not too difficult to show that the random variable $N(t)$ is a proper random variable for every $t \geq 0$, so that the probability of an infinite number of releases occurring during a finite time interval is zero. As such

$$(52) \qquad V_1(t, z) = \sum_{k=0}^{\infty} V_1(k, t, z).$$

Again taking into account the first release, if it occurs, it is easy to establish the following system of recurrence relations for the V:

$$(53) \qquad V_1(0, t, z) = \exp \{-[\mu(z) + \delta f(z)]t\},$$

$$(54) \quad V_1(k, t, z)$$

$$= \mu(z) \int_0^t \exp \{-[\mu(z) + \delta f(z)]u\} \left[\int_0^z \beta \exp \{-\beta y\} V_1(k - 1, t - u, z - y) \, dy \right.$$

$$\left. + \exp \{-\beta z\} V(k - 1, t - u, 0) \right], \qquad k \geq 1.$$

Let

$$(55) \qquad \begin{aligned} V_1^*(k, \theta, z) &= \int_0^\infty \exp \{-\theta t\} V_1(k, t, z) \, dt, \\ V^*(k, \theta, z) &= \int_0^\infty \exp \{-\theta t\} V(k, t, z) \, dt, \end{aligned}$$

where $\mathrm{Re} \, \theta > 0$. Then from (53) and (54), we have

$$(56) \quad V_1^*(0, \theta, z) = [\theta + \mu(z) + \delta f(z)]^{-1},$$

$$(57) \quad V_1^*(k, \theta, z) = \mu(z)[\mu(z) + \delta f(z) + \theta]^{-1} \left[\exp \{-\beta z\} V^*(k - 1, \theta, 0) \right.$$

$$\left. + \beta \int_0^z \exp \{-\beta y\} V_1^*(k - 1, \theta, z - y) \, dy \right], \qquad k \geq 1.$$

Clearly,

$$(58) \qquad V(k, t, 0) = \frac{[\mu(0)t]^k}{k!} \exp \{-\mu(0)t\},$$

so that

$$(59) \qquad V^*(k, \theta, 0) = [\mu(0)]^k[\mu(0) + \theta]^{-k-1}.$$

Using this, one can easily solve the system (56) and (57) recursively. However, our aim is to obtain $\psi(z)$, the probability of no response. To this end, summing (56) and (57) over the possible values of k, we obtain

$$(60) \quad V_1^*(\theta, z)$$

$$= [\theta + \mu(z) + \delta f(z)]^{-1} \left[1 + \mu(z) \exp \{-\beta z\} \{\theta^{-1} + \beta \int_0^z \exp \{\beta v\} V_1^*(\theta, v) \, dv\} \right].$$

We assume now, for simplicity, that besides $f(z)$, the risk function $\mu(z)$ is also differentiable for $z \geq 0$. With this (60) can be easily transformed into the differential equation

$$(61) \quad \frac{\partial V_1^*}{\partial z} + [\mu(\delta f' + \beta \theta + \beta \delta f) - \mu'(\theta + \delta f)][\mu(\theta + \mu + \delta f)]^{-1} V_1^*$$

$$= \left[\beta - \frac{\mu'}{\mu} \right] [\theta + \mu + \delta f]^{-1},$$

where f' and μ' denote, respectively, the derivatives of f and μ. Here we have suppressed, for convenience, the arguments of all the functions such as f, μ, and so forth. Equation (61) can be solved easily subject to the initial condition $V_1^*(\theta, 0) = 1/\theta$, yielding

$$(62) \quad V_1^*(\theta, z) = \frac{\mu(z)(\theta + \mu_0)}{\mu_0[\theta + \mu(z) + \delta f(z)]} \exp\{-\beta B(z)\}$$

$$\left[\frac{1}{\theta} + \frac{\mu_0}{\theta + \mu_0} \int_0^z (\beta\mu(s) - \mu'(s))(\mu(s))^{-2} \exp\{\beta B(s)\} ds\right],$$

where $\mu_0 = \mu(0)$ and

$$(63) \qquad\qquad B(s) = \int_0^s \frac{\theta + \delta f(v)}{\theta + \mu(v) + \delta f(v)} dv.$$

Finally, since $\psi(z) = \lim_{\theta \to 0} \theta V_1^*(\theta, z)$, it follows from (62), that

$$(64) \quad \psi(z) = \mu(z)[\mu(z) + \delta f(z)]^{-1} \exp\left\{-\beta \int_0^z \delta f(v)[\mu(v) + \delta f(v)]^{-1} dv\right\}.$$

This then is the generalization of formula (32), where $\mu(z)$ is assumed to be a positive constant. Finally, for the special case with $f(x) = x$ and $\mu(x) = \mu_0 + \nu x$ such that $\mu_0 + \nu x > 0$ for $0 \leq x \leq z$, we have

$$(65) \quad \psi(z) = \exp\left\{-\frac{\beta\delta}{\nu + \delta} z\right\}\left(1 + \frac{\nu z}{\mu_0}\right)\left(1 + \frac{\delta + \nu}{\mu_0} z\right)^{-1 + \beta\delta\mu_0(\delta + \nu)^{-2}}, \quad z \geq 0.$$

6. Discussion

The present work is inspired by an earlier work of one of the authors (Puri [16]) and by the need of giving a fresh look to the classical theory of quantal response assays (see Finney [7]), which, in the opinion of the authors, appears to have certain unappealing features. Most of the mathematical models of random phenomena incorporate assumptions, which tend to simplify the real situation, yet, by now, it is evident that there are certain fundamental differences in the approach adopted here from the one classically used. For instance, the present approach permits the consideration of the response time, while the classical one does not. Unlike the classical approach, the present one is based on a nonthreshold hypothesis which appears more appealing. Most importantly, however, the present model allows ample room for the consideration of the mechanism of the causation of the response, while the classical theory does not. The mechanism incorporated in the model studied here may be oversimplified for certain situations. However, this, in general, can easily be rectified by incorporating more complicated yet realistic mechanisms into the present theory, usually, of course, at the cost of making the algebra more involved.

In the present model the only input allowed is at the start of the experiment. However, this can easily be extended to cover the general case, where the input pattern over time is controlled and determined ahead of time by the experimenter (see Neyman and Scott [12]). Also situations such as exposure to natural radiation, or to specific chemicals as part of certain occupational hazards, involve perhaps a random mechanism for the input process. Such models involving more elaborate input and release processes are reported elsewhere (see Senturia [23]).

The classical theory of quantal response assays has been extended to the case of multiple responses to one or several drugs (see [1]) or to the case of a single response to a mixture of drugs (see [2]). It appears worthwhile to examine and extend the present approach to cover these cases. Also, deeper models along the present lines, while incorporating the role of the defense mechanism utilized by the subject in order to cope with the drug, are very much needed. This mechanism, of course, may vary considerably from one situation to another. In several situations, to gain knowledge of this mechanism itself would need a considerable amount of further experimentation.

Again, in many situations, it may appear realistic to consider the risk function f not only dependent on the level $Z(t)$ of the drug but also on some other relevant functionals of the process $Z(t)$. (See, for instance, [16], [17], and the work done at the Statistical Laboratory, University of California, Berkeley [24], [25].)

In the present model, a special form (8) of the common distribution of $Y_1, Y_2, \cdots$, the amounts released, was assumed. This can be generalized to the case with an arbitrary distribution function, say $H(y)$, for the random variables Y. One can easily set up the integral equations analogous to (19) and (21) for this case. For instance, equation (21) now takes the form

$$(66) \quad [\mu + \theta + \delta f(z)]\phi_1(\theta, z)$$
$$= 1 + \mu[1 - H(z)][\theta + \delta f(0)]^{-1} + \mu \int_0^z \phi_1(\theta, z - y) \, dH(y).$$

Unfortunately, however, the solution of these equations becomes relatively cumbersome.

Finally, it is hoped that, in due course, the approach adopted here will find its proper place in its usefulness in comparison to the classical approach. This will emerge even more when the experimenter wishes to use the data on response times of the subjects for an appropriate analysis, rather than only on whether the subject does or does not respond in a given period of time.

7. Summary

The classical theory of quantal response assays (see [7]) is based on the hypothesis of existence of a threshold level T (tolerance limit), such that if the injected dose z of the drug is smaller than T, the subject does not respond, and it does respond if $z \geq T$. The threshold level T is assumed to vary randomly over the population of subjects with a common distribution, usually with an arbitrarily chosen form. As it stands, the classical theory has several unattractive features. First, the hypothesis of existence of a threshold level may not be strictly correct. Second, the classical model does not lend itself to the consideration of any biological mechanism leading to the subject's response. And third, it does not allow for consideration of the time when the response actually occurs, if it does. In view of these objections, the present paper gives a fresh look to the problem. As a result, a new stochastic model is constructed along the more realistic lines (see [16], [17]) adopted elsewhere for a similar situation. Here it is assumed that

$$(67) \qquad P\{\chi(t + \tau) = 0 | \chi(t) = 1, Z(t) = x\} = \delta f(x)\tau + o(\tau),$$

where $\chi(t)$ is one if the subject has not responded until time t, and is zero otherwise; the random variable $Z(t)$ denotes the level of the drug at time t; $\delta > 0$ and f is a nonnegative risk function defined for all $x \geqq 0$ and is assumed to satisfy certain mild regularity conditions. The process $\{Z(t)\}$ is assumed to involve a certain random release mechanism. Here $Z(0)$ is the dose administered at time $t = 0$. Under these assumptions, the joint distribution of $\chi(t)$ and $Z(t)$ is studied for an arbitrary risk function f. In particular with $f(0) = 0$, the probability of no response is obtained. Assuming $f(x) = x$, this probability is then fitted to certain observed data. Finally, an indirect comparison of this model is made with the classical one.

REFERENCES

[1] J. R. ASHFORD, "Quantal responses to mixtures of poisons under conditions of similar action—the analysis of uncontrolled data," *Biometrika*, Vol. 45 (1958), pp. 74–88.

[2] J. R. ASHFORD and C. S. SMITH, "General models for quantal response to the joint action of a mixture of drugs," *Biometrika*, Vol. 51 (1964), pp. 413–428.

[3] R. BELLMAN, "Some mathematical aspects of chemotherapy—II: The distribution of a drug in a body," *Bull. Math. Biophys.*, Vol. 22 (1960), pp. 309–322.

[4] ———, "Topics in pharmacokinetics I. Concentration dependent rates," *Math. Biosci.*, Vol. 6 (1970), pp. 13–17.

[5] J. BERKSON, "A statistically precise and relatively simple method of estimating the bioassay with quantal response, based on the logistic function," *J. Amer. Statist. Assoc.*, Vol. 48 (1953), pp. 565–599.

[6] C. I. BLISS, *The Statistics of Bioassay with Special Reference to the Vitamins*, New York, Academic Press, 1952 (reprinted with additions from *Vitamin Methods*, Vol. 2).

[7] D. J. FINNEY, *Statistical Method in Biological Assay*, London, Charles Griffin, 1952.

[8] ———, *Probit Analysis. A Statistical Treatment of the Sigmoid Response Curve*, Cambridge, Cambridge University Press, 1947.

[9] J. GANI, "Some problems in the theory of provisioning and of dams," *Biometrika*, Vol. 42 (1955), pp. 179–200.

[10] J. T. MARTIN, "The problem of the evaluation of rotenone-containing plants VI. The toxicity of *l*-elliptone and of poisons applied jointly with further observations on the rotenone equivalent method of assessing the toxicity of derris root," *Ann. Appl. Biol.*, Vol. 29 (1942), pp. 69–81.

[11] P. A. P. MORAN, "A theory of dams with continuous input and a general release rule," *J. Appl. Probability*, Vol. 6 (1969), pp. 88–98.

[12] J. NEYMAN and E. L. SCOTT, "Statistical aspect of the problem of carcinogenesis," *Proceedings of the Fifth Berkeley Symposium on Mathematical Statistics and Probability*, Berkeley and Los Angeles, University of California Press, 1967, Vol. 4, pp. 745–776.

[13] R. L. PLACKETT and P. S. HEWLETT, "A comparison of two approaches to the construction of models for quantal responses to mixtures of drugs," *Biometrics*, Vol. 23 (1967), pp. 27–44.

[14] ———, "A unified theory for quantal responses to mixture of drugs: the fitting of data of certain models for two non-interactive drugs with complete positive correlation of tolerances," *Biometrics*, Vol. 19 (1963), pp. 517–531.

[15] N. U. PRABHU, *Queues and Inventories*, New York, Wiley, 1965.

[16] P. S. PURI, "A class of stochastic models of response after infection in the absence of defense mechanism," *Proceedings of the Fifth Berkeley Symposium on Mathematical Statistics and Probability*, Berkeley and Los Angeles, University of California Press, 1967, Vol. 4, pp. 511–535.

[17] ———, "Some new results in the mathematical theory of phage reproduction," *J. Appl. Probability*, Vol. 6 (1969), pp. 493–504.

[18] ———, "A quantal response process associated with integrals of certain growth processes," *Proc. Symp. Mathematical Aspects of Life Sciences*, Queens University Press, 1971, pp. 95–125.

[19] ———, "A method for studying the integral functionals of stochastic processes with applications: I. Markov chain case.," *J. Appl. Probability*, Vol. 8 (1971), pp. 331–343.

[20] ———, "A method for studying the integral functionals of stochastic processes with applications: II. Sojourn time distributions for Markov chains," *Z. Wahrscheinlichkeitstheorie und verw. Gebiete*, 1972, in press.

[21] ———, "A method for studying the integral functionals of stochastic processes with applications: III. Birth and death processes," *Proceedings of the Sixth Berkeley Symposium on Mathematical Statistics and Probability*, Berkeley and Los Angeles, University of California Press, 1972, Vol. 3, pp. 481–500.

[22] L. A. SAPIRSTEIN, D. G. VIDT, J. J. MANDEL, and G. HANUSEK, "Volume of distribution and clearances of intravenously injected creatinine in the dog," *Amer. J. Physiol.*, Vol. 181 (1955), pp. 330–336.

[23] J. SENTURIA, "On a mathematical theory of quantal response assays and some new models in dam theory," Ph.D. thesis, Purdue University, 1971.

[24] M. R. WHITE, "Studies of the mechanism of induction of pulmonary adenoma in mice," *Proceedings of the Sixth Berkeley Symposium on Mathematical Statistics and Probability*, Berkeley and Los Angeles, University of California Press, 1972, Vol. 4, pp. 287–307.

[25] C. GUILLIER, "Evaluation of the internal exposure due to various administered dosages of urethane to mice," *Proceedings of the Sixth Berkeley Symposium on Mathematical Statistics and Probability*, Berkeley and Los Angeles, University of California Press, 1972, Vol. 4, pp. 309–315.

ESTIMATING THE MEAN OF A RANDOM BINOMIAL PARAMETER

G. MORRIS SOUTHWARD

INTERNATIONAL PACIFIC HALIBUT COMMISSION

and

J. VAN RYZIN

UNIVERSITY OF WISCONSIN

1. Introduction

In studying biological phenomenon, one often observes random variables which are the result of other randomly occurring unobservable events. This is usually the case in the observation of genetic traits. The measurable trait in question has a probability distribution for the population of animals under study. Each individual member of the population of animals carries a value of the measurable trait, but it may or may not (and often is not) directly observable. It is not difficult to envision the probability distribution of the trait in the population as being continuous, while the distribution of the visible expression of the trait is a discrete count depending on the value of the measurable trait.

Such a problem came to the authors' attention during discussion with a poultry scientist who was interested in the probability distribution governing the frequency with which blood spotted eggs occur. Poultrymen wish to determine from examination of a small number of eggs laid early in the life of each hen what the average probability of laying blood spotted eggs is for the flock.

The problem can be conceptualized as follows. The distribution of blood spots in eggs for a given chicken is taken as binomial. That is, if p represents the probability of a given chicken to lay a blood spotted egg and m eggs are laid, then $X =$ number of blood spotted eggs is binomially distributed with parameters m and p assuming the eggs are laid independently. However, the probability p (or propensity) for laying blood spotted eggs (the trait in question), differs from chicken to chicken and can be thought of as having a continuous distribution on the unit interval. The probability distribution of the blood spotting trait p in the population is not directly observable. That is, one might postulate that the binomial parameter p (or trait) has a distribution on the unit interval and that the values of this probability carried by each bird in the flock are independently allocated according to this distribution, denoted $G(p)$. Rarely, if ever, are values of p directly observable.

The investigation of J. Van Ryzin was supported in part by USPHS Research Grant No. GM-10525-08, National Institute of Health, Public Health Service, and in part by NSF Contract No. GP-9324.

Thus, the model is written as

(1.1)
$$f(x; m) = \int_0^1 \binom{m}{x} p^x(1 - p)^{m-x} \, dG(p),$$

$x = 0, \cdots, m$, where m is the size of the sample examined and $G(p)$ is the distribution of the probability p.

The problem we consider here is that of estimating the mean μ_p of the probability distribution $G(p)$, that is, $\mu = \mu_p = \int p \, dG(p)$, based on a random sample $X_1, \cdots, X_n$ from $f(x; m)$, where X_i is the number of blood spotted eggs among the m eggs sampled from the ith chicken. The moment estimator of μ_p and its large sample properties along with confidence intervals are developed in Section 2.

It is clear that the above type of sampling, when we wish to estimate μ_p, occurs in many setups similar to that of our chicken example. Also, the allied problem, when the sample size m is allowed to vary from individual to individual, is discussed in Sections 3, 4, and 5. In that case, the distribution of each X_i is given by equation (1.1), where m is now replaced by m_i; that is, X_i is distributed with discrete density $f(x_i; m_i)$ in (1.1), $x_i = 0, \cdots, m_i, i = 1, \cdots, n$.

Theorems 5.1 and 5.2 develop the consistency and asymptotic distribution theory for the case of differing sample sizes (m_i different). These theorems concern an estimator μ_0^* for μ which behaves asymptotically like the minimum variance unbiased linear (in the X_i) estimator of μ which is studied in Section 3.

Some aspects of this general problem are covered by Pearson [2] who discusses Bayes theorem in the light of experimental sampling. However, no attack on the above problem is made therein.

2. Estimation of the mean of $G(p)$

Let $X_1, \cdots, X_n$ be a random sample from the model

(2.1)
$$f(x; m) = \int_0^1 \binom{m}{x} p^x(1 - p)^{m-x} \, dG(p).$$

We consider the problem of estimating the mean

(2.2)
$$\mu = \int_0^1 p \, dG(p)$$

based *only* on the observations $X_1, \cdots, X_n$. Note that in fact there exists a bivariate random sample $\{(X_i, P_i), i = 1, \cdots, n\}$, where we assume that X_i conditional on $P_i = p$ is binomially distributed with m trials and success probability p and the P_i are independent marginally distributed as $G(p)$. We write $X_i | P_i = p \sim b(m, p)$ and $P_i \sim G(p), i = 1, \cdots, n$.

We employ the method of moments to obtain our estimator. Observe that

(2.3)
$$E(X_1) = E\{E[X_1 | P_1]\} = mE(P_1) = m\mu.$$

From (2.3) and the fact that $X_1, \cdots, X_n$ are independent and identically distributed with distribution (2.1), we have $E\overline{X} = m\mu$. Hence, the method of moments yields the estimator $\hat{\mu}$ of μ given by

$$(2.4) \qquad \hat{\mu} = \frac{\overline{X}}{m} = \frac{1}{mn} \sum_{i=1}^{n} X_i.$$

From the strong law of large numbers, we have immediately that $\hat{\mu}$ is a strongly consistent estimator of μ. That is,

$$(2.5) \qquad P(\lim_{n \to \infty} \hat{\mu} = \mu) = 1.$$

Next we will obtain the large sample distribution of $\hat{\mu}$ quite directly from the central limit theorem. First, observe that the variance of $\hat{\mu}$ is given by

$$(2.6) \qquad \mathrm{Var}\,(\hat{\mu}) = \mathrm{Var}\left(\frac{\overline{X}}{m}\right) = \frac{\sigma_1^2}{m^2 n},$$

where $\sigma_1^2 = \mathrm{Var}\,(X_1)$. Therefore, by the central limit theorem for independent, identically distributed random variables with finite variance, we have as $n \to \infty$

$$(2.7) \qquad \mathcal{L}\left(\frac{m\sqrt{n}(\hat{\mu} - \mu)}{\sigma_1}\right) \to N(0, 1),$$

where $\mathcal{L}(Z_n) \to N(\mu, \sigma^2)$ means $\{Z_n\}$ converges in distribution to a random variable Z which is normally distributed with mean μ and variance σ^2.

Besides $\hat{\mu}$ being strongly consistent as in (2.5) and asymptotically normal as in (2.7), we note that $\hat{\mu}$ in (2.4) is the minimum variance unbiased linear (in the X_i) estimator of μ. This is a direct result of Theorem 3.1 in Section 3.

Furthermore, by defining

$$(2.8) \qquad S^2 = (n - 1)^{-1} \sum_{i=1}^{n} (X_i - \overline{X})^2,$$

we have S^2 in an unbiased, consistent estimator of σ_1^2. That is,

$$(2.9) \qquad S^2 \xrightarrow{P} \sigma_1^2$$

as $n \to \infty$. Using (2.9) and (2.7), we obtain (see for example, Rao [3], $(x) - (b)$, p. 102) as $n \to \infty$

$$(2.10) \qquad \mathcal{L}\left(\frac{m\sqrt{n}(\hat{\mu} - \mu)}{S}\right) \to N(0, 1).$$

From (2.10), we can immediately give a $100(1 - \alpha)$ per cent, $0 < \alpha < 1$, large sample confidence interval for μ, since

$$(2.11) \quad \lim_{n \to \infty} P\left\{\frac{1}{m}\left(\overline{X} - \frac{1}{\sqrt{n}} Z_{\alpha/2} S\right) < \mu < \frac{1}{m}\left(\overline{X} + \frac{1}{\sqrt{n}} Z_{\alpha/2} S\right)\right\} = 1 - \alpha,$$

where $Z_{\alpha/2}$ is defined by the equation

$$(2.12) \qquad \int_{-Z_{\alpha/2}}^{Z_{\alpha/2}} \left(\frac{1}{2\pi}\right)^{\frac{1}{2}} \exp\left\{-\frac{t^2}{2}\right\} dt = 1 - \alpha.$$

For example, if we want a 95 per cent confidence interval for the mean probability of the flock for laying a blood spotted egg, we would choose $\alpha = 0.05$ yielding an approximate large sample confidence interval

$$(2.13) \qquad \left(\frac{1}{m} \left(\overline{X} - \frac{1.96S}{\sqrt{n}} \right), \frac{1}{m} \left(\overline{X} + \frac{1.96S}{\sqrt{n}} \right) \right).$$

Some sample intervals are constructed for data randomly generated by a simulation process involving varying sample sizes and are here included.

The density given by (2.1) was computed for the case of $G(p)$ being a beta distribution. That is, assume $dG(p) = g(p) \, dp$, where the density $g(p)$ is given by

$$(2.14) \qquad g(p) = \{\beta(r, s)\}^{-1} p^{r-1} (1 - p)^{s-1}, \qquad 0 < p < 1, \qquad r > 0, \qquad s > 0,$$

and $\beta(r, s) = \int_0^1 p^{r-1}(1 - p)^{s-1} \, dp$. A range of values of m, r, and s was chosen and μ computed for each set of values thereof. Random samples were drawn and $\hat\mu$ and Var $(\hat\mu)$ estimated. Table I gives μ, $\hat\mu$, and the estimated standard error of $\hat\mu$, $S/(m\sqrt{n})$, for a few selected values of m, r, and s. The entry on the first line is for a sample of $n = 50$ and on the second line for a sample of $n = 200$. In most instances $\hat\mu$ estimates μ well; $\hat\mu \pm 1.96S/m\sqrt{n}$ fails to contain μ only three times out of the 40 cases presented. That is, when $m = 10$, $r = s = 1$, $n = 50$; $m = 15$, $r = 1$, $s = 5$, $n = 200$; and $m = 15$, $r = 2$, $s = 15$, $n = 200$. Many other values of m, r, s, and n were also tried with similar good results.

3. The case of differing sample sizes

Often times in applications the number of trials m connected with each observation may not be the same. That is, consider the case where each X_i is distributed as (2.1) with m replaced by m_i, $i = 1, \cdots, n$. We assume the m_i are all known, fixed, positive integers, but not necessarily equal.

To estimate μ, we again use the method of moments. Similar to (2.3), we have

$$(3.1) \qquad\qquad E(X_i) = m_i\mu, \qquad\qquad i = 1, \cdots, n.$$

Since (3.1) implies both $E\{\sum_{i=1}^n (X_i/m_i)\} = n\mu$ and $E(\sum_{i=1}^n X_i) = (\sum_{i=1}^n m_i)\mu$, we have as possible moment estimators of μ both

$$(3.2) \qquad\qquad \hat\mu_1 = \frac{1}{n} \sum_{i=1}^n \frac{X_i}{m_i}$$

and

$$(3.3) \qquad\qquad \hat\mu_2 = \frac{\overline{X}}{\overline{m}},$$

where $\overline{m} = (1/n) \sum_{i=1}^n m_i$.

In order to discuss the relative merits of the estimators $\hat\mu_1$ and $\hat\mu_2$, we compute their variances. With

$$(3.4) \qquad\qquad \sigma^2 = \text{Var}(P_1) = \int (p - \mu)^2 \, dG(p)$$

and

$$(3.5) \qquad\qquad \tau = E\{P_1(1 - P_1)\} = \int p(1 - p) \, dG(p),$$

TABLE I

COMPARISON OF μ AND $\hat{\mu}$ FOR CASE OF BETA
DISTRIBUTION, $n = 50$ AND $n = 200$

m	r	s	μ_p	$\hat{\mu}_p$	$S/(m\sqrt{n})$
10	1	1	.500	.594	.0411
				.505	.0217
		2	.333	.314	.0366
				.342	.0198
		5	.167	.170	.0241
				.158	.0125
		10	.091	.100	.0204
				.093	.0087
		15	.063	.060	.0121
				.060	.0068
	2	1	.667	.698	.0366
				.688	.0177
		2	.500	.548	.0388
				.482	.0181
		5	.286	.314	.0287
				.298	.0146
		10	.167	.178	.0225
				.154	.0106
		15	.118	.120	.0232
				.116	.0082
15	1	1	.500	.489	.0470
				.474	.0218
		2	.333	.295	.0397
				.327	.0179
		5	.167	.197	.0268
				.190	.0129
		10	.091	.116	.0209
				.096	.0082
		15	.063	.052	.0107
				.062	.0057
	2	1	.667	.653	.0341
				.657	.0183
		2	.500	.449	.0386
				.485	.0165
		5	.286	.320	.0306
				.285	.0136
		10	.167	.192	.0225
				.167	.0102
		15	.118	.112	.0175
				.118	.0075

we have

(3.6)
$$\mathrm{Var}\,(\hat{\mu}_2) = (\bar{m}n)^{-2} \sum_{i=1}^{n} \mathrm{Var}\,(X_i)$$

$$= n^{-1}(a_n\sigma^2 + b_n\tau),$$

where $a_n = (\bar{m}^2 n)^{-1} \sum_{i=1}^{n} m_i^2$, $b_n = (\bar{m})^{-1}$, $\bar{m} = n^{-1} \sum_{i=1}^{n} m_i$.

Also, we obtain

$$(3.7) \qquad \mathrm{Var}\,(\hat\mu_1) = n^{-2} \sum_{i=1}^{n} \mathrm{Var}\,(X_i) = n^{-1}(\sigma^2 + c_n\tau),$$

where $c_n = n^{-1} \sum_{i=1}^{n} m_i^{-1}$.

From the Cauchy-Schwarz inequality, it is easy to show that

$$(3.8) \qquad a_n \geqq 1 \quad \text{and} \quad b_n \leqq c_n,$$

where the inequalities are strict unless $m_i = m$ for all i. Hence, it is clear that neither $\hat\mu_1$ nor $\hat\mu_2$ is for all G relatively more efficient than the other. In fact, from (3.8) we see that if $\sigma^2 = 0$ and $\tau > 0$, $\hat\mu_2$ is more efficient, $\mathrm{Var}\,(\hat\mu_2) \leqq \mathrm{Var}\,(\hat\mu_1)$, than $\hat\mu_1$, while the reverse is true if $\sigma^2 > 0$ and $\tau = 0$.

Note the case $\sigma^2 = 0$ implies that $G(p)$ is degenerate at, say, p_0, and hence that $S_n = \sum_{i=1}^{n} X_i$ is binomially distributed with parameter $\sum_{i=1}^{n} m_i$ and p_0. Thus, $\hat\mu_2$ in this case becomes the classical (maximum likelihood, moment and minimum variance unbiased estimator) solution to the problem of estimating $\mu = p_0$. *In the remainder of the paper, we omit this case from consideration and shall assume $\sigma^2 > 0$.*

We consider now the question of the existence of an optimal solution in the minimum variance sense. The following theorem gives a solution to the problem for unbiased linear (in X_i) estimators.

Let M_n be the class of all unbiased linear estimators of μ based on $X_1, \cdots, X_n$. That is,

$$(3.9) \qquad M_n = \left\{ \hat\mu \Big| \hat\mu = \sum_{i=1}^{n} c_{in} \frac{X_i}{m_i}, \sum_{i=1}^{n} c_{in} = 1 \right\}.$$

Observe that the condition $\sum_{i=1}^{n} c_{in} = 1$ implies that $\hat\mu$ is unbiased by (3.1). Also, $\hat\mu \in M_n$ is clearly linear in the X_i as well as in the X_i/m_i by taking $c'_{in} = c_{in}/m_i$ and defining $\hat\mu = \sum_{i=1}^{n} c'_{in} X_i$ in M_n.

THEOREM 3.1. *The minimum variance unbiased linear estimate of μ (that is, the $\hat\mu \in M_n$ of minimum variance) is given by*

$$(3.10) \qquad \hat\mu_0 = \sum_{i=1}^{n} c_{in}^{\circ} \frac{X_i}{m_i},$$

where

$$(3.11) \qquad c_{in}^{\circ} = c_{in}^{\circ}(\sigma^2, \tau) = \left\{ \sigma^2 + \frac{\tau}{m_i} \right\}^{-1} \Big/ \sum_{i=1}^{n} \left\{ \sigma^2 + \frac{\tau}{m_i} \right\}^{-1},$$

with σ^2 and τ as in (3.4) and (3.5).

REMARK. In particular, $\hat\mu_0 = \hat\mu_1 = \hat\mu_2$ if all $m_i = m$ (see Section 1), and $\hat\mu_0 = \hat\mu_1$ if $\sigma^2 > 0$, $\tau = 0$, and $\hat\mu_0 = \hat\mu_2$ if $\sigma^2 = 0$, $\tau > 0$.

PROOF. Let $\sigma_i^2 = \mathrm{Var}\,(X_i/m_i) = \sigma^2 + \tau/m_i$. Then, for $\hat\mu \in M_n$, we have $\mathrm{Var}\,(\hat\mu) = \sum_{i=1}^{n} c_{in}^2 \sigma_i^2$, which is minimized by taking $c_{in} = c_{in}^{\circ}$ as in (3.11). (See for example, Rao [3], 2.2, p. 249.)

THEOREM 3.2. *If $\sigma^2 > 0$, then $P\{\lim_{n \to \infty} \hat\mu_0 = \mu\} = 1$ for any sequence $\{m_n\}$ of positive integers.*

PROOF. Let $Y_i = \sigma_i^{-2}(X_i/m_i)$, where $\sigma_i^2 = \text{Var}(X_i/m_i) = \sigma^2 + \tau/m_i$. Let $b_n = \sum_{i=1}^n \sigma_i^{-2}$ and observe that (see Loève [1], 16.3, II, A, p. 238) $\hat{\mu}_0 - \mu = b_n^{-1} \sum_{i=1}^n (Y_i - EY_i) \to 0$ with probability 1 as $n \to \infty$ provided

$$(3.12) \qquad \sum_{n=1}^\infty b_n^{-2} \text{Var}(Y_n) < \infty.$$

But since $b_n \geq n(\sigma^2 + \tau)^{-1}$ and $\text{Var}(Y_i) = \sigma_i^{-2} \leq \sigma^{-2}$, we see that (3.12) holds since $\sum_{n=1}^\infty n^{-2} < \infty$.

THEOREM 3.3. *If $\sigma^2 > \sigma$, then for any sequence of positive integers $\{m_n\}$,*

$$(3.13) \qquad \mathcal{L}\left(\frac{\hat{\mu}_0 - \mu}{(\text{Var}(\hat{\mu}_0))^{1/2}}\right) \to N(0, 1)$$

as $n \to \infty$, where

$$(3.14) \qquad \text{Var}(\hat{\mu}_0) = \left\{\sum_{i=1}^n \sigma_i^{-2}\right\}^{-1} = \left\{\sum_{i=1}^n (\sigma^2 + \tau/m_i)^{-1}\right\}^{-1}.$$

PROOF. Let $Y_{in} = c_{in}^\circ(m_i^{-1}X_i - \mu)$, $\sigma_{in}^2 = \text{Var}(Y_{in})$, and $s_n^2 = \sum_{i=1}^n \sigma_{in}^2$. Then, by an extended version of the Liapounov theorem (Loève [1], 20.1, a, p. 277), we have

$$(3.15) \qquad \mathcal{L}\left(\frac{\hat{\mu}_0 - \mu_0}{(\text{Var}(\hat{\mu}_0))^{1/2}}\right) = \mathcal{L}\left(\frac{\sum_{i=1}^n Y_{in}}{s_n}\right) \to N(0, 1)$$

as $n \to \infty$ provided

$$(3.16) \qquad s_n^{-3} \sum_{i=1}^n E|Y_{in}|^3 \to 0$$

as $n \to \infty$. But since $s_n^2 = \{\sum_{i=1}^n \sigma_i^{-2}\}^{-1}$ and $c_{in}^\circ = s_n^2 \sigma_i^{-2}$ with $\sigma_i^2 = \sigma^2 + \tau/m_i$, we have

$$(3.17) \qquad s_n^{-3} \sum_{i=1}^n E|Y_{in}|^3 = s_n^3 \sum_{i=1}^n \sigma_i^{-6} E\left|\frac{X_i}{m_i} - \mu\right|^3$$

$$\leq s_n^3 \sum_{i=1}^n \sigma_i^{-4}$$

$$\leq n^{-1/2}(\sigma^2 + \tau)^{3/2}\sigma^{-4},$$

where the last inequality follows by using $(\sigma^2 + \tau)^{-1} \leq \sigma_i^{-2} \leq \sigma^{-2}$. Hence, (3.16) holds and the theorem is proved.

We note that Theorem 3.3 immediately yields large sample confidence intervals on μ provided σ^2 and τ are known. Under the condition of Theorem 3.3 a $100(1 - \alpha)$ per cent large sample approximate confidence interval for μ is given by

$$(3.18) \qquad (\hat{\mu}_0 - \varepsilon_n, \hat{\mu}_0 + \varepsilon_n),$$

where $\varepsilon_n = Z_{\alpha/2}\{\sum_{i=1}^n (\sigma^2 + \tau/m_i)^{-1}\}^{-1/2}$ and $\hat{\mu}_0 = \sum_{i=1}^n c_{in}^\circ(X_i/m_i)$. However, in most applications σ^2 and τ remain unknown and we must therefore concern ourselves with this case. Section 4 discusses the question of estimating σ^2 and τ, while Section 5 develops the necessary large sample results for estimating μ when σ^2 and τ are unknown and the sample sizes m_i differ.

4. Estimation of σ^2 and τ

Define the random variables Y_i, Z_i and the indicator variables δ_i, $i = 1, \cdots,$ n, as follows:

$$(4.1) \qquad Y_i = \frac{X_i}{m_i},$$

$$(4.2) \qquad Z_i = \begin{cases} \dfrac{X_i(m_i - X_i)}{m_i(m_i - 1)} & \text{if } m_i > 1, \\ 0 & \text{if } m_i = 1, \end{cases}$$

and

$$(4.3) \qquad \delta_i = \begin{cases} 1 & \text{if } m_i > 1, \\ 0 & \text{if } m_i = 1. \end{cases}$$

Observing that $EX_i^2 = EX_i(X_i - 1) + EX_i = m_i^2 E(P_1^2) + m_i\tau$, one obtains

$$(4.4) \qquad EZ_i = \delta_i\tau.$$

Furthermore, using the relationship

$$(4.5) \qquad \sum_{i=1}^{n} (Y_i - \bar{Y})^2 = \sum_{i=1}^{n} (Y_i - \mu)^2 - n(\bar{Y} - \mu)^2,$$

it can easily be shown that

$$(4.6) \qquad E\left\{ \sum_{i=1}^{n} (Y_i - \bar{Y})^2 \right\} = (n - 1)\left\{ \sigma^2 + \left(\frac{1}{n} \sum_{i=1}^{n} \frac{1}{m_i} \right)\tau \right\}.$$

From equations (4.4) and (4.6) and defining

$$(4.7) \qquad S_1^2 = (n - 1)^{-1} \sum_{i=1}^{n} (Y_i - \bar{Y})^2$$

and

$$(4.8) \qquad a_n = \max\left\{ \sum_{i=1}^{n} \delta_i, 1 \right\},$$

we obtain as moment estimators of τ and σ^2, when $\sum_{i=1}^{n} \delta_i > 0$,

$$(4.9) \qquad \hat{\tau} = a_n^{-1} \sum_{i=1}^{n} Z_i$$

and

$$(4.10) \qquad (\sigma^*)^2 = S_1^2 - \hat{\tau} \left(\frac{1}{n} \sum_{i=1}^{n} \frac{1}{m_i} \right).$$

Note that from (4.4) and (4.6) the unbiasedness of τ and $(\sigma^*)^2$ follows. That is, when $\sum_{i=1}^{n} \delta_i > 0$,

$$(4.11) \qquad E(\hat{\tau}) = \tau, \qquad E\{(\sigma^*)^2\} = \sigma^2.$$

The estimator $(\sigma^*)^2$ in (4.9) may be negative as an estimator of $\sigma^2 > 0$. We shall find it convenient to modify $(\sigma^*)^2$ for later purposes and we define $\hat{\sigma}^2$ as the following positive truncation of $(\sigma^*)^2$,

$$(4.12) \qquad \hat{\sigma}^2 = \max \{(\sigma^*)^2, n^{-1}\}.$$

The following theorem gives the consistency properties of $\hat{\tau}$, $\hat{\sigma}^2$ (and $(\sigma^*)^2$).

THEOREM 4.1.   *Let $\sigma^2 > 0$. If $\{m_n\}$ is any sequence of positive integers for which $a_n \to \infty$ as $n \to \infty$ (see (4.8)), then as $n \to \infty$, $\hat{\tau} \to \tau$ and $\hat{\sigma}^2 \to \sigma^2$ (or $(\sigma^*)^2 \to \sigma^2$) in probability. Furthermore, if $\{m_n\}$ is such that $\sum_{n=1}^{\infty} a_n^{-2} < \infty$, the convergences hold with probability one.*

PROOF.   Observe that since $0 \leq Z_i \leq \frac{1}{2}$, we have

$$(4.13) \qquad \mathrm{Var}\,(\hat{\tau}) = a_n^{-2} \sum_{i=1}^{n} \delta_i \,\mathrm{Var}\,(Z_i) \leq (4a_n)^{-1}.$$

Hence, $\hat{\tau} \to \tau$ in probability as $n \to \infty$ by Chebyshev's inequality. To prove convergence with probability one for $\hat{\tau}$, it suffices (by Loève [1], 16.3, II, A, p. 238) to verify that $\sum_{n=1}^{\infty} a_n^{-2}\,\mathrm{Var}\,(Z_n) < \infty$, which clearly holds in $\sum_{n=1}^{\infty} a_n^{-2} < \infty$, since $\mathrm{Var}\,(Z_n) \leq \frac{1}{4}$.

Observe that $(\sigma^*)^2$ is linear in $\hat{\tau}$ in (4.10). Thus, convergence of $(\sigma^*)^2$ to σ^2 in probability ($\overset{P}{\to}$) or with probability one ($\overset{a.s.}{\to}$) as $n \to \infty$ follows from Theorem 3.2 provided

$$(4.14) \qquad S_1^2 - \left(\sigma^2 + \frac{\tau}{n} \sum_{i=1}^{n} \frac{1}{m_i}\right) \overset{a.s.}{\to} 0$$

as $n \to \infty$. But (4.14) follows immediately from (4.5), (4.6), and (4.7) provided as $n \to \infty$,

$$(4.15) \qquad \frac{1}{n} \sum_{i=1}^{n} (Y_i - \mu)^2 - \left(\sigma^2 + \frac{\tau}{n} \sum_{i=1}^{n} \frac{1}{m_i}\right) \overset{a.s.}{\to} 0.$$

Let $X_i' = (Y_i - \mu)^2$ in (4.15) and write the left side of (4.15) as $n^{-1} \sum_{i=1}^{n} (X_i' - EX_i')$. Now, applying a version of the Kolmogorov strong law of large numbers (see Loève [1], 16.3, II, A, p. 238), we see (4.15) holds provided

$$(4.16) \qquad \sum_{n=1}^{\infty} n^{-2}\,\mathrm{Var}\,(X_n') < \infty.$$

But the convergence of the series in (4.16) is an immediate consequence of the boundedness of X_n' by one. Thus, the theorem is proved.

REMARK.   We observe that the condition $a_n \to \infty$ is necessary in Theorem 4.1. To see this consider the case where all the m_i are 1 or 2. Then $a_n \nrightarrow \infty$ implies there exist n_0 such that $\delta_n = 0$ ($m_n = 1$) for $n \geq n_0$. Thus $\hat{\tau} = a_{n_0}^{-1} \sum_{i=1}^{n_0} Z_i$ for all $n \geq n_0$ and clearly $\hat{\tau} \overset{P}{\nrightarrow} \tau$ as $n \to \infty$.

5. Estimation of μ when σ^2 and τ are unknown in the differing sample size case

The minimum variance unbiased linear estimate of μ in Theorem 3.1 depends on *knowing* σ^2 and τ for the optimal choice of the constants c_{in}° in (3.11). To overcome this problem when σ^2 and τ are unknown, we propose and study an estimator of μ, denoted μ_0^*, which chooses the c_{in}° in (3.11) based on the estimators $\hat{\sigma}^2$, $\hat{\tau}$ of σ^2, τ given in the previous section. Theorems 5.1 and 5.2 give the large sample properties of the proposed estimator.

Specifically, let

$$(5.1) \qquad \hat{c}_{in} = c_{in}^\circ(\hat{\sigma}^2, \hat{\tau}) = \begin{cases} \dfrac{1}{n} & \text{if } \hat{\tau} = 0, \\[2ex] \dfrac{\left(\hat{\sigma}^2 + \dfrac{\hat{\tau}}{m_i}\right)^{-1}}{\displaystyle\sum_{i=1}^{n}\left(\hat{\sigma}^2 + \dfrac{\hat{\tau}}{m_i}\right)^{-1}} & \text{if } \hat{\tau} > 0, \end{cases}$$

where $\hat{\tau}$ and $\hat{\sigma}^2$ are defined by (4.9), (4.10), and (4.12). Now define

$$(5.2) \qquad \mu_0^* = \sum_{i=1}^{n} \hat{c}_{in} \frac{X_i}{m_i}.$$

It will be shown that under appropriate conditions $\mu_0^* \to \mu$ in probability as $n \to \infty$ (see Theorem 5.1). Before proving this theorem, however, we develop the following lemma.

LEMMA 5.1.   *If $\sigma^2 > 0$ and $a_n \to \infty$ as $n \to \infty$ (see (4.3) and (4.8)), then*

$$(5.3) \qquad \mu_0^* = \hat{\mu}_0 + (\hat{\sigma}^2 - \sigma^2) \sum_{i=1}^{n} \alpha_{in}\left(\frac{X_i}{m_i} - \mu\right)$$

$$+ (\hat{\tau} - \tau) \sum_{i=1}^{n} \beta_{in}\left(\frac{X_i}{m_i} - \mu\right)$$

$$+ [|\hat{\sigma}^2 - \sigma^2| + |\hat{\tau} - \tau|]^2 O_p(1)\hat{\mu}_1,$$

where α_{in} and β_{in} are nonrandom coefficients such that $\sum_{i=1}^{n} \alpha_{in} = \sum_{i=1}^{n} \beta_{in} = 0$ and $O_p(1)$ indicates a random factor which is bounded in probability.

PROOF.   Let

$$c_{in}(u, v) = \left\{\sum_{i=1}^{n}\left(u + \frac{v}{m_i}\right)^{-1}\right\}^{-1}\left(u + \frac{v}{m_i}\right)^{-1},$$

$$(5.4) \qquad \alpha_{in} = \left.\frac{\partial c_{in}}{\partial u}\right|_{u=\sigma^2, v=\tau},$$

$$\beta_{in} = \left.\frac{\partial c_{in}}{\partial v}\right|_{u=\sigma^2, v=\tau}.$$

Observe that $c_{in}(u, v)$ has continuous second order partial (and mixed partial) derivatives on the set $\{(u, v): 0 < u < \infty, 0 \leq v < \infty\}$, where the partial derivative is defined from the right at $v = 0$. Hence, we have the following second order Taylor expansion for $c_{in}(\hat{\sigma}^2, \hat{\tau})$,

$$(5.5) \qquad c_{in}(\hat{\sigma}^2, \hat{\tau}) = c_{in}(\sigma^2, \tau) + (\hat{\sigma}^2 - \sigma^2)\alpha_{in} + (\hat{\tau} - \tau)\beta_{in}$$

$$+ \frac{(\hat{\sigma}^2 - \sigma^2)^2}{2} \left.\frac{\partial^2 c_{in}}{\partial u^2}\right|_{u=u_i^*, v=v_i^*}$$

$$+ (\hat{\sigma}^2 - \sigma^2)(\hat{\tau} - \tau) \frac{\partial^2 c_{in}}{\partial u\, \partial v}\bigg|_{u=u_i^*, v=v_i^*}$$

$$+ \frac{(\hat{\tau} - \tau)^2}{2} \frac{\partial^2 c_{in}}{\partial v^2}\bigg|_{u=u_i^*, v=v_i^*},$$

where $\min (\sigma^2, \hat{\sigma}^2) \leqq u_i^* \leqq \max (\sigma^2, \hat{\sigma}^2)$ and $\min (\tau, \hat{\tau}) \leqq v_i^* \leqq \max (\tau, \hat{\tau})$. Observe that

(5.6) $\quad \dfrac{\partial c_{in}}{\partial u} = \dfrac{\left\{\left(u + \dfrac{v}{m_i}\right)^{-1} \sum\limits_{j=1}^{n} \left(u + \dfrac{v}{m_j}\right)^{-2}\right\} - \left\{\left(u + \dfrac{v}{m_i}\right)^{-2} \sum\limits_{j=1}^{n} \left(u + \dfrac{v}{m_j}\right)^{-1}\right\}}{\left\{\sum\limits_{j=1}^{n} \left(u + \dfrac{v}{m_j}\right)^{-1}\right\}^2},$

(5.7)

$\dfrac{\partial c_{in}}{\partial v} = \dfrac{\left\{\left(u + \dfrac{v}{m_i}\right)^{-1} \sum\limits_{j=1}^{n} \dfrac{1}{m_j}\left(u + \dfrac{v}{m_j}\right)^{-2}\right\} - \left\{\dfrac{1}{m_i}\left(u + \dfrac{v}{m_i}\right)^{-2} \sum\limits_{j=1}^{n} \left(u + \dfrac{v}{m_j}\right)^{-1}\right\}}{\left\{\sum\limits_{j=1}^{n} \left(u + \dfrac{v}{m_j}\right)^{-1}\right\}^2},$

(5.8) $\quad \dfrac{\partial^2 c_{in}}{\partial u^2} = \dfrac{2\left(u + \dfrac{v}{m_i}\right)^{-3}}{\sum\limits_{j=1}^{n} \left(u + \dfrac{v}{m_i}\right)^{-1}} - \dfrac{2\left(u + \dfrac{v}{m_i}\right)^{-1} \sum\limits_{j=1}^{n} \left(u + \dfrac{v}{m_j}\right)^{-3}}{\left\{\sum\limits_{j=1}^{n} \left(u + \dfrac{v}{m_j}\right)^{-1}\right\}^2}$

$\quad + \dfrac{2\left(u + \dfrac{v}{m_i}\right)^{-1} \left\{\sum\limits_{j=1}^{n} \left(u + \dfrac{v}{m_j}\right)^{-2}\right\}^2}{\left\{\sum\limits_{j=1}^{n} \left(u + \dfrac{v}{m_j}\right)^{-1}\right\}^3} - \dfrac{2\left(u + \dfrac{v}{m_i}\right)^{-2} \sum\limits_{j=1}^{n} \left(u + \dfrac{v}{m_j}\right)^{-2}}{\left\{\sum\limits_{j=1}^{n} \left(u + \dfrac{v}{m_j}\right)^{-1}\right\}^2},$

(5.9) $\quad \dfrac{\partial^2 c_{in}}{\partial v^2} = \dfrac{\dfrac{2}{m_i^2}\left(u + \dfrac{v}{m_i}\right)^{-3}}{\sum\limits_{j=1}^{n} \left(u + \dfrac{v}{m_j}\right)^{-1}} - \dfrac{2\left(u + \dfrac{v}{m_i}\right)^{-1} \sum\limits_{j=1}^{n} \dfrac{1}{m_j^2}\left(u + \dfrac{v}{m_j}\right)^{-3}}{\left\{\sum\limits_{j=1}^{n} \left(u + \dfrac{v}{m_j}\right)^{-1}\right\}^2}$

$\quad + \dfrac{2\left(u + \dfrac{v}{m_i}\right)^{-1} \left\{\sum\limits_{j=1}^{n} \dfrac{1}{m_j}\left(u + \dfrac{v}{m_j}\right)^{-2}\right\}^2}{\left\{\sum\limits_{j=1}^{n} \left(u + \dfrac{v}{m_j}\right)^{-1}\right\}^3} - \dfrac{\dfrac{2}{m_i}\left(u + \dfrac{v}{m_i}\right)^{-2} \sum\limits_{j=1}^{n} \dfrac{1}{m_j}\left(u + \dfrac{v}{m_j}\right)^{-2}}{\left\{\sum\limits_{j=1}^{n} \left(u + \dfrac{v}{m_j}\right)^{-1}\right\}^2},$

and

(5.10) $\quad \dfrac{\partial^2 c_{in}}{\partial u\, \partial v} = \dfrac{\dfrac{2}{m_i}\left(u + \dfrac{v}{m_i}\right)^{-3}}{\sum\limits_{j=1}^{n} \left(u + \dfrac{v}{m_j}\right)^{-1}} - \dfrac{2\left(u + \dfrac{v}{m_i}\right)^{-1} \sum\limits_{j=1}^{n} \dfrac{1}{m_j}\left(u + \dfrac{v}{m_j}\right)^{3}}{\left\{\sum\limits_{j=1}^{n} \left(u + \dfrac{v}{m_j}\right)^{-1}\right\}^2}$

$\quad + \dfrac{\left(u + \dfrac{v}{m_i}\right)^{-2} \sum\limits_{j=1}^{n} \dfrac{1}{m_j}\left(u + \dfrac{v}{m_j}\right)^{-2}}{\left\{\sum\limits_{j=1}^{n} \left(u + \dfrac{v}{m_j}\right)^{-1}\right\}^2} - \dfrac{\dfrac{1}{m_i}\left(u + \dfrac{v}{m_i}\right)^{-2} \sum\limits_{j=1}^{n} \left(u + \dfrac{v}{m_j}\right)^{-2}}{\left\{\sum\limits_{j=1}^{n} \left(u + \dfrac{v}{m_j}\right)^{-1}\right\}^2}$

$$+ \frac{2\left(u + \dfrac{v}{m_i}\right)^{-1}\left\{\displaystyle\sum_{j=1}^{n}\left(u + \dfrac{v}{m_j}\right)^{-2}\right\}\left\{\displaystyle\sum_{j=1}^{n}\dfrac{1}{m_j}\left(u + \dfrac{v}{m_j}\right)^{-2}\right\}}{\left\{\displaystyle\sum_{j=1}^{n}\left(u + \dfrac{v}{m_j}\right)^{-1}\right\}^3}$$

$$- \frac{2\left(u + \dfrac{v}{m_i}\right)^{-2}\displaystyle\sum_{j=1}^{n}\dfrac{1}{m_j}\left(u + \dfrac{v}{m_j}\right)^{-2}}{\left\{\displaystyle\sum_{j=1}^{n}\left(u + \dfrac{v}{m_j}\right)^{-1}\right\}^2}.$$

Note that from (5.6) and (5.7), we see that $\sum_{i=1}^{n}\alpha_{in} = \sum_{i=1}^{n}\beta_{in} = 0$. Thus, we have from (5.2) and the Taylor expansion (5.5),

$$(5.11) \quad \mu_0^* - \left\{\hat{\mu}_0 + (\hat{\sigma}^2 - \sigma^2)\sum_{i=1}^{n}\alpha_{in}\left(\frac{X_i}{m_i} - \mu\right) + (\hat{\tau} - \tau)\sum_{i=1}^{n}\beta_{in}\left(\frac{X_i}{m_i} - \mu\right)\right\}$$

$$= \frac{(\hat{\sigma}^2 - \sigma^2)^2}{2}\sum_{i=1}^{n}\frac{X_i}{m_i}\left(\frac{\partial^2 c_{in}}{\partial u^2}\bigg|_{u=u_i^*, v=v_i^*}\right)$$

$$+ (\hat{\sigma}^2 - \sigma^2)(\hat{\tau} - \tau)\sum_{i=1}^{n}\frac{X_i}{m_i}\left(\frac{\partial^2 c_{in}}{\partial u\, \partial v}\bigg|_{u=u_i^*, v=v_i^*}\right)$$

$$+ \frac{(\hat{\tau} - \tau)^2}{2}\sum_{i=1}^{n}\frac{X_i}{m_i}\left(\frac{\partial^2 c_{in}}{\partial v^2}\bigg|_{u=u_i^*, v=v_i^*}\right).$$

But the right side of (5.11) is bounded by

$$(5.12) \qquad \{|\hat{\sigma}^2 - \sigma^2| + |\hat{\tau} - \tau|\}^2 \left\{\frac{5(\underline{u})^{-3}}{(\bar{u} + \bar{v})^{-1}}\right\}\hat{\mu}_1,$$

where $\bar{u} = \max_i u_i^*$, $\underline{u} = \min_i u_i^*$, and $\bar{v} = \max_i v_i^*$, since from (5.8) through (5.10) and repeated use of the inequalities

$$(5.13) \qquad (u_i^* + v_i^*)^{-1} \leqq \left(u_i^* + \frac{v_i^*}{m_i}\right)^{-1} \leqq (u_i^*)^{-1}, \qquad \frac{1}{m_i} \leqq 1,$$

it is easy to show that

$$(5.14) \qquad \left|\left(\frac{\partial^2 c_{in}}{\partial u^2}\bigg|_{u=u_i^*, v=v_i^*}\right)\right| \leqq \frac{8(u_i^*)^{-3}}{n(u_i^* + v_i^*)^{-1}},$$

$$\left|\left(\frac{\partial^2 c_{in}}{\partial v^2}\bigg|_{u=u_i^*, v=v_i^*}\right)\right| \leqq \frac{8(u_i^*)^{-3}}{n(u_i^* + v_i^*)^{-1}},$$

and

$$(5.15) \qquad \left|\left(\frac{\partial^2 c_{in}}{\partial u\, \partial v}\bigg|_{u=u_i^*, v=v_i^*}\right)\right| \leqq \frac{10(u_i^*)^{-3}}{n(u_i^* + v_i^*)^{-1}}.$$

Bounding the right side of (5.11) by (5.12) and noting that Theorem 4.1 implies that as $n \to \infty$,

$$(5.16) \qquad \frac{(\underline{u})^{-3}}{(\bar{u} + \bar{v})^{-1}} \overset{P}{\longrightarrow} \frac{\sigma^{-6}}{(\sigma^2 + \tau)^{-1}} > 0,$$

we have that $5(\underline{u})^{-3}(\bar{u} + \bar{v})$ is $O_p(1)$. Hence, the lemma is proved.

THEOREM 5.1. *If $\sigma^2 > 0$ and $a_n \to \infty$ as $n \to \infty$ (see (4.3) and (4.8)), then μ_0^* defined by (5.1) and (5.2) is such that $\mu_0^* \xrightarrow{P} \mu$ as $n \to \infty$.*

PROOF. Repeated use of $(\sigma^2 + \tau)^{-1} \le (\sigma^2 + \tau/m_i)^{-1} \le \sigma^{-2}$ and $m_i^{-1} \le 1$ in (5.6) and (5.7) imply $\sum_{i=1}^{n} |\alpha_{in}|$ and $\sum_{i=1}^{n} |\beta_{in}|$ are bounded by $\sigma^{-4}(\sigma^2 + \tau)^{-1}$. Hence, bounding $|(X_i/m_i) - \mu| \le 1$ in (5.3) and invoking the convergences in Theorems 3.2 and 4.1, expansion (5.3) yields the result.

LEMMA 5.2. *If $n^{1/2}a_n^{-1} \to 0$ as $n \to \infty$, then $n^{1/4}(\hat{\sigma}^2 - \sigma^2) \xrightarrow{P} 0$ and $n^{1/4}(\hat{\tau} - \tau) \xrightarrow{P} 0$ as $n \to \infty$.*

PROOF. From (4.2) we have $0 \le Z_i \le \frac{1}{2}$ and $\text{Var}(Z_i) \le \frac{1}{4}$ and therefore,

$$(5.17) \qquad \text{Var}(n^{1/4}\hat{\tau}) = n^{1/2}a_n^{-2} \sum_{i=1}^{n} \delta_i \text{Var}(Z_i) \le \frac{1}{4}n^{1/2}a_n^{-1}.$$

Thus, by Chebyshev's inequality, we have

$$(5.18) \qquad n^{1/4}(\hat{\tau} - \tau) \xrightarrow{P} 0$$

as $n \to \infty$.

Next, in (4.5) and (4.7) observe that

$$(5.19) \qquad (n - 1)S_1^2 = \sum_{i=1}^{n} (Y_i - \mu)^2 - n(\bar{Y} - \mu)^2 \le 2n(\bar{Y} - \mu)^2.$$

Since S_1^2 is a nonnegative random variable and $|\bar{Y} - \mu| \le 1$, it follows that

$$(5.20) \qquad \text{Var}(S_1^2) \le ES_1^4 \le \left(\frac{2n}{n-1}\right)^2 \text{Var}(\bar{Y})$$

$$= \left(\frac{2n}{n-1}\right)^2 \frac{1}{n}\left(\sigma^2 + \frac{1}{n}\sum_{i=1}^{n} \frac{\tau}{m_i}\right).$$

But this inequality together with $m_i^{-1} \le 1$ imply that $\text{Var}(n^{1/4}S_1^2)$ is $O(n^{-1/2}(\sigma^2 + \tau))$. Hence, again by Chebyshev's inequality and (4.6), we have

$$(5.21) \qquad n^{1/4}\left\{S_1^2 - \left[\sigma^2 + \tau\left(\frac{1}{n}\sum_{i=1}^{n} \frac{1}{m_i}\right)\right]\right\} \xrightarrow{P} 0$$

as $n \to \infty$. This result together with (5.18) combine in (4.10) to yield $n^{1/4}[(\sigma^*)^2 - \sigma^2] \xrightarrow{P} 0$ as $n \to \infty$ which completes the proof of the lemma by using the definition of $\hat{\sigma}^2$.

THEOREM 5.2. *If $a_n \to \infty$ and $n^{1/2}a_n^{-1} \to 0$ as $n \to \infty$ (see (4.3) and (4.8)) and $\sigma^2 > 0$, then*

$$(5.22) \qquad \mathcal{L}\left(\frac{\mu_0^* - \mu}{(\text{Var}(\hat{\mu}_0))^{1/2}}\right) \to N(0, 1)$$

as $n \to \infty$. Furthermore, replacing

$$\text{Var}(\hat{\mu}_0) = 1 \bigg/ \left[\sum_{i=1}^{n} \left(\sigma^2 + \frac{\tau}{m_i}\right)^{-1}\right]$$

by

$$(5.23) \qquad U^2 = 1 \bigg/ \left[\sum_{i=1}^{n} \left(\hat{\sigma}^2 + \frac{\hat{\tau}}{m_i}\right)^{-1}\right],$$

the result (5.22) still holds.

PROOF. Using the Taylor expansion (5.3) of Lemma 5.1, write

$$(5.24) \quad \frac{\mu_0^* - \mu}{(\text{Var}\,(\hat{\mu}_0))^{1/2}} = \frac{\hat{\mu}_0 - \mu}{(\text{Var}\,(\hat{\mu}_0))^{1/2}} + \frac{n^{1/4}(\hat{\sigma}^2 - \sigma^2)\left[n^{1/4} \sum_{i=1}^{n} \alpha_{in}\left(\frac{X_i}{m_i} - \mu\right)\right]}{(n\,\text{Var}\,(\hat{\mu}_0))^{1/2}}$$

$$+ \frac{n^{1/4}(\hat{\tau} - \tau)\left[n^{1/4} \sum_{i=1}^{n} \beta_{in}\left(\frac{X_i}{m_i} - \mu\right)\right]}{(n\,\text{Var}\,(\hat{\mu}_0))^{1/2}}$$

$$+ \frac{\{n^{1/4}|\hat{\sigma}^2 - \sigma^2| + n^{1/4}|\hat{\tau} - \tau|\}^2 O_p(1)\hat{\mu}_1}{(n\,\text{Var}\,(\hat{\mu}_0))^{1/2}}.$$

From (5.24) and Theorem 3.3, the theorem will be completed provided the last three terms on the right side of (5.24) converge to zero in probability as $n \to \infty$. However, such is the case from Lemma 5.2 provided

$$(5.25) \qquad\qquad \lim\inf \{n\,\text{Var}\,(\hat{\mu}_0)\} \geq c > 0$$

and that as $n \to \infty$,

$$(5.26) \qquad\qquad \left\{n^{1/4} \sum_{i=1}^{n} \alpha_{in}\left(\frac{X_i}{m_i} - \mu\right)\right\} \xrightarrow{P} 0$$

and

$$(5.27) \qquad\qquad \left\{n^{1/4} \sum_{i=1}^{n} \beta_{in}\left(\frac{X_i}{m_i} - \mu\right)\right\} \xrightarrow{P} 0.$$

The result (5.25) follows by noting that

$$(5.28) \quad n\,\text{Var}\,(\hat{\mu}_0) = n\left\{\sum_{i=1}^{n} \left(\sigma^2 + \left(\frac{\tau}{m_i}\right)\right)^{-1}\right\}^{-1} \geq \sigma^2 > 0 \qquad \text{for all } n.$$

The result (5.26) follows immediately from Chebyshev's inequality upon observing from (5.6) we have $|\alpha_{in}| \leq 2\sigma^{-4}/n(\sigma^2 + \tau)^{-1}$, which implies

$$(5.29) \qquad\qquad \text{Var}\left\{\alpha_{in}\left(\frac{X_i}{m_i} - \mu\right)\right\} = \alpha_{in}^2\left(\sigma^2 + \frac{\tau}{m_i}\right)$$

$$\leq \frac{4\sigma^{-6}}{n^2(\sigma^2 + \tau)^{-2}}.$$

A similar argument implies (5.27) holds. This completes the proof of the theorem.

REMARK. A $100(1 - \alpha)$ per cent, $0 < \alpha < 1$, large sample confidence interval for μ when σ^2 and τ are *unknown* which is close to being optimal in the sense that asymptotically it is the same as that based on $\hat{\mu}_0$ in (3.10) (the minimum variance unbiased linear estimator of μ) is given from (5.22) and (5.23) by

$$(5.30) \qquad\qquad \lim_{n \to \infty} P\{\mu_0^* - Z_{\alpha/2}U < \mu < \mu_0^* + Z_{\alpha/2}U\} = 1 - \alpha,$$

where μ_0^*, U, and $Z_{\alpha/2}$ are defined in (5.2), (5.23), and (2.12), respectively.

6. Summary

This paper has examined the question of estimating the mean μ in (2.2) of a random binomial parameter having distribution $G(p)$. Such a problem arose in the context of measuring an unobservable genetic trait in flocks of chickens. The sampling scheme upon which our procedures are based involves observations X_i from a density $f(x_i; m_i)$ given by (1.1), $i = 1, \cdots, n$, where the m_i are known, fixed, positive integers. The case in which $m_i = m$ for $i = 1, \cdots, n$ is treated in Section 2 with the confidence intervals for μ being given by (2.11) based on the estimator $\hat{\mu}$ in (2.4).

The case in which the m_i differ is developed in Sections 3, 4, and 5 with the corresponding confidence interval for μ given by (3.18) based on $\hat{\mu}_0$ in (3.10) of σ^2 and τ are known and by (5.30) based on μ_0^* in (5.2) if σ^2 and τ are unknown.

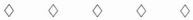

The authors would like to thank Mr. Min-Chiang Wang for doing the computer programming of the simulation results in Section 2.

REFERENCES

[1] M. Loève, *Probability Theory*, Princeton, Van Nostrand, 1960 (2nd ed.).
[2] E. S. Pearson, "Bayes theorem in the light of experimental sampling," *Biometrika*, Vol. 17 (1925), pp. 388–442.
[3] C. R. Rao, *Linear Statistical Inference and Its Applications*, New York, Wiley, 1965.

NONTHRESHOLD MODELS OF THE SURVIVAL OF BACTERIA AFTER IRRADIATION

PETER CLIFFORD
BRISTOL UNIVERSITY
and
UNIVERSITY OF TEL-AVIV

1. Introduction

The purpose of this paper is to investigate a certain class of nonthreshold models for the survival of the bacteria *E. coli* following exposure to X-ray and ultraviolet radiation. The threshold or multihit model contains two assumptions —that the effect of radiation is a process of accumulation of hits or irreversible structural defects in the cell and that death occurs when exactly n hits have accumulated. Woodbury [17] suggested a general method of modifying the model to include the possibility of repair during the irradiation period. Although the purport of the method is clear, some of the generality has to be abandoned to resolve the conflict between the first two sets of equations on p. 77 of [17]. The second assumption in the threshold model is retained, changing its form slightly so that the cell will die if more than n unrepaired hits have been accumulated at the end of the dose.

A fruitful approach to threshold problems in general has been suggested by L. LeCam and developed by Puri [13] in connection with a situation in which a host is infected with a parasite which multiplies and eventually kills the host. If we call the underlying process, be it the accumulation of hits in a cell or parasites in a host, $\{X(s): 0 \leq s \leq t\}$, where t is the time interval considered, then the LeCam-Puri approach is that the probability of dying in a time period $(s, s + \tau)$ is proportional to $\tau g(X(s)) + o(\tau)$, where g may be, for example, the identity function. It follows that the probability $S(t)$ of surviving a time t is of the form $f(X(s): 0 \leq s \leq t)$, for example, $\exp\left\{-\int_0^t X(s)\, ds\right\}$. In a seminar given at the University of California in 1967, the author applied this approach to radiation problems and showed that repair could be incorporated quite naturally in this context.

For the present purposes this approach is too general. In most cases the

This research was prepared with the partial support of the United States Public Health Service Grant GM-10525(06). Part of this work appears in the author's Ph.D. thesis, University of California, Berkeley.

radiation damage is accumulated almost immediately and repair, if any, takes place after irradiation. For these cases, it appears natural to consider only the class of survival models for which $f(X(s): 0 \leq s \leq t)$ depends only on $X(t)$, the total amount of damage after the dose. This is equivalent to a suggestion of Haynes [8] that a cell with k hits following irradiation has some probability $0 \leq Q(k) \leq 1$ of survival. If hits are accumulated in a Poisson process, it follows that both the multihit and multitarget models, which have been used extensively in the past [1], [11], [16] are special cases of the preceding. Properties of the theoretical model are discussed, in particular the property that the rate parameter of the Poisson process and the function $Q(k)$ are not jointly identifiable.

In the second half of the paper, the idea is developed that the bacteria survive because of enzyme systems which are capable of repairing structural defects [8]. The general model is interpreted in terms of repair and a more specific model is proposed based on Harm's ideas [6]. In a series of experiments, Harm has shown that E. coli can survive large doses of ultraviolet radiation if the exposure is at a low dose rate. The implication is that repair takes place during the irradiation period. Harm has suggested also that certain configurations of lesions on the chromosome may be more difficult to repair, particularly defects at approximately the same location on opposing strands. The enhanced survival for low dose rate exposure is then the result of the continual repair of the DNA molecule during the radiation period which minimizes the chances of overlapping structural defects. The mathematical model based on these ideas is shown to agree well with the empirical data for high dose rate survival and to predict "liquid-holding recovery". For low dose rate exposure with the largest total dose, there is some indication of an interaction between the radiation and the repair mechanism.

In a further application of this model, the interaction between X-ray and ultraviolet radiation is considered as in the experiments of Haynes [7]. It was shown that the previous application of X-ray altered the shape of the ultraviolet survival curve. A similar effect was observed by reversing the order of radiation. In general, there appears to be a synergism between the two types of radiation. By postulating that the presence of X-ray structural defects may block the repair of ultraviolet damage, a mathematical model is constructed. The predictions of this model compare favorably with the empirical data.

2. Mathematical description of the model

A cell is exposed to a dose d (ergs/mm^2) of radiation. During the radiation period a number of events occur in the cell. An event may be the absorption of a photon in the case of ultraviolet radiation or the initiation of a chain of ionizations in the case of X-ray or hard radiation. The number of these primary events is assumed to be Poisson distributed with a mean ηd, where η is some unknown constant. At the site of each primary event a certain amount of damage is formed. In the case of ultraviolet radiation, it may be reasonable to say that one lesion or abnormal photoproduct is formed randomly and independently with probability π at each primary event, so that the number of lesions formed in a cell would have a Poisson distribution with mean λd where, $\lambda = \eta\pi$. The probability $Q(n)$ that a cell will survive n lesions is assumed to be independent of the dose which caused the lesions. In general, it will depend on many factors including the experimental conditions, the presence of a repair mechanism in the cell and any delay in replication which the n lesions may produce. The probability that a cell will survive a dose d of ultraviolet light is evidently

$$(1) \qquad S(d) = \sum_{k=0}^{\infty} \frac{e^{-\lambda d}(\lambda d)^k}{k!} Q(k).$$

From biological considerations, it appears natural that the class should be restricted by

$$(2) \qquad \begin{aligned} Q(k) &\geq Q(k+1), \qquad\qquad k = 0, 1, 2 \cdots, \\ Q(0) &= 1, \\ \lim_{k\to\infty} Q(k) &= 0. \end{aligned}$$

That is, the chance that a cell will survive cannot increase as the number of lesions increases; the cell will survive if no lesions are present and the cell is certain to die if the number of lesions exceeds all bounds. The class of survival curves satisfying both (1) and (2) will be called the class A.

The first observation is that the class contains the multihit survivor curve in the case

$$(3) \qquad Q(k) = \begin{cases} 1 & k = 0, 1, \cdots, n-1, \\ 0 & \text{otherwise.} \end{cases}$$

It also contains the multitarget model. The multitarget model with m targets each with a mean number $\lambda d/m$ lesions has a survivor function

$$(4) \qquad S(d) = 1 - \left(1 - \exp\left\{-\frac{\lambda d}{m}\right\}\right)^m.$$

By expanding the terms of (4), it follows that $S(d)$ is in the class A with parameters λ and

$$(5) \qquad Q(j) = \sum_{k=1}^{m} (-1)^{k+1} \binom{m}{k} \left(\frac{m-k}{m}\right)^j.$$

We recognize $Q(k)$ to be the occupancy probability that out of m boxes in which k balls are distributed at random, at least one box will be empty. In general, any occupancy model where the lethal configuration becomes increasingly likely as the number of lesions increases will have a survivor function in the class A.

The second observation is that the class is equivalent to the class of multihit mixtures. Fowler [5] gives an example of fitting a multihit mixture to radiation survival data. A multihit mixture survivor function is of the form

$$(6) \qquad S(d) = \sum_{j=1}^{\infty} p_j \sum_{k=0}^{j-1} \frac{e^{-\lambda d}(\lambda d)^k}{k!},$$

where $p_j \geq 0$, $j = 1, 2, 3, \cdots$, and $\sum_{j=1}^{\infty} p_j = 1$. Note that this class excludes the possibility of surviving an infinite number of lesions. By changing the order of summation, we have the result that $S(d)$ satisfies condition (1) with parameters λ and $Q^*(k)$, where $Q^*(k) = \sum_{j=k+1}^{\infty} p_j$. Since $Q^*(0) = 1$, $Q^*(k) \geq Q^*(k+1)$ and $\lim_{k \to \infty} Q^*(k) = 0$, the function (6) is a member of the class A. Conversely, setting $p_{k+1} = Q(k) - Q(k+1)$, that is $Q(k) = \sum_{j=k+1}^{\infty} p_j$, $k = 0, 1, 2, \cdots$, and substituting in (1), it is evident, after changing the order of summation, that any member of the class is a finite multihit mixture.

Instead of assuming that the primary event causes only a single lesion, it may be assumed, more generally, that there will be a random and independent distribution of damage $X \geq 0$, at each event. If the accumulation of damage is additive and if $Q(x)$, the probability that the cell will survive an amount x of damage, is restricted to be nonincreasing such that $Q(0) = 1$ and $\lim_{x \to \infty} Q(x) = 0$, then it can be shown that the class is not increased. This more general description of the class is not used here since the emphasis will be placed on the interpretation of ultraviolet survival data, where the simplifying assumptions leading to the class A may be approximately valid.

3. Properties of the theoretical model

Before considering the problem of estimating $Q(k)$ and λ from an empirical survivor function, it is important to know whether $Q(k)$ and λ are identifiable from a theoretical survivor function in the class A and for an arbitrary theoretical survivor function it is useful to have a criterion for deciding whether the function is in the class A.

PROPOSITION 1. *If $S(d)$ is a member of the class A with the parameters λ and $Q(k)$, then $S(d)$ and λ determine $Q(k)$ uniquely.*

PROOF. This result is contained in the work of Teicher [16] concerning general problems of identifiability. More directly, consider the function $S(d)e^{\lambda d}$. This is an entire function with a unique power series expansion. The coefficient $Q(k)\lambda^k/k!$ of d^k is therefore determined by $S(d)e^{\lambda d}$, and hence $S(d)$ and λ determine $Q(k)$ uniquely. This concludes the proof.

PROPOSITION 2. *If $S(d)$ is an arbitrary nonincreasing survivor function and $\mu > 0$, then the transform*

$$(7) \qquad f(u, \mu) = \int_0^\infty \exp\left\{\frac{x(u-1)}{u}\right\} dF\left(\frac{x}{\mu}\right)$$

is analytic for $u \in C$, where $F(d) = 1 - S(d)$ and C is the interior of the circle with radius $\frac{1}{2}$ and center $\frac{1}{2}$ in the complex plane.

PROOF. Since $F(x/\mu) = 1 - S(x/\mu)$ is a distribution function, it has a Laplace transform $g(\theta)$ which is analytic for $\Re(\theta) > 0$. Since $f(u, \mu) = g((1-u)/u)$ and since the function $\theta = (1-u)/u$ is analytic in C and maps $C \to \Re(\theta) > 0$, the result follows.

PROPOSITION 3. *If $S(d)$ is an arbitrary nonincreasing survivor function and $\mu > 0$, then $f(u, \mu)$, $u \in C$, determines $S(d)$ uniquely.*

PROOF. For $\mu > 0$, arbitrary, $S(x)$ is determined by $S(x/\mu)$ which in turn is determined by its Laplace transform $f((1 + \theta)^{-1}, \mu)$, $\Re(\theta) > 0$. Since $(1 - u)/u$ is analytic in C and the mapping $C \to \Re(\theta) > 0$ is one to one, it follows that $f((1 + \theta)^{-1}, \mu)$, $\Re(\theta) > 0$, is determined by $f(u, \mu)$, $u \in C$, which concludes the proof.

THEOREM 1. *Let $S(d)$, $d > 0$ be an arbitrary nonincreasing survivor function and let $F(d) = 1 - S(d)$.*

A necessary and sufficient condition for the function $S(d)$ to be in the class A is that for some $\mu > 0$ function (7) has an analytic continuation which is a probability generating function (p.g.f.).

If the p.g.f. generates the quantities $\{\eta_k, k = 1, 2, \cdots\}$, then

$$(8) \qquad S(d) = \sum_{k=0}^{\infty} \sum_{j=k}^{\infty} \eta_{j+1} \frac{e^{-\mu d}(\mu d)^k}{k!}.$$

PROOF. Let $S(d)$ be in the class A with parameters λ and $Q(k)$, then

$$(9) \qquad \begin{aligned} S\left(\frac{x}{\lambda}\right) &= \sum_{k=0}^{\infty} Q(k) \frac{e^{-x}x^k}{k!}, \\ \frac{d}{dx} F\left(\frac{x}{\lambda}\right) &= \sum_{k=1}^{\infty} q_k \frac{e^{-x}x^k}{k!}, \end{aligned}$$

where $q_k = Q(k - 1) - Q(k)$, $k = 1, 2, \cdots$. The integral

$$(10) \qquad f(u, \lambda) = \int_0^{\infty} \exp\left\{-\frac{x(1 - u)}{u}\right\}\left(\sum_{k=1}^{\infty} q_k \frac{e^{-x}x^k}{k!}\right) dx$$

converges for $u \in C$; hence $f(u, \lambda) = \sum_{k=1}^{\infty} u^k q_k$, $u \in C$. Since $q_k > 0$, $k = 1, 2, \cdots$ and $\sum_{k=1}^{\infty} q_k = 1$, $f(u, \lambda)$ has an analytic continuation which is a p.g.f. The second part of the theorem follows with $q_k = \eta_k$, $k = 1, 2, \cdots$.

Let $S(d)$ be a nonincreasing survivor function and suppose that for some $\mu > 0$, $f(u, \mu) = \int_0^{\infty} \exp\{-x(1 - u)/u\} dF(x/\mu)$ has an analytic continuation which is a p.g.f. Let $f(u, \mu) = \sum_{k=1}^{\infty} u^k \eta_k$. Then the function

$$(11) \qquad S^*(x) = \sum_{k=0}^{\infty} \sum_{j=k}^{\infty} \eta_{j+1} \frac{e^{-\mu x}(\mu x)^k}{k!}$$

is in the class A. For this function $f^*(u, \mu) = \sum_{k=1}^{\infty} u^k \eta_k$ for $u \in C$. From Proposition 3 it follows that $S(x) = S^*(x)$, $x > 0$ so that $S(x)$ is in the class A.

COROLLARY 1. *If $S(d)$ is a member of the class A with parameters λ and $Q(k)$, then for each $\mu > \lambda$ there exists a $Q^*(k)$ satisfying condition (2) such that*

$$(12) \qquad S(d) = \sum_{k=0}^{\infty} Q(k) \frac{e^{-\lambda d}(\lambda d)^k}{k!} = \sum_{k=0}^{\infty} Q^*(k) \frac{e^{-\mu d}(\mu d)^k}{k!}.$$

PROOF. Let $\mu > \lambda$. Since $S(d)$ is in the class A it is nonincreasing so that from Proposition 2, $f(u, \mu) = \int_0^{\infty} \exp\{-x(1 - u)/u\} d[1 - S(x/\mu)]$ is analytic,

$u \in C$. After integration, we have $f(u, \mu) = g(\lambda u/(\mu - u(\mu - \lambda)))$, $u \in C$, where $g(u) = f(u, \lambda)$ is a p.g.f. It follows that $f(u, \mu)$, $\mu > \lambda$, is the p.g.f. of a negative binomial mixture. Therefore, $S(d)$ is also in the class A with parameters μ and $Q^*(k) = \sum_{j=k}^{\infty} q_{j+1}^*$, $k = 0, 1, 2, \cdots$, where

$$(13) \qquad \sum_{k=1}^{\infty} u^k q_k^* = g\left(\frac{\lambda\mu}{\mu - u(\mu - \lambda)}\right), \qquad\qquad |u| \leq 1.$$

This concludes the proof.

For some purposes, it may be useful to have a relationship between $Q(k)$ and $Q^*(k)$ directly. From the equation in Corollary 1 after multiplying both sides by $e^{\mu d}$ and equating coefficients of d^k, it is easy to verify that

$$(14) \qquad Q^*(k) = \sum_{m=0}^{k} Q(m)\binom{k}{m}\left(\frac{\lambda}{\mu}\right)^m\left(1 - \frac{\lambda}{\mu}\right)^{k-m}.$$

EXAMPLE 1. In the case $Q(k) = 1_{[k<n]}$, $S(d) = \sum_{k=0}^{\infty} Q(k)e^{-\lambda d}(\lambda d)^k/k!$ has the form of the classical n hit survival function. From the corollary, it follows that the function $S(d)$ has an infinite number of alternative representations in the class A with parameters $\mu > \lambda$ and $Q^*(k)$, where

$$(15) \qquad Q^*(k) = \begin{cases} \displaystyle\sum_{j=k-n+1}^{\infty} \frac{\dbinom{j+n+1}{j}(\mu/\lambda - 1)^j}{(\mu/\lambda)^{j+n}}, & k \geq n, \\[2ex] \displaystyle\sum_{j=0}^{n-1} \binom{k}{j}((\mu - \lambda)/\mu)^{k-i}(\lambda/\mu)^i, & k \geq n, \\[2ex] 1 & k < n \text{ for all } \mu > \lambda. \end{cases}$$

Provided $\mu > \lambda$, $Q^*(k)$ is always positive and decreasing. This function may be a more acceptable explanation of the survival curve than the function $Q(k) = 1_{[k<n]}$ which implies that the cell survives with $n - 1$ lesions but not with n lesions. As an illustration, for the "5 hit" function $S(d) = \sum_{k=0}^{4} e^{-d}d^k/k!$ the equivalent $Q^*(k)$ are drawn for $\mu = 1, 2, 4, 10$ in Figure 1. Thus, a cell which appears to have a 5 hit survivor function may have a 50 per cent chance of surviving 50 lesions if the equivalent representation with $\mu = 10$ is used. In general if $S(d) = \sum_{k=0}^{\infty} Q(k)e^{-\mu d}(\mu d)^k/k!$, then it is necessary to know μ before we can determine $Q(k)$. An equivalent result in terms of multihit mixtures has been obtained by Teicher [16] and Dittrich [3].

It also follows from Theorem 1 that if $S(d)$ is in the class A with parameters μ and $Q(k)$ and if $q_k = Q(k-1) - Q(k)$ for $k = 1, 2, \cdots$, then the factorial moments of the distribution $\{q_k: k = 1, 2, \cdots\}$ are given by

$$(16) \qquad \mu_{[j]} = \sum_{k=1}^{\infty} k(k+1) \cdots (k+j)q_k$$

$$= (j+1) \int_0^{\infty} x^j S(x/\mu) \, dx, \qquad j = 0, 1, 2, \cdots.$$

If μ is known and $Q(k)$ has some theoretical form depending on unknown parameters, it may be feasible to use a "method of moments" to estimate $Q(k)$.

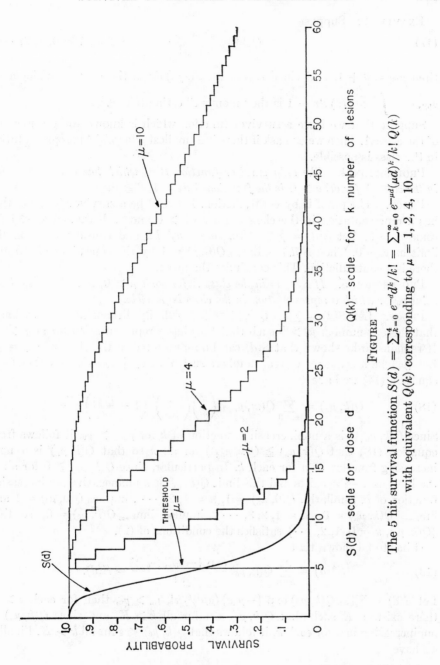

FIGURE 1

The 5 hit survival function $S(d) = \sum_{k=0}^{4} e^{-d} d^{k} / k! = \sum_{k=0}^{\infty} e^{-\mu d} (\mu d)^{k} / k! \, Q(k)$
with equivalent $Q(k)$ corresponding to $\mu = 1, 2, 4, 10$.

EXAMPLE 2. Suppose

$$(17) \qquad\qquad Q(k) = \sum_{j=k}^{\infty} \frac{e^{-\theta}\theta^j}{j!}, \qquad \theta > 0, \, k = 0, 1, 2, \cdots,$$

then $\mu_{[0]} = \theta + 1$, and since $m_{[0]} = \int_0^{\infty} \hat{S}(x/\mu) \, dx$ is the sample analogue of $\mu_{[0]}$, $\hat{\theta} = \int_0^{\infty} \hat{S}(x/\mu) \, dx - 1$ is the "moment" estimate of θ.

Suppose that we have a survivor function which is known to be a member of the class A. Then we can ask if there is a smallest μ for which a representation in the class is possible.

PROPOSITION 4. *The only survivor function $S(d)$ which has a representation in the class A for all $\mu > 0$ is the function $S(d) = 1$, $d \geqq 0$.*

PROOF. The proof is by contradiction. Let $S(d)$ be a survivor function that has a representation in the class A for all $\mu > 0$ and such that $S(d_0) < 1$ for some $d_0 > 0$. Let $S(d) = \sum_{k=0}^{\infty} Q(k, \mu)e^{-\mu d}(\mu d)^k/k!$, and consider $S(d_0)$ in the limit as $\mu \to 0$. Then $S(d_0) \to \lim_{\mu \to 0} Q(0, \mu) = 1$ by the conditions of (2) and there is a contradiction. This concludes the proof.

PROPOSITION 5. *If $S(d)$ is in the class A for some $\mu > 0$, then there is a least value μ_0 for which a representation in the class is possible.*

PROOF. Let $S(d) = \sum_{k=0}^{\infty} Q(k, \mu)e^{-\mu d}(\mu d)^k/k!$. By Proposition 4, we know that there is number $\mu_0 > 0$ such that $S(d)$ has a representation for all $\mu > \mu_0$. It remains to be shown that $S(d)$ can be represented in the class with $\mu = \mu_0$. Let $\{\mu_n\}$ be a sequence of real numbers such that $\mu_n \downarrow \mu_0$ as $n \to \infty$ then from equation (14) we have

$$(18) \qquad Q(k, \mu_n) = \sum_{m=0}^{k} Q(m, \mu_{n+1}) \binom{k}{m} \left(\frac{\mu_{n+1}}{\mu_n}\right)^m \left(1 - \frac{\mu_{n+1}}{\mu_n}\right)^{k-m}.$$

Since $Q(k, \mu_{n+1})$ is a nonincreasing function of k for $\mu_{n+1} > \mu_0$, it follows from equation (18) that $Q(k, \mu_n) \geqq Q(k, \mu_{n+1})$ for all n so that $Q(k, \mu_n)$ is a nonincreasing function of n for each k. In particular, since $Q(k, \mu_n) \geqq 0$ for all n, the limit as $n \to \infty$ exists and this limit $Q(k, \mu_0)$ is a nonnegative nonincreasing function of k. Similarly, $Q(0, \mu_n) = 1$, $n = 1, 2, \cdots$, implies $Q(0, \mu_0) = 1$ and $\lim_{k \to \infty} Q(k, \mu_n) = 0$, $n = 1, 2, 3, \cdots$, implies $\lim_{k \to \infty} Q(k, \mu_0) = 0$, so that $\{Q(k, \mu_0), k = 0, 1, 2, \cdots\}$ satisfies the conditions of (2).

It has to be shown that

$$(19) \qquad\qquad S^*(d) = \sum_{k=0}^{\infty} Q(k, \mu_0) \frac{\exp\{-\mu_0 d\} (\mu_0 d)^k}{k!} = S(d).$$

Let $S(d) = \sum_{k=0}^{\infty} Q(k, \mu_n) \exp\{-\mu_n d\} (\mu_n d)^k/k!$, $\mu_n > \mu_0$, then for each $\varepsilon > 0$, there exists a K such that $Q(k, \mu_n) < \varepsilon$ for all $k > K$, and since $Q(k, \mu_n)$ is nonincreasing in n for each k, it follows that $Q(k, \mu_0) < \varepsilon$ for all $k > K$. Finally, we have

$$(20) \quad |S^*(d) - S(d)|$$

$$\leqq \left| \sum_{k=0}^{K} \left\{ Q(k, \mu_0) \frac{\exp\{-\mu_0 d\} (\mu_0 d)^k}{k!} - Q(k, \mu_n) \frac{\exp\{-\mu_n d\} (\mu_n d)^k}{k!} \right\} \right| + 2\varepsilon.$$

Since there are a finite number of terms in the summation and each converges to zero as $n \to \infty$, we have shown that $S(d) \to S^*(d)$ for each $d \geq 0$. Since $S(d)$ is independent of n, it follows that $S(d) = S^*(d)$ for $d \geq 0$. This concludes the proof.

PROPOSITION 6. *If $S(d)$ is a function of the class A, then the parameter μ is restricted by the following inequalities:*

(21)
$$\mu \geq -S'(0),$$

(22)
$$\mu \geq \frac{\int_0^\infty S(x)\, dx}{2 \int_0^\infty x S(x)\, dx - \left(\int_0^\infty S(x)\, dx\right)^2}.$$

PROOF. For (21), let $S(d) = \sum_{k=0}^\infty Q(k) e^{-\mu d}(\mu d)^k/k!$. Then $S'(0) = -\mu(1 - Q(1))$. Since $0 \leq Q(1) \leq 1$, we have $-S'(0)/\mu \leq 1$ or $\mu \geq -S'(0)$.

For (22), since the variance of the q_k distribution must be nonnegative, from (16) we have

(23)
$$2\mu^2 \int_0^\infty x S(x)\, dx - \mu \int_0^\infty S(x)\, dx - \left(\mu \int_0^\infty S(x)\, dx\right)^2 \geq 0,$$

that is,

(24)
$$\mu \left\{ 2 \int_0^\infty x S(x)\, dx - \left(\int_0^\infty S(x)\, dx\right)^2 \right\} \geq \int_0^\infty S(x)\, dx$$

or

(25)
$$\mu \left\{ \int_0^\infty x^2\, dF(x) - \left(\int_0^\infty x\, dF(x)\right)^2 \right\} \geq \int_0^\infty x\, dF(x),$$

where $F(x) = 1 - S(x)$ is a distribution function. It follows that $\int_0^\infty x^2\, dF(x) - \left(\int_0^\infty x\, dF(x)\right)^2$ is positive provided the distribution function $F(x)$ is nondegenerate. The result then follows from equation (24).

If we consider T the lethal dose, a random variable for each cell, with distribution $P(T > d) = S(d)$, then (25) says that the Poisson rate of arrival of damage per unit dose cannot be less than $E(T)/\mathrm{Var}\,(T)$.

EXAMPLE 3. For the multihit class, $S(d) = \sum_{k=0}^{n-1} e^{-\lambda d}(\lambda d)^k/k!$, we have

(26)
$$-\int_0^\infty x\, dS(x) = \int_0^\infty x \frac{e^{-\lambda x}(\lambda x)^{n-1}}{(n-1)!}\, dx = \frac{n}{\lambda},$$
$$-\int_0^\infty x^2\, dS(x) = \int_0^\infty x^2 \frac{e^{-\lambda x}(\lambda x)^{n-1}}{(n-1)!}\, dx = \frac{n(n+1)}{\lambda^2},$$

so that from (21) and (22), $\mu \geq n\lambda^2/n\lambda = \lambda$.

If $S(d)$ is identical to a multihit survivor function with parameter λ, then the only other possible representations of $S(d)$ in the class A have $\mu \geq \lambda$.

From (26), it follows that the value of the parameter λ for which $S(d)$ has the multihit representation is given by

$$(27) \qquad \lambda = \frac{\int_0^\infty S(x)\, dx}{2 \int_0^\infty x S(x)\, dx - \left(\int_0^\infty S(x)\, dx\right)^2},$$

and the value of the parameter n, the threshold number of lesions, is given by

$$(28) \qquad n = \lambda \int_0^\infty S(x)\, dx.$$

By substituting the sample analogues of $\int_0^\infty S(x)\, dx$ and $\int_0^\infty x S(x)\, dx$, equations (27) and (28) can be used to provide estimates of n and λ. This procedure has been advocated by Kellerer [10].

DEFINITION 1. *In radiation biology, it is customary to plot* $\log S(d)$ *versus dose and consider the limiting slope of* $\log S(d)$ *as* d *increases. If there is such a limiting slope and the asymptotic tangent is extrapolated back to intersect the ordinate at* $\log (N)$, *then* N *is called the extrapolation number.*

DEFINITION 2. *If* $F(x)$ *is a positive nonincreasing function of* $x > 0$ *and if there exists* $0 < \rho < 1$ *such that* $F(x)/\rho^x$ *converges to a finite nonzero limit, say* N, *as* $x \to \infty$, *then* $F(x)$ *is asymptotic to* $N\rho^x$. *This is written as* $F(x) \sim N\rho^x$.

Let $S(d)$ be a member of the class A with parameters $Q(k)$ and λ, then

$$(29) \qquad \frac{d}{dx} \log S(x) = -\lambda \frac{\sum\limits_{k=0}^\infty (Q(k) - Q(k+1)) e^{-\lambda d} (\lambda d)^k / k!}{\sum\limits_{k=0}^\infty Q(k) e^{-\lambda d} (\lambda d)^k / k!}.$$

If $Q(k_0) = 0$ for some particular integer value k_0, then

$$(30) \qquad \lim_{x \to \infty} \frac{d}{dx} \log S(x) = -\lambda.$$

Thus, the asymptotic slope of $\log S(d)$ is $-\lambda$. The extrapolation number N is given by

$$(31) \qquad \lim_{x \to \infty} e^{\lambda x} S(x) = \lim_{x \to \infty} \sum_{k=0}^{k_0 - 1} \frac{Q(k)(\lambda x)^k}{k!},$$

if $k_0 = 1$, $N = 1$. If $k_0 > 1$, the limit diverges to $+\infty$.

PROPOSITION 7. *If* $Q(k) > 0$ *for all* $k > 0$ *and if* $Q(k) \sim N\rho^k$ *for* $N > 0$ *and* $0 < \rho < 1$, *then* $S(x) \sim N \exp \{-\lambda(1 - \rho)\}$.

PROOF. Let $Q(k) \sim N\rho^k$ for $N > 0$, $0 < \rho < 1$. Then $N = \lim_{k \to \infty} Q(k)/\rho^k$. Consider

$$(32) \qquad S(x) \exp \{\lambda(1 - \rho)x\} = \sum_{k=0}^\infty Q(k) \frac{e^{-\lambda \rho x}(\lambda x)^k}{k!}$$

$$= \sum_{k=0}^\infty \frac{Q(k)}{\rho^k} \frac{e^{-\lambda \rho x}(\lambda \rho x)^k}{k!}.$$

This is $E(Q(X)/\rho^X)$, where X is a Poisson variable with mean $\lambda \rho x$. Let $\varepsilon > 0$; then there exists a K such that $|Q(k)/\rho^k - N| < \varepsilon$ for $k > K$. From (32) we have

$$(33) \qquad |S(x) \exp \{\lambda(1 - \rho)x\} - N| \leq \sum_{k=0}^{\infty} \left| \frac{Q(k)}{\rho^k} - N \right| \frac{e^{-\lambda \rho x}(\lambda \rho x)^k}{k!}$$

$$\leq \sum_{k=0}^{K} \left| \frac{Q(k)}{\rho^k} - N \right| \frac{e^{-\lambda \rho x}(\lambda \rho x)^k}{k!} + \varepsilon$$

$$\leq \max \left(N, \frac{1}{\rho^K} \right) \Pr (X \leq K) + \varepsilon.$$

For x sufficiently large $\Pr (X \leq K)$ is arbitrarily small so that we have $S(x) \exp \{\lambda(1 - p)x\} \to N$ as $x \to \infty$. This concludes the proof.

EXAMPLE 4.   In the case of the m target model where $S(d) = 1 - (1 - \exp \{-\lambda d/m\})^m$ it was shown in (4) that $Q(j) = \sum_{k=1}^{m} (-1)^{k+1} \binom{m}{k} ((m - k)/m)^j$, $j = 0, 1, 2, \cdots$. It follows that

$$(34) \qquad \lim_{j \to \infty} \frac{Q(j)}{((m - 1)/m)^j},$$

that is, $Q(j) \sim m((m - 1)/m)^j$. From Proposition 7, we have $S(d) \sim m \exp \{-\lambda d/m\}$.

If $S(d)$ is hypothesized to be a multitarget survivor function, the asymptotic behavior of $S(d)$ can be exploited to provide quick estimates of m and λ. In practice, information on $S(d)$ is only available for a finite range of d and estimates of this type can be criticized for the assumption made that the asymptotic behavior of $S(d)$ can be deduced from the finite dose range.

4. The implications of repair for the general damage dependent survivor function

From this point, it is assumed that λ and $Q(k)$ are known and the theoretical survivor function is $S(d) = \sum_{k=0}^{\infty} (e^{-\mu d}(\mu d)^k/k!)Q(k)$. If repair can take place, a certain number of lesions formed will be removed. It is assumed that all lesions have been removed if the cell survives [8]. Let $M(d)$ be the mean number of lesions repaired after a dose d. This will be called the repair function. It is possible to observe experimentally the amount of new material incorporated into a cell following irradiation [9]. It is assumed that the amount of new material is proportional to $M(d)$. The problem is to relate $M(d)$ to $S(d)$. Since d is the mean number of lesions formed at dose d, Haynes [8] has suggested the rule

$$(35) \qquad M(d) = \log S(d) + \mu d.$$

The exact relationship between $M(d)$ and $S(d)$ depends on the mechanism of repair. To see this, first note that if the repair of all lesions is essential for survival, then $Q(k)$ is the probability that k lesions are removed from a cell which has k lesions after irradiation. It does not say anything about the probability $p(k, n)$ that n lesions are removed from a cell with k units of damage where $n < k$. Three general repair mechanisms are described before introducing a specific model. These mechanisms are chosen so that $M(d)$ and $S(d)$ have a simple relationship and are intended to be examples of the diverse types of relationship possible.

4.1. *The minimum repair mechanism.* If the survivor function is $S(d) = \sum_{k=0}^{\infty} (e^{-\mu d}(\mu d)^k/k!)Q(k)$ and the cell is repairing a minimum of its damage, then given that it has k lesions it will repair all and survive with probability $Q(k)$ or repair none and die. Then the mean number of lesions repaired for a cell with k lesions is $kQ(k)$ and after a dose d the mean number of lesions repaired is

$$(36) \qquad \min(d) = \sum_{k=0}^{\infty} kQ(k) \frac{e^{-\mu d}(\mu d)^k}{k!}$$

$$= \mu d \sum_{k=0}^{\infty} Q(k+1) \frac{e^{-\mu d}(\mu d)^k}{k!}$$

$$= d(S'(d) + \mu S(d)).$$

4.2. *Maximum repair mechanism.* If the cell is repairing a maximum of its damage, then given it has k lesions, it will repair all and survive with probability $Q(k)$ or repair $k - 1$ lesions and die with probability $1 - Q(k)$. The mean number of lesions repaired is then $kQ(k) + (k-1)(1 - Q(k))$ and after a dose d the mean number of lesions repaired is

$$(37) \qquad \max(d) = \sum_{k=0}^{\infty} \{kQ(k) + (k-1)(1 - Q(k))\} \frac{e^{-\mu d}(\mu d)^k}{k!}$$

$$= \mu d - 1 + S(d).$$

4.3. *Mechanism with mixture of repair capacity.* Define the repair capacity of a cell at a particular time as the maximum number R of lesions it can remove regardless of the number of lesions present. Suppose that R is a random variable. For example, following irradiation the cell will have a certain number n of lesions. As each lesion is removed by repair there is a probability that an event may occur which will render the cell incapable of division. Let $1 - \eta_k$ be the probability that such an event occurs during the removal of the kth lesion, given that it has not occurred previously. Then the probability that a cell will survive n lesions is $\eta_1 \cdots \eta_n$. If $Q(n)$ is an arbitrary function in the class (2) then $\{\eta_k, k = 1, 2, \cdots\}$ can be chosen so that $Q(n) = \eta_1 \cdots \eta_n, n = 1, 2, \cdots$. That is, a survivor function in the class A can be interpreted as having arisen from this mechanism.

If the cell has n lesions the probability that it will repair k lesions is then $\eta_1 \cdots \eta_k(1 - \eta_{k+1})$ for $0 \leq k \leq n - 1$, and $\eta_1 \cdots \eta_n$ for $k = n$. Further, since $\eta_1 \cdots \eta_k(1 - \eta_{k+1}) = Q(k+1) - Q(k) = q_k$, we have the mean number of lesions repaired in a cell with n lesions after irradiation is

$$(38) \qquad 0q_1 + 1q_2 + \cdots + kq_{k+1} + \cdots (n-1)q_n + nQ(n).$$

This is evidently equivalent to considering a repair capacity distribution with $\Pr(R = k) = q_{k+1}$, since if a cell has a repair capacity k it will repair a maximum of k lesions and the mean number of lesions repaired for all cells with n lesions after irradiation is then given by (38).

It is also possible to consider that the probability of the successful removal of a lesion depends on the number of lesions remaining in the cell, but in general no simple relationship between $M(d)$ and $S(d)$ results from this mechanism.

Returning to (38), we have

$$(39) \qquad 0q_1 + 1q_2 + \cdots + (n-1)q_n + nQ(n) = \sum_{j=1}^{k} Q(j),$$

so that the mean number of lesions removed after dose d is then

$$(40) \qquad \text{mix}(d) = \sum_{k=1}^{\infty} \frac{e^{-\mu d}(\mu d)^k}{k!} \sum_{j=1}^{k} Q(j)$$

$$= S(d) + \mu \int_0^d S(x)\, dx - 1.$$

As a first example consider the 1 hit survivor function $S(d) = e^{-d}$. In the class A, $S(d)$ may have equivalent representations of the form

$$(41) \qquad S(d) = e^{-d} = \sum_{k=0}^{\infty} Q(k)\frac{e^{-\mu d}(\mu d)^k}{k!}, \qquad\qquad \mu > 1.$$

For the case $\mu = 1$ the repair functions for $d \geq 0$ are

$$(42) \qquad \begin{aligned} \text{Haynes rule} &= 0, \\ \text{min}(d) &= 0, \\ \text{max}(d) &= e^{-d} - 1 + d, \\ \text{mix}(d) &= 0. \end{aligned}$$

For the case $\mu > 1$ the repair functions for $d \geq 0$ are

$$(43) \qquad \begin{aligned} \text{Haynes rule} &= (\mu - 1)d, \\ \text{min}(d) &= de^{-d}(\mu - 1), \\ \text{max}(d) &= \mu d - 1 + e^{-d}, \\ \text{mix}(d) &= (\mu - 1)(1 - e^{-d}). \end{aligned}$$

EXAMPLE 5.   Harm [6] has shown that the function $\exp\{-d^2/\sigma^2\}$ approximates the empirical survivor function of E. coli B/r, following ultraviolet irradiation over the range 0 to 1500 ergs/mm². Using Harm's value of σ, and a value for μ given by Setlow [14], the repair functions are computed in Figure 2.

5. A particular model of the effect of ultraviolet radiation on E. coli

In the preceding theory a function $Q(k)$ was introduced. The value $Q(k)$ was defined to be the probability a cell would survive k lesions under some fixed experimental condition. This general formulation does not permit any inference to be made on the form of this function under different experimental conditions. In order to proceed further than the fitting of an isolated survivor function it is necessary to construct a more detailed model of the biological system. Such a model is described below.

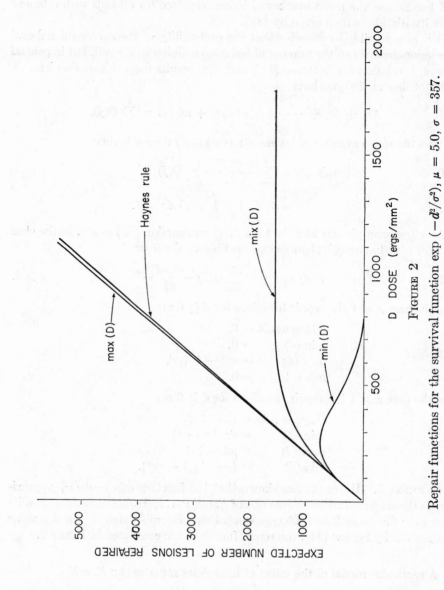

FIGURE 2

Repair functions for the survival function $\exp(-d^2/\sigma^2)$, $\mu = 5.0$, $\sigma = 357$.

5.1. *General assumptions.* Three general assumptions are made. The first is that the irradiated cells are homogeneous in their response to radiation. The second is that the principal effect of ultraviolet light for considerations of survival is the formation of lesions on the chromosome of the cell. The chromosome of *E. coli* consists of a long double strand of DNA. Each strand contains approximately 4.5 million nucleotides of four different types A, C, G, and T. The information coded by the whole sequence of nucleotides is vital to the survival of a cell. If only a section of the DNA is damaged there is some probability that the cell will lose its reproductive ability. Fortunately, the two strands of DNA are complementary to each other, so that damage to one strand may not result in a loss of information. The third basic assumption is that the cell can repair damaged sections of the DNA molecule by copying from the complementary strand.

5.2. *Specific assumptions.* (i) It is assumed that an ultraviolet dose d produces a Poisson distribution of lesions with mean d. These lesions are assumed to be formed randomly along the length of both strands of DNA. The term lesion is used to describe any kind of abnormal product of radiation. There is evidence [15] that these lesions may be the formation of dimers between adjacent T nucleotides in the DNA molecule. If all lesions were of this type, we would be led into an occupancy problem. Preliminary calculations show that in this case the Poisson assumption and the assumption that lesions are formed at random along the DNA would still be approximately valid.

(ii) The chromosome is assumed to consist of a large number N of repairable sections. For a particular section, repair is accomplished by removing the damaged strand within that section and copying from the complement. If only one strand is damaged in a particular section, it is assumed that the section will be successfully repaired. If both strands are damaged, then when one of the damaged strips is removed there is a loss of information and it will only be by chance that the correct information is recovered from the remaining damaged strip. There is also the possibility that faulty repair may physically damage the chromosome. It has been suggested by Harm [6] that breaks in the chromosome may occur. We will assume that if a faulty repair occurs in any section of the chromosome, then no matter what the subsequent history of the cell is, it will not reproduce. The probability of such a faulty repair will in general depend on the medium in which the bacteria are held. Let the probability of faulty repair for a section with both strands damaged be π for plating medium and ν for non-nutrient medium. It is assumed that this probability is independent of the success of repair of any other section.

If the bacteria are irradiated at a high dose rate, repair will not be possible in the irradiation period. The preceding assumptions enable the theoretical probability of survival $S(d)$ to be obtained. Let $s(d)$ be the probability that a particular section successfully repairs whatever lesions are formed after dose d, then

(44) $$S(d) = s(d)^N.$$

If the number of sections N is large, then for reasonable dose ranges $1 - s(d)$ will be small. Taking logarithms in (44), we have

$$(45) \qquad \log S(d) = N \log s(d) \cong -N(1 - s(d)).$$

If the bacteria are immediately transferred to a plating medium, we have

$$(46) \qquad\qquad 1 - s(d) = \pi \left(1 - \exp\left\{-\frac{\lambda d}{2N}\right\}\right)^2, \qquad\qquad d > 0,$$

where $\lambda d/2N$ is the mean number of lesions formed on a single strand in each section. Thus, provided N is large, from (45), we have

$$(47) \qquad\qquad \log S(d) \cong -N\pi \left(1 - \exp\left\{-\frac{\lambda d}{2N}\right\}\right)^2 \cong -\frac{\pi \lambda^2 d^2}{4N}.$$

Harm [6] was led to a function of this form by similar reasoning. This function is fitted to empirical data for the survival of *E. coli* B/r exposed to ultraviolet light. The value of $\pi \lambda^2/N$ is estimated to be $(2.44 \pm 0.10) \times 10^{-5}$, where the dose d is measured in ergs/mm².

6. The repair function $M(d)$

For the mechanism described above, it is possible to obtain the repair function or the expected number of nucleotides which are replaced as a function of dose. For each section, we have the following events and probabilities

no damage:	$\exp\{-\lambda d/N\}$,
1 strip repaired:	$2(\exp\{-\lambda d/2N\} - \exp\{-\lambda d/N\})$,
2 strips repaired:	$(1 - \pi)(1 - \exp\{-\lambda/2N\})^2$.

If it is assumed that no nucleotides are replaced if repair is unsuccessful, then for the cell

$$(48) \quad M(d) = 2Nn_0 \left[\left(\exp\left\{-\frac{\lambda d}{2N}\right\} - \exp\left\{-\frac{\lambda d}{N}\right\}\right) \right.$$
$$\left. + (1 - \pi)\left(1 - \exp\left\{-\frac{\lambda d}{2N}\right\}\right)^2\right],$$

where $2n_0$ is the number of nucleotides per section. Assuming the same number of nucleotides are replaced even if repair is unsuccessful, then $M(d)$ is given by (48) with $\pi = 0$. In Figure 3, empirical data for the function $M(d)$ are plotted against dose. The bacteria *E. coli* 干 differs from the bacteria used to obtain the estimate of $\pi \lambda^2/N$. It has been suggested that the apparent drop in $M(d)$ as d increases may be an experimental artifact. A theoretical curve with parameters $\lambda/N = 0.0032$ and $\pi = 0.3$ is drawn to illustrate that equation (48) can represent the observed type of function. However, using these parameters and the estimate for $\pi \lambda^2/N$ obtained previously, we have $\lambda = 0.011$, $N = 3.4$, and $\pi = 0.3$. These values are not consistent with values available elsewhere and this experiment will be ignored in what follows.

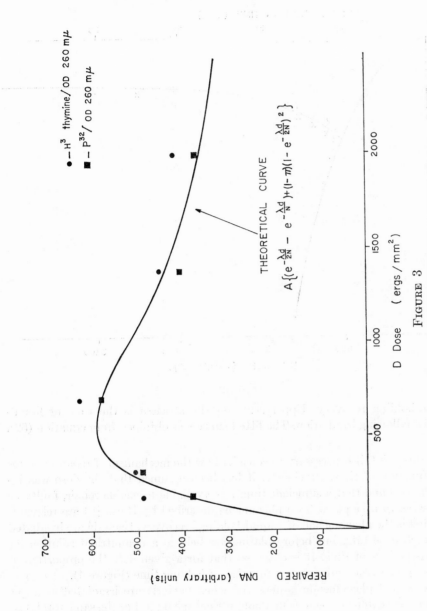

FIGURE 3

Repair function for *E. coli τ*. Data from Haynes [8].

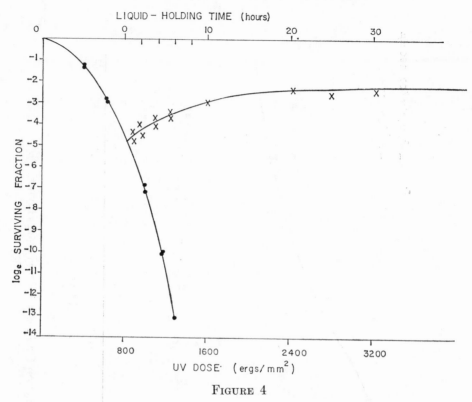

FIGURE 4

Liquid-holding recovery. Upper scale on the abscissa is the time of liquid-holding following irradiation. The fitted curve was obtained from equation (52).

At this point, it is necessary to consider how the mechanism of repair operates as a function of time. Previously, it has been assumed that the dose was instantaneous and that a sufficient time was available to enable repair, faulty or otherwise, to take place. Two phenomena described by Harm [6] are relevant. The first is the phenomenon of "liquid-holding" recovery. Bacteria are irradiated at a high dose rate, but before plating are held in a nonnutrient solution for various periods of time. It is observed that for a given dose the proportion of surviving bacteria increases as a function of holding time (Figure 4).

The second phenomenon is observed when bacteria are irradiated at a low dose rate for extensive periods in a nonnutrient medium. For the same total dose the proportion of survivors is markedly higher for low dose rate exposure than for high dose rate exposure (Figure 5).

The preceding model is readily modified to predict these observations. It is assumed that lesions are formed on the chromosome at a Poisson rate $\lambda\rho$ per hour. The dose rate parameter ρ is in units of ergs/mm^2/hr. For each section, the waiting time before a damaged strand is detected is assumed to be an exponential random variable with mean $1/\mu$. It is assumed that repair is instanta-

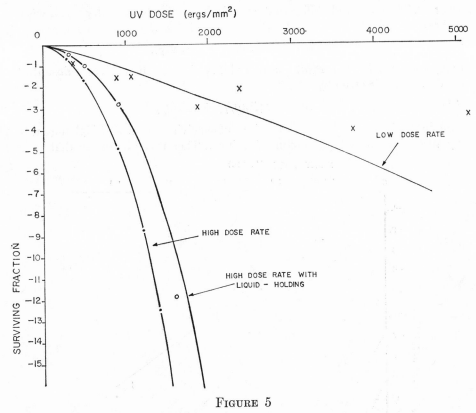

FIGURE 5

Comparison of survival for low dose rate and high dose rate exposure.
The fitted curves were obtained from equations (47), (51), and (52).

neous once the damage is detected. The probabilities of faulty repair of sections
in which both strands are damaged remain π in plating medium, ν in nonnutrient
medium. At some time t in the low dose rate experiment each section will be in
one of four states:

(0) no damage,
(1) damage on one strand,
(2) damage on both strands,
(3) faulty repair has taken place.

Let $P_n(t)$ be the probability of being in state n at time t. Since irradiation takes
place in a nonnutrient medium, we have

(49)
$$
\begin{aligned}
P_0'(t) &= -P_0(t)\lambda\rho/N + P_1(t)\mu, \\
P_1'(t) &= +P_0(t)\lambda\rho/N - P_1(t)(\mu + (\lambda\rho/2N)) + P_2(t)2\mu(1-\pi), \\
P_2'(t) &= \qquad\qquad\qquad + P_1(t)\lambda\rho/2N \qquad\quad - P_2(t)2\mu, \\
P_3'(t) &= \qquad\qquad\qquad\qquad\qquad\qquad\qquad\quad + P_2(t)2\mu\pi.
\end{aligned}
$$

Suppose that the cells are irradiated for a time t_0 and then plated. It is assumed
that in the plating medium, replication is delayed until all possible repair has

occurred. Thus, the probability that a particular section has a faulty repair when replication begins is $P_3(t_0) + \pi P_2(t_0)$. In terms of dose $d = \rho t_0$, we have

$$(50) \qquad 1 - s(d) = P_3(d/\rho) + \pi P_2(d/\rho).$$

Using relationship (45), $S_\rho(d)$ the probability that a cell survives a dose d at the dose rate ρ is given by

$$(51) \qquad \log S_\rho(d) \cong N\{P_3(d/\rho) + \pi P_2(d/\rho)\}.$$

Similarly, let $H(d, t)$ be the probability of surviving a dose d at high dose rate exposure followed by liquid-holding for time t. Then it can be shown that

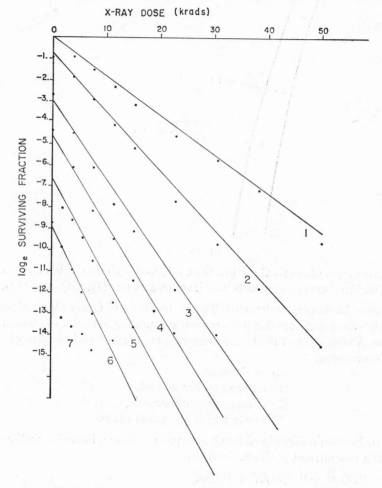

FIGURE 6

Effect of X-ray dose following ultraviolet exposure
(fitted curves are obtained from equation (54)).
Pre-U.V. exposure: 1: 0; 2: 400 ergs/mm²; 3: 800 ergs/mm²;
4: 1,000 ergs/mm²; 5: 1,200 ergs/mm²; 6: 1,400 ergs/mm²; 7: 1,600 ergs/mm².

$$(52) \qquad \log H(d, t) \cong -\frac{\lambda^2 d^2}{4N} \{\pi e^{-\mu\rho t} + \nu(1 - e^{-\mu\rho t})\}.$$

In the particular case $t = 0$, we have the case of immediate plating. To demonstrate the effect of low dose rate exposure as distinct from liquid-holding recovery, Harm also considers $H(d, d/\rho)$, that is, the effect of liquid-holding for the same time as low dose rate exposure. Three empirical sets of survival data corresponding to instantaneous dose, low dose rate exposure, and instantaneous dose followed by liquid-holding for the same time as the low dose rate exposure are given in Figure 5. Theoretical curves with the parameters $\pi = 0.25$, $p = 0.15$, $N = 2 \times 10^5$, $\lambda = 5.4$, and $\mu = 0.173$ are drawn for comparison. For larger values of total dose with low dose rate the model is inadequate since $\log S_\rho(d)$ must decrease steadily in this dose range whereas the empirical data suggest that the proportion surviving has reached a minimum. This effect could possibly be due to a process of damage reversal in which radiation is involved.

The data for liquid-holding recovery as a function of time should be fitted by the function $H(d, t)$. In Figure 4, the theoretical curve with the same parameters as above is superimposed upon the empirical data points.

In a series of experiments Haynes [7] irradiated the bacteria *E. coli* B/r at a relatively high dose rate with one dose of ultraviolet light and one dose of X-ray, alternating the order of exposure. Although there are indications that the order of exposure does affect the probability of survival, it is possible that this is an experiment artifact. With this possibility in mind, an extension of the previous mechanism is proposed. In this model there is no effect of the order of exposure. It is assumed that X-ray ionizations produce a Poisson distribution of X-ray lesions which are uniformly distributed along the chromosome. The X-ray lesions are considered to be large compared with ultraviolet lesions. They are assumed to damage both strands and may be extreme enough to cause chromosome breaks. Let $\eta\theta$ be the mean number of X-ray lesions on the chromosome after a dose θ of X-ray. Let p be the probability that a section containing an X-ray lesion and no other damage has a faulty repair. Let π be the probability that a section with either X-ray damage or ultraviolet damage on both strands will have a faulty repair. In all other cases it is assumed that repair is successful. Then the probability a section has a faulty repair after a dose d of ultraviolet and a dose θ of X-ray is given by

$$(53) \quad 1 - s(d, \theta) = \left(1 - \exp\left\{-\frac{\eta\theta}{N}\right\}\right)\left(\pi - (\pi - p)\exp\left\{-\frac{\lambda d}{N}\right\}\right)$$

$$+ \pi \exp\left\{-\frac{\eta\theta}{N}\right\}\left(1 - \exp\left\{-\frac{\lambda d}{2N}\right\}\right)^2$$

$$\cong \frac{\pi p \theta}{N} + \frac{(\pi - p)\eta\lambda\theta d}{N^2} + \frac{\lambda^2 \pi d^2}{4N^2}.$$

The probability $S(d, \theta)$ that a cell will survive a dose d of ultraviolet and a dose θ of X-ray is given by

$$(54) \qquad \log S(d, \theta) \cong -\left\{\eta p\theta + \frac{(\pi - p)\eta\lambda\theta d}{N} + \frac{\lambda^2 \pi d^2}{4N}\right\}.$$

This function can be readily fitted to the empirical data of Haynes [7]. With parameters $\eta = 49.3$, $p = 0.0037$, $N = 2 \times 10^5$, $\lambda = 3.84$, and $\pi = 0.25$; the fitted curves are superimposed upon the empirical data in Figure 6. The fitted curves compare favorably with the empirical data.

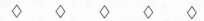

Dr. R. H. Haynes sparked my interest in this subject in the course of several discussions I had with him. In the preparation of the paper I have received encouragement and many helpful suggestions from Professors J. Neyman and L. LeCam.

REFERENCES

[1] J. A. CROWTHER, "Some considerations relative to the action of X-rays on tissue cells," *Proc. Roy. Soc. London Ser. B*, Vol. 96 (1924), pp. 207–211.
[2] H. DÄNZER, "Über einege Wirkungen von Strählen VII," *Z. Physik.*, Vol. 89 (1934), pp. 421–425.
[3] W. DITTRICH, "Treffermischkurven," *Z. Naturforsch.*, Vol. 15b (1960), pp. 261–266.
[4] W. FELLER, *An Introduction to Probability Theory and Its Applications*, Vol. 2, New York, Wiley, 1964.
[5] J. F. FOWLER, "Differences in survival curve shapes for formal multi-target and multi-hit models," *Phys. Med. Biol.*, Vol. 9 (1964), pp. 177–188.
[6] W. HARM, "Effects of dose fractionation and ultraviolet survival of *Escherichia coli*," *Photochemistry and Photobiology*, Vol. 7 (1968), pp. 73–86.
[7] R. H. HAYNES, "Role of DNA repair mechanisms in microbial inactivation and recovery phenomena," *Photochemistry and Photobiology*, Vol. 3 (1964), pp. 429–450.
[8] ———, "Interpretation of microbial inactivation and recovery phenomena," *Radiation Res. Supp.*, No. 6 (1966), pp. 1–29.
[9] R. H. HAYNES, R. M. BAKER, and G. E. JONES, "Genetic implications of DNA repair," Lawrence Radiation Laboratory Report UCRL-17964, 1967.
[10] A. M. KELLERER, *Stochastik der Strahlenwirkung*, Berlin-Heidelberg-New York, Springer-Verlag, 1966.
[11] A. NORMAN, "The nuclear role in the U.V. inactivation of *Neurospora conidia*," *J. Cell. Comp. Physiol.*, Vol. 44 (1954), pp. 1–10.
[12] E. H. PORTER, "Multi-hit v. multi-target curves," *Brit. J. Radiol.*, Vol. 37, No. 444 (1964), p. 958.
[13] P. S. PURI, "A class of stochastic models of response after infection in the absence of defense mechanism," *Proceedings of the Fifth Berkeley Symposium on Mathematical Statistics and Probability*, Berkeley and Los Angeles, University of California Press, 1966, Vol. 4, pp. 511–536.
[14] R. B. SETLOW, P. A. SWENSON, and W. L. CARRIER, "Thymine dimers and inhibitions of DNA synthesis by ultraviolet irradiation of cells," *Science*, Vol. 142 (1963), pp. 1464–1466.
[15] R. B. SETLOW and J. K. SETLOW, "Evidence that U.V. induced thymine dimers in DNA cause biological damage," *Proc. Nat. Acad. Sci., U.S.A.*, Vol. 48 (1962), pp. 1250–1257.
[16] H. TEICHER, "Identifiability of mixtures," *Ann. Math. Statist.*, Vol. 31 (1960), pp. 55–73.
[17] M. A. WOODBURY, "Some mathematical and statistical methods in radiation therapy," *Nat. Canc. Inst. Monograph*, No. 24 (1965).
[18] K. G. ZIMMER, *Studies on Quantitative Radiation Biology* (translated by H. D. Griffith), Edinburgh, Oliver and Boyd, 1961.

STUDIES OF THE MECHANISM OF INDUCTION OF PULMONARY ADENOMAS IN MICE

MARGARET R. WHITE

LAWRENCE BERKELEY LABORATORY

1. Introduction

The present paper is related to the frequently discussed question as to whether urethane tumorigenesis is a one stage or a multistage process. In either case, the tumorigenic process is assumed to begin with what may be called an *initial event*, a change in a single normal cell (*mutation*) resulting from a single *hit* by a tumorigenic molecule (one hit theory) or from several such hits (multihit theory). If the initial event is followed by the growth of the tumor studied, then the mechanism is described as a one stage mechanism. However, as explicitly suggested by Brues [5], the growth (of *first order mutants*) following an initial event may well be "benign" in the sense of being destined to disappear, except for the possibility of a second mutation in one of its cells creating *second order mutants*. If this second mutation in a cell of the benign growth turns into a tumor cell, then the process of tumorigenesis is called a two stage mechanism. It is easy to visualize three or four or, generally, multistage mechanisms of tumorigenesis. Naturally, there is the possibility that, with respect to some particular tumors, say pulmonary adenomas in mice, the tumorigenic process is a one stage process while, with respect to some other tumors, say pulmonary carcinomas, it is a multistage mechanism.

Some years ago a private communication from M. B. Shimkin to J. Neyman raised the question as to whether an experiment could be devised to decide whether a particular tumorigenesis, say of pulmonary adenomas in mice, is a one stage or a multistage phenomenon. The experiment contemplated was to consist of injecting mice with specified doses of urethane and counting adenomas. Briefly, the investigation by Neyman and Scott [18] resulted in the finding that, with a two stage mechanism, the fractionation of a given dose of urethane may influence the ultimate number of tumors. On the other hand, with a one stage mechanism, they concluded that the ultimate number of tumors must be independent of the time pattern in which the given fixed dose of the tumorigenic

This work was supported by the U.S. Atomic Energy Commission, by Cancer Research Funds of the University of California, and by Research Grant GM-10525 from the NIH, USPHS, to the Statistical Laboratory, University of California, Berkeley.

material is administered, since the *given fixed dose* should produce the same number of initial events, irrespective of the time pattern in which this material is administered.

In the cited paper Neyman and Scott took it for granted that the average number of initial events is proportional to the dose of urethane in milligrams per gram of body weight of the mice (mg/g). A number of experiments performed in several laboratories [11], [21], [24], with fractionation of the total doses measured in these units (mg/g), indicated unambiguously that the presumed ultimate number of pulmonary adenomas in mice depends on the time patterns in which the same dose of urethane is administered to mice. This, then, suggested that the mechanism of this particular tumorigenesis cannot consist of just one stage. However, certain circumstances suggested doubts as to whether the average number of initial events generated by varying doses $D_1, D_2, \cdots, D_s$ of urethane is really proportional to these doses. In particular, two points of doubt emerged. One is the question whether the rate at which the urethane is catabolized into some nontumorigenic material is or is not dependent upon the dose D injected. The second point of doubt concerns the identity of the chemical entity that is actually tumorigenic: is this the intact urethane molecule or, possibly, some other molecule originating in the process of catabolism of urethane? The present study is intended to provide some information on these two particular points. The details of the background follow.

The tumor system in which pulmonary adenomas are induced in mice by administration of the carcinogen urethane (ethyl carbamate) is a useful system for quantitative studies of tumorigenesis. Urethane has been shown to produce tumors in animals other than mice and to produce a variety of types of tumors. It appears to be a true carcinogen. Pulmonary adenomas can be induced by other carcinogens and occur spontaneously in some strains of mice. They grow as small, round, white nodules which usually protrude from the surface of the lungs and are easily identifiable with the naked eye. An occasional tumor occurs deeper in the lung tissue, but the lungs of mice are very thin and somewhat translucent, so that if they are counted not too soon after urethane administration, most of the tumors are visible without the need for serial sectioning and tedious microscope work. A dose as small as $\frac{1}{16}$ mg/g induces significant numbers of tumors, and abundant tumors are induced by a dose of 1.0 mg/g.

Some aspects of urethane catabolism have been investigated in other laboratories. Some of these studies, including those done in this laboratory, used urethane labeled with radionuclides. Urethane has been synthesized with ^{14}C in either of two positions in the molecule and with ^{3}H in one position as follows:

$$CH_3-CH_2-O-{}^{*}C\overset{O}{\underset{NH_2}{<}} \qquad CH_3-{}^{*}CH_2-O-C\overset{O}{\underset{NH_2}{<}}$$

Ethyl Carbamate (carbonyl-^{14}C)   Ethyl (1-^{14}C) Carbamate

$$\text{*HCH}_2\text{—CH}_2\text{—O—C} \overset{\displaystyle O}{\underset{\displaystyle NH_2}{\big<}}$$

Ethyl (2-³H) Carbamate

*C=¹⁴C   *H=³H

Bryan, Skipper, and White [6] and Skipper, Bennett, Bryan, White, Newton, and Simpson [22] reported that, within 24 hours after the administration of ethyl carbamate (carbonyl-¹⁴C), 90 to 95 per cent of the ¹⁴C was exhaled as ¹⁴CO₂ in the breath of mice and five to ten per cent was excreted in the urine. They postulated that urethane was hydrolyzed in the body to carbon dioxide, ethyl alcohol, and ammonia, that is,

$$CH_3\text{—CH}_2\text{—O—C}\overset{\displaystyle O}{\underset{\displaystyle NH_2}{\big<}} + H_2O \xrightarrow[\text{catalyzed}]{\text{enzymatically}} CO_2 + CH_3\text{—CH}_2\text{—OH} + NH_3.$$

Boyland and Rhoden [4], using rats and doing chemical analyses of blood and tissues, and Berenblum, Haran-Ghera, R. Winnick, and T. Winnick [1], administering ethyl carbamate (carbonyl-¹⁴C) to mice, also concluded that the intact urethane molecule disappeared from the blood and tissues of animals within 24 hours. Both Skipper and co-workers [22] and Berenblum and co-workers [1] found that when ethyl (1-¹⁴C) carbamate was administered, the rate of appearance of ¹⁴C in the breath was slower than when ethyl carbamate (carbonyl-¹⁴C) was administered. There seemed to be no selective concentration of urethane in any of the organs analyzed by these investigators.

Kaye [14], using ethyl carbamate (carbonyl-¹⁴C), found that two-week-old Swiss mice catabolized urethane more slowly than those six months old, and that C3H mice catabolized it more rapidly than did Swiss mice. Mirvish, Cividalli, and Berenblum [16], by chemical analysis of livers for urethane content, found that adult Swiss mice catabolized urethane at approximately ten times the rate of newborn Swiss mice. Cividalli and co-workers [7], by blood analysis for ¹⁴C from ethyl carbamate (carbonyl-¹⁴C), found that there was a rapid increase in the rate of catabolism of urethane in SWR mice as age increased from 1 to 30 days, and that newborn mice of five other strains also eliminated it slowly as compared to adult SWR mice. The rates of urethane elimination in these five strains did not seem well correlated with the differences in susceptibility of the adult animals of these strains to tumor induction.

Skipper and co-workers [22] inferred from their data that the rate of hydrolysis of urethane decreased with time after administration, whereas Kaye [14] stated that urethane was catabolized at a constant rate. After administration of ethyl carbamate (carbonyl-¹⁴C), Grogan, Lane, Liebelt, and Smith [10] measured the concentration of ¹⁴C in blood and liver of intact mice and of partially hepatectomized mice that were sacrificed at 1, 2, 4, 8, or 24 hours after urethane administration. They reported that the disappearance of urethane from blood and liver was approximately linear for 8 hours and appeared to be more rapid in the next 16 hours.

As stated above, it is not known whether urethane or some metabolite of urethane is the active carcinogen. N-hydroxy urethane was thought to be a possible carcinogenic metabolite of urethane since it is chemically closely related and is carcinogenic. Studies by Mirvish [15] and Biota, Mirvish, and Berenblum [2] suggested that the carcinogenicity of N-hydroxy urethane is due to its conversion to urethane rather than the reverse. Nery [17] proposed that urethane is metabolically activated *in vivo* and that an intermediary metabolite which can be formed from either urethane or N-hydroxy urethane is probably the proximate carcinogen.

None of the cited experiments investigated the possible differences in results from administration of various dosages. The various investigators used different dosages and different strains and ages of animals. In order to investigate the relationship of dose to tumor induction, it is important to know whether internal exposure of the animals to the molecule (and thus risk of producing initial events in the cell) is proportional to the administered dose over a fairly wide dosage range in animals of the same strain, sex, and age. We know of no direct means of determining internal exposure to the intact urethane molecule, but we can assert that the exposure cannot exceed the lesser of the two values of exposure calculated from the body retention times of the ethyl moiety and the carbonyl moiety. If the tumor yield correlates closely with the smaller of these calculated internal exposures, it would seem likely that the intact molecule is responsible for the tumorigenic process. If, on the other hand, the tumor yield is more nearly proportionate to the larger exposure value, it is likely that some metabolite of urethane that contains the corresponding fraction of the molecule is the key to the tumorigenic process. We therefore undertook studies on the rate of catabolism of urethane given in various dosages and labeled with ^{14}C in either the ethyl or carbonyl position.

2. Materials and methods

Female A/Jax mice were obtained from Jackson Laboratory when they were three to four weeks old. The mice were numbered with metal ear tags and randomized into dosage categories by use of tables of random numbers. They were housed ten to a large plastic cage, with wood shavings for bedding, but no two animals of the same dose category were housed together. They were fed Simonsen's white diet to which terramycin was added during milling with the aim of keeping them as disease free as possible. Their water was chlorinated and HCl was added to pH 2.5 in order to discourage *Pseudomonas aeruginosa* infections. The mice were ten to eleven weeks old and their mean weight was 20.3 g (range, 15 to 26 g) when urethane was administered. They were sacrificed for tumor counts exactly 24 weeks after urethane administration. Tumors were counted as previously described [25]. Untreated control animals were housed with the experimental animals. One hundred and thirty controls and 259 urethane treated animals were sacrificed for tumor counts.

Ethyl carbamate (carbonyl-^{14}C) and ethyl (1-^{14}C) carbamate were obtained from Schwarz Bioresearch. Nonradioactive urethane was obtained from Eastman Organic Chemicals. Injection solutions combining radioactive and nonradioactive urethane to the desired total urethane concentrations were made up in sterile distilled water such that each solution contained 1 μCi/ml. Measurements of the exact radioactivity in each solution were made by diluting aliquots with scintillation solution and counting in a Nuclear-Chicago Mark I scintillation counter. The scintillation solution used for these tests and for counting urine and feces samples consisted of 12.5 g PFO, 0.31 g FOPOP, and 125 g naphthalene diluted to 1 liter with p-dioxane. The urethane concentration of the injection solutions was adjusted to a set of values ranging from 1.25 to 14.00 per cent. The mice were injected with 0.01 ml of the appropriate solution per gram of body weight. Thus, for example, to administer a dose of 0.125 mg/g to a 20 g mouse, we injected 0.20 ml of 1.25 per cent solution of urethane, which contained 0.2 μCi of ^{14}C.

Each of the 70 experimental groups was comprised of four animals. When a group was treated, the mice were injected as rapidly as possible (usually less than a minute between the first and fourth injections) and quickly put into the metabolism cage. The cages were of plastic with raised wire screen bottoms which allowed most of the urine and feces to fall through to the cage floor. Food and water were available. Air from a tank of compressed air, aged to reduce its natural radioactivity, was passed through a calibrated flowmeter and into the metabolism cages at a rate of approximately 300 cc/min. The air, which now included the expired breath of the animals, flowed from the metabolism cage through a U-tube filled with water absorber (Drierite) and into a 250 cc ionization chamber. The charge collected in the ionization chamber because of ionization caused by radioactive decay of ^{14}C was measured with a vibrating reed electrometer [23]. The potential in millivolts produced by this charge was recorded every 20 seconds on a 12 channel Leeds and Northrup recorder. The air leaving the ionization chamber passed through soda lime to remove the radioactive CO_2, through a second flowmeter to monitor for leaks in the system, and into a wet test meter. Readings were taken from the wet test meter periodically to accurately measure the air flow. The radioactivity in the breath of the animals was followed in this manner for approximately 24 hours in most experiments and for 48 hours in a few experiments. Three sets of the above described equipment were used and each was standardized with gas containing trace amounts of $^{14}CO_2$. The concentration of $^{14}CO_2$ in the gas was determined by the method of Jeffay and Alvarez [12]: measured volumes of gas were passed through fritted glass dispersion tubes into CO_2 absorber solutions; aliquots of the absorber solution were diluted with scintillation fluid and counted. A calibration curve relating millivolts recorded to the amount of ^{14}C in the ionization chamber was then plotted.

After the mice were removed, at the end of a run, urine and feces were quantitatively washed from the metabolism chamber, diluted to an exact volume, homogenized with a magnetic stirrer, and centrifuged, and an aliquot was added to scintillation fluid for counting. Duplicate samples were taken and each was counted at least twice.

The areas under the curves relating ^{14}C in the breath to time after administration of urethane were measured with a Bendix Data Digitizer in order to obtain the time integral of internal exposure. Mathematical and computer methods for handling these data were worked out by Claude Guillier of Neyman and Scott's group and are described in a companion paper [9]. The end result of these calculations is a value called *milligram-hours per gram weight of mouse* (mg-hrs/g), a measure of the apparent internal exposure of the animal to that part of the molecule in which the ^{14}C atom was located. These calculations assume that at any instant the amount of unrecovered ^{14}C is still in the animal. There was no reason to believe that the experimental procedure allowed loss of any of the ^{14}C eliminated by the animals. However, if some of the difference between injected and recovered ^{14}C was due to experimental error, the internal exposure calculations would lead to values higher than the true values.

3. Results

Urethane acts as an anesthetic at a dosage of about 1 mg/g. The animals used in these experiments showed slight grogginess at dosages of 0.5 and 0.75 mg/g. Dosage of 1.0 mg/g produced unconsciousness for an hour or two; 1.2 mg/g, four to six hours; and 1.4 mg/g, eight or more hours. In animals that received 1.2 mg/g, 3 of 40 did not survive the anesthesia, and in those receiving 1.4 mg/g, 14 of 40 did not survive. During the 24 week holding period, there were a few deaths in other dosage groups from causes apparently unrelated to urethane administration. Though there were five experiments performed at each dosage, some of these are not included in the data because of the deaths.

The rates of catabolism of urethane were obtained using Guillier's calculations [9] of urethane exhaled/g mouse (based on either carbon label) over small time intervals to obtain rates at particular times after the injection of urethane.

Figure 1 shows the rates of catabolism of various doses of urethane as computed from the rates at which the carbonyl carbon is eliminated in the breath of the animals. With a dose of 0.125 mg/g, the rate of catabolism drops off very rapidly after three hours. When 0.25 mg/g is administered, the rate reaches a peak at two to three hours, decreases slightly for the next four hours and then a rapid decrease begins. When the dose is 0.5 to 1.2 mg/g, the rate gradually rises for eight to nine hours and then, after an interval which increases with dose,

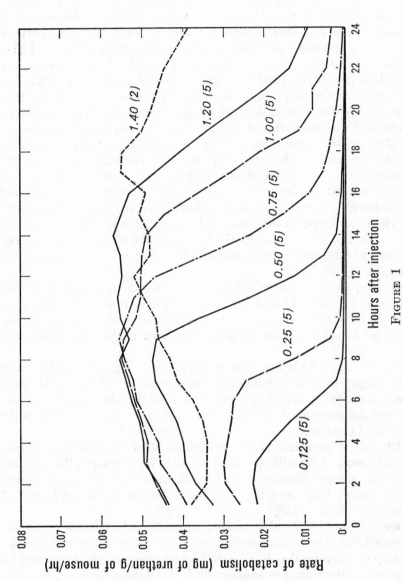

FIGURE 1

Rate of catabolism of urethane as measured with ethyl carbamate (carbonyl-^{14}C). Each curve is labeled with the injected dose in mg/g. Numbers in parentheses are the numbers of experiments used to obtain the curves.

the rate rapidly declines. When 1.4 mg/g is given, there is a slight decline in rate which persists for three hours, and the rate stays lower than that for doses of 0.5 to 1.2 mg/g for at least nine hours. A possible explanation of the variations in rates of elimination at these doses is that the normal enzyme system responsible for converting the carbonyl radical to CO_2 is saturated at the blood level of urethane produced by a dose between 0.25 and 0.5 mg/g, that doses between 0.5 and 1.2 mg/g stimulate additional production of enzyme to a new, higher level which then becomes saturated, and that doses of 1.4 mg/g temporarily partially poison the enzyme producing system. Slowed respiration, circulation, and metabolism, due to deep anesthesia, probably also contribute to the relatively low rate of catabolism at this high dosage. The maximum rate of catabolism as measured with the carbonyl tracer is approximately 0.056 mg/g/hr.

Figure 2 shows the rates of catabolism of various dosages of urethane as measured by the rates at which the ethyl carbon is eliminated. The situation here is somewhat more complicated since ethyl alcohol, into which this part of the urethane molecule supposedly is metabolized [22], is more slowly hydrolyzed and degraded to CO_2 than is the carbonyl radical. Thus, this part of the molecule probably circulates longer in the blood, and so more of it is likely to enter the normal metabolic pathways than is the CO_2 from the carbonyl carbon. The maximum rate of catabolism as measured with the ethyl carbon is approximately 0.045 mg/g/hr.

In some cases, the data used to obtain Figures 1 and 2 differ from those used in the other figures and tables. If the animals lived more than 48 hours after the end of the metabolism experiment, they were used in these figures. If they died before the time for sacrifice, they were not used in the other figures and the tables.

In the experiments with lower doses (0.125 and 0.25 mg/g), in which it was possible to roughly estimate the long lived component at the end of the curve (not shown), it was found that the amount of ^{14}C from the ethyl labeled urethane which entered this component was about twice the corresponding portion of the carbonyl labeled urethane.

Table I tabulates the results of the measurements for integrated internal exposure at 24 hours, along with the numbers of tumors induced. The relative errors of the means are reasonably small for the integrated internal exposure; for induced tumors, they are larger. The mean number of tumors in control animals was 0.41 (S.E. = 0.08).

In Figure 3, two estimates of integrated internal exposure, based on the different carbon labels, are plotted against the injected doses. The relationships are obviously curvilinear; that is, as injected dose increases, the integrated internal exposure of the animal to urethane (or its breakdown products) increases more than proportionately.

In Figure 4a, tumors in animals injected with carbonyl labeled urethane are plotted against injected dose; in Figure 4b, they are plotted against internal

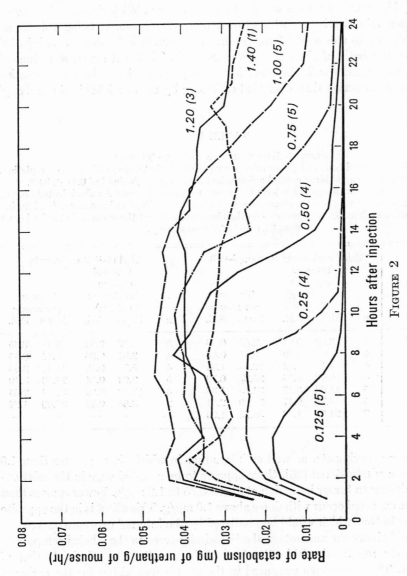

FIGURE 2

Rate of catabolism of urethane as measured with ethyl (1-^{14}C) carbamate. Each curve is labeled with the injected dose in mg/g. Numbers in parentheses are the numbers of experiments used to obtain the curves.

exposure. (The marked dip in the curve at a dose of 0.5 mg/g is probably due to random biological variability, since we have not seen this effect in other experiments and it did not occur in the animals used in the experiments in which the ^{14}C was in the ethyl group.) Figures 5a and 5b show the corresponding relationships when the label was in the ethyl carbon. With either carbon label, the tumor induction *versus* internal exposure comes nearer to being a linear relationship (up to a dose of 1.0 mg/g) than does tumor induction *versus* injected dose. On the basis of these data, it appears that internal exposure estimated from measurements with the label in the ethyl group has a better correlation with tumor induction than does that estimated by use of a label in the carbonyl group.

TABLE I

INTERNAL EXPOSURE AND INDUCED TUMORS

n = number of experiments, with four mice per experiment, that were continued to completion.
One hundred and thirty control animals had mean tumors/animal of 0.41 ± 0.08.
No measurements for integrated internal exposure could be obtained for the injected dose of 1.40 mg/g in the ethyl (1-^{14}C) carbamate case due to the death of at least one animal during each experiment. Tumors were counted on the nine survivors and the mean and standard error were 31.1 and 3.27 respectively.

| Injected dose | Ethyl carbamate (carbonyl-^{14}C) | | | | Ethyl (1-^{14}C) carbamate | | | |
| | | Internal exposure (mg-hrs/g) (24 hrs) | | Tumors per mouse | | Internal exposure (mg-hrs/g) (24 hrs) | | Tumors per mouse |
	n	Mean	S.E.	Mean	S.E.	n	Mean	S.E.	Mean	S.E.
0.125	4	0.60	0.01	2.45	0.40	5	1.07	0.02	2.45	0.35
0.25	4	1.64	0.09	6.44	0.44	4	2.32	0.06	6.12	0.85
0.50	4	4.14	0.13	10.13	1.34	4	5.24	0.16	14.31	2.08
0.75	4	6.97	0.18	24.87	0.76	5	9.09	0.14	23.10	3.10
1.00	5	11.03	0.47	34.15	1.38	4	12.92	0.29	32.56	2.63
1.20	5	14.78	0.47	38.00	2.11	2	18.64	0.32	39.00	1.22
1.40	2	21.66	1.36	36.75	1.00	—	—	—	—	—

In these experiments, as well as in another in which doses greater than 1.0 mg/g were administered [26], there appears to be a real change in the relationship of dosage to tumor induction at about 0.75 to 1.0 mg/g. Fewer tumors than would be expected occur with doses above 1.0 mg/g. This effect is in the opposite direction to that which would be predicted by the internal exposure curves.

Table II shows the amounts of the ^{14}C administered in the labeled compounds which were recovered within the first 24 hours after the administration of urethane. The percentage measured in the breath was higher for the carbonyl label than for the ethyl label. In the urine and feces, this situation was reversed.

For most dosages, one experiment was performed in which the run was continued for 48 hours rather than being stopped at approximately 24 hours.

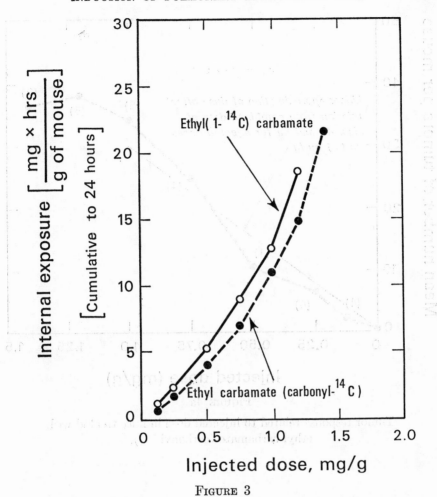

FIGURE 3

Internal exposure *versus* injected dose as measured with ^{14}C label in two positions
in the urethane molecule.

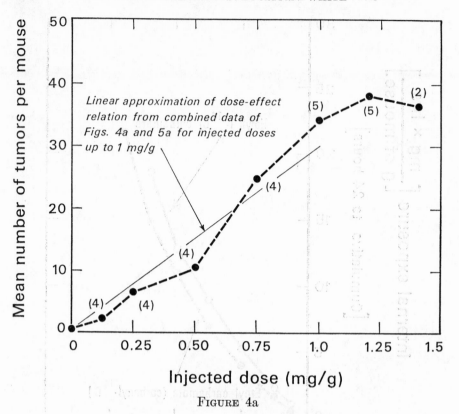

FIGURE 4a

Tumor response related to injected dose in mice treated with
ethyl carbamate (carbonyl-^{14}C).

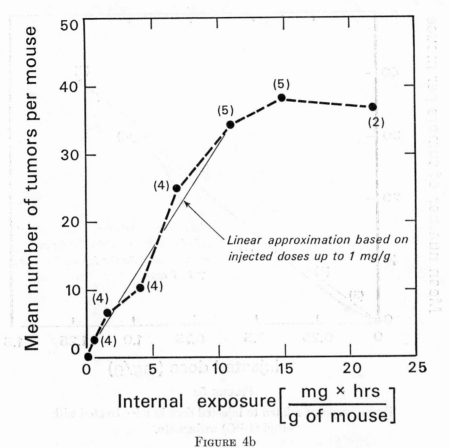

FIGURE 4b

Tumor response related to internal exposure as measured with
ethyl carbamate (carbonyl-^{14}C).

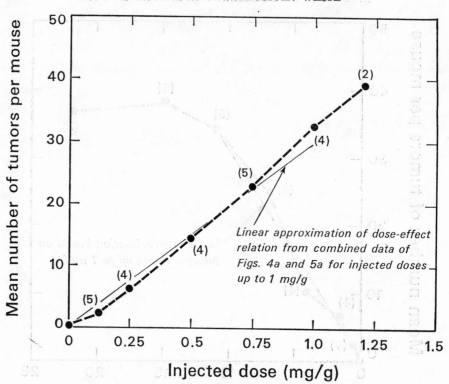

FIGURE 5a

Tumor response related to injected dose in mice treated with
ethyl (1-¹⁴C) carbamate.

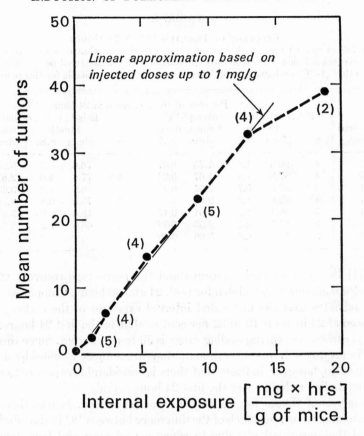

FIGURE 5b

Tumor response related to internal exposure as measured with
ethyl (1-14C) carbamate.

TABLE II

RECOVERY OF INJECTED ^{14}C AT 24 HOURS

n = number of experiments, with four mice per experiment, that continued to completion. At least one animal died in each of the experiments with administered dose 1.40 mg/g in the ethyl (1-^{14}C) carbamate case. Therefore no data are available for this point.

Administered dose (mg/g)		Per cent of ^{14}C recovered at 24 hours								
		Ethyl carbamate (carbonyl-^{14}C)				Ethyl (1-^{14}C) carbamate			
		Breath		Urine and feces			Breath		Urine and feces	
	n	Mean	S.E.	Mean	S.E.	n	Mean	S.E.	Mean	S.E.
0.125	4	90.6	1.0	1.75	0.07	5	76.6	0.5	3.23	0.19
0.25	4	87.3	1.1	1.67	0.24	4	77.9	1.0	2.87	0.24
0.50	4	87.2	0.7	2.05	0.25	4	80.6	1.3	3.63	0.16
0.75	4	89.8	1.2	2.09	0.35	5	76.5	0.8	3.70	0.12
1.00	5	86.1	1.7	2.01	0.12	4	78.5	1.6	3.66	0.18
1.20	5	85.5	0.5	2.55	0.38	2	66.6	2.2	3.62	0.22
1.40	2	73.1	6.4	3.06	0.39	—	—	—	—	—

Table III lists the internal exposures and the percentage recovery of ^{14}C for the labeled compounds calculated for both 24 and 48 hours. Comparison of these values indicates that the integrated internal exposure to the carbonyl carbon in the second 24 hours is 19 to 32 per cent of that in the first 24 hours; and for the ethyl carbon, the corresponding range is 26 to 54 per cent. Since these measurements are for only one experiment, they are subject to considerable error. These data do, however, indicate that there is considerable exposure to urethane or its metabolic products after the first 24 hour period.

No analysis of tissues for ^{14}C content was performed. It was therefore not possible to determine how much of the difference between ^{14}C in the administered dose and that recovered was due to experimental error and how much to retention by the animals. The 48-hour experiments indicate that there certainly are long lived components into which these carbon atoms enter. Further experiments will be necessary to assess more accurately the magnitude of the long lived components.

4. Discussion

The rate at which urethane is catabolized is neither exponential nor constant as has been proposed by other investigators [14], [22]. The system is more complicated than can be explained by either of these simple descriptions and is dependent on the size of the dose. Administered doses of 0.125 and 0.25 mg/g appear not to saturate the system responsible for breaking off the carbonyl group from the molecule. Doses of 0.50 mg/g and above do appear to saturate this system initially and, since the rate of catabolism continues to rise for some hours, probably stimulate production of the enzyme [13] responsible for this process.

Since the ethyl carbon must go through at least two steps before it appears

TABLE III

COMPARISON OF VALUES OBTAINED AT 24 HOURS WITH THOSE OBTAINED AT 48 HOURS AFTER URETHANE ADMINISTRATION

These data pertain to one experiment at each dosage.

The figures for the per cent recovery of injected ^{14}C are for ^{14}C in breath plus that in urine and feces.

No experiment was continued for 48 hours in the ethyl carbamate (carbonyl-^{14}C) case for injected dose 0.25 mg/g.

One animal died in the experiment with injected dose 1.40 mg/g in the ethyl (1-^{14}C) carbamate case, so no data are available.

| Injected dose | Internal exposure (mg-hrs/g) | | | | | | Per cent recovery of injected ^{14}C | | | | | |
| | Ethyl carbamate (carbonyl-^{14}C) | | | Ethyl (1-^{14}C) carbamate | | | Ethyl carbamate (carbonyl-^{14}C) | | | Ethyl (1-^{14}C) carbamate | | |
	24 hr	48 hr	Ratio of 48 to 24	24 hr	48 hr	Ratio of 48 to 24	24 hr	48 hr	Difference	24 hr	48 hr	Difference
0.125	0.61	0.79	1.31	1.11	1.71	1.54	92.8	94.7	1.9	77.9	81.2	3.3
0.25	—	—	—	2.44	3.64	1.49	—	—	—	78.4	81.8	3.4
0.50	4.31	5.67	1.32	5.30	7.12	1.34	88.0	89.3	1.3	82.8	86.5	3.7
0.75	7.42	8.80	1.19	9.42	13.05	1.39	91.0	94.1	3.1	77.6	81.7	4.1
1.00	12.46	14.88	1.19	13.00	16.33	1.26	87.9	91.3	3.4	83.0	87.9	4.9
1.20	15.21	19.08	1.25	18.99	26.07	1.37	86.0	86.8	0.8	67.2	78.2	11.0
1.40	23.02	27.74	1.21	—	—	—	68.7	89.4	20.7	—	—	—

in the breath as CO_2, the curves for its catabolism are more complicated than those for the carbonyl carbon. The initial rise in the rate is more prolonged, and the "plateau" is flatter and somewhat more prolonged, indicating a slower and hence probably more complicated catabolism process. No attempt has been made in these studies to analyze the curves into their various components except for some rough measurements on the tail (not shown) of the curves of animals given low dosages. Further studies on individual animals are planned. Such curves should be easier to analyze than those obtained from each run in this investigation, since each is a composite of the breath of four animals. The more prolonged stay in the animals of the ethyl moiety of urethane as compared with the carbonyl moiety is in agreement with findings of Skipper and co-workers [22] and Berenblum and co-workers [1].

Internal exposure of the animals to the urethane molecule, based on the length of stay of either the carbonyl or ethyl carbon, is not linearly related to administered dose. At doses of 1.0 mg/g and below, the internal exposure values appear to have a more linear relationship to tumor induction than does administered dose. The fact that small doses give disproportionately less internal exposure than large ones may be the explanation for the phenomenon, found in earlier experiments, of the induction of fewer tumors with fractionated doses as compared with the corresponding single dose; that is, the risk of inducing an initial event in the cell is smaller if a total dose is divided into fractions.

The internal exposure based on the persistence of the ethyl carbon in the body tentatively appears to be a better fit to tumor incidence than does that based on the carbonyl carbon. If this holds true in more extensive experiments, it may mean that the ethyl part of the molecule is more intimately involved in the process responsible for tumorigenic action. This would, however, not necessarily rule out the possibility that the intact molecule is necessary for the primary reaction with tissue components. Once reacted, the carbonyl carbon might be hydrolyzed from a larger molecule, leaving the ethyl part of the molecule attached.

Some experiments performed in other laboratories on the binding of the ^{14}C from labeled urethane to cellular constituents are of interest with regard to our findings on integrated internal exposure. Boyland and Williams [3] found ^{14}C in RNA and DNA of liver and lungs after giving either ethyl (1-^{14}C) carbamate or ethyl carbamate (carbonyl-^{14}C). The liver fractions were labeled equally well regardless of which carbon of urethane was labeled; however, ethyl (1-^{14}C) carbamate was more efficient in labeling lung nucleic acids than was ethyl carbamate (carbonyl-^{14}C). They state that this was probably mainly due to metabolic incorporation of ^{14}C released in the catabolism of urethane, but that the results were noteworthy in view of the fact that urethane is more carcinogenic for lungs than liver. Grogan and co-workers [10], working with partially hepatectomized mice, found no significant labeling of either DNA or RNA when they gave ethyl carbamate (carbonyl-^{14}C). Prodi, Rocchi, and Grilli [19] gave rats tracer doses of ethyl (1-^{14}C) carbamate, ethyl carbamate (carbonyl-^{14}C), or ethyl (2-³H) carbamate. They found ¹⁴C from ethyl (1-¹⁴C) carbamate in DNA, RNA, cytoplasmic proteins, and nuclear proteins of liver, spleen, lung, kidney, and skin. Essentially the same components were labeled when ethyl (2-³H) carbamate was used, except that skin and kidney were not analyzed in this case. Negligible activity was found in the organs of animals to which ethyl carbamate (carbonyl-¹⁴C) had been administered. They concluded from their experiments that there is true binding of the ethyl moiety of the urethane molecule to RNA and DNA rather than metabolic utilization of the ethyl alcohol resulting from hydrolysis of urethane. Thus, the preponderance of evidence is that the ethyl moiety is more permanently fixed in the tissues.

Acute deaths in the groups receiving 1.2 and 1.4 mg/g indicate that these doses are definitely in the toxic range. There may be competing risks here in that the less vigorous animals, which did not survive these high doses, may also have been the least resistant of the group to tumor induction. Another possibility is that, in the animals that did survive these doses, there may be considerable cell death as compared to lower doses, and this factor may be involved in the lower than expected tumor incidence. There may also be some cell death, though at a diminished level, in the animals receiving smaller doses. This may explain the increased cell proliferation, as measured by the incorporation of thymidine, without increased cellularity seen in several laboratories [8], [20], [26], that is, proliferation to replace dead or dying cells.

In summary, with regard to the two questions posed in the introduction, it appears that the rate at which urethane is catabolized is dependent upon dose size, and that the number of initial events in the cell (first order mutants) might not be strictly proportional to administered dose. The question of the identity of the proximal carcinogen is still unanswered, but the data presented here seem to indicate that the ethyl moiety may be more intimately involved with the tumorigenic activity than is the carbonyl moiety.

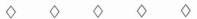

I wish to thank Mr. James W. Lieb for very able technical assistance, Mr. Alexander Grendon and Dr. Hardin B. Jones for their helpful discussions and encouragement, and Drs. J. Neyman and E. L. Scott whose theories were the inspiration for this work.

REFERENCES

[1] I. BERENBLUM, N. HARAN-GHERA, R. WINNICK, and T. WINNICK, "Distribution of C¹⁴-labeled urethans in tissues of the mouse and subcellular localization in lung and liver," *Cancer Res.*, Vol. 18 (1958), pp. 181–185.

[2] L. BOIATO, S. S. MIRVISH, and I. BERENBLUM, "The carcinogenic action and metabolism of N-hydroxyurethane in newborn mice," *Internat. J. Cancer*, Vol. 1 (1966), pp. 265–269.

[3] E. BOYLAND and K. WILLIAMS, "Reaction of urethane with nucleic acids *in vivo*," *Biochem. J.*, Vol. 111 (1969), pp. 121–127.

[4] E. BOYLAND and E. RHODEN, "The distribution of urethane in animal tissues, as deter-

mined by a microdiffusion method, and the effect of urethane treatment on enzymes,"
Biochem. J., Vol. 44 (1949), pp. 528–531.

[5] A. M. BRUES, "Critique of linear theory of carcinogenesis," *Science*, Vol. 128 (1958), pp. 693–699.

[6] C. E. BRYAN, H. E. SKIPPER, and L. WHITE, JR., "Carbamates in the chemotherapy of leucemia. IV. The distribution of radioactivity in tissues of mice following injection of carbonyl-labeled urethane," *J. Biol. Chem.*, Vol. 177 (1949), pp. 941–950.

[7] G. CIVIDALLI, S. S. MIRVISH, and I. BERENBLUM, "The catabolism of urethan in young mice of varying age and strain, and in x-irradiated mice, in relation to urethan carcinogenesis," *Cancer Res.*, Vol. 25 (1965), pp. 855–858.

[8] W. A. FOLEY, L. J. COLE, B. J. INGRAM, and T. T. CROCKER, "X-ray inhibition of urethan-stimulated proliferation of lung cells of the mouse as estimated by incorporation of tritiated thymidine," *Nature*, Vol. 199 (1963), pp. 1267–1268.

[9] C. GUILLIER, "Evaluation of the internal exposure due to various administered dosages of urethane to mice," *Proceedings of the Sixth Berkeley Symposium on Mathematical Statistics and Probability*, Berkeley and Los Angeles, University of California Press, 1972, Vol. 4, pp. 309–315.

[10] D. E. GROGAN, M. LANE, R. A. LIEBELT, and F. E. SMITH, "The effect of partial hepatectomy on the metabolism of urethan in young adult mice," *Cancer Res.*, Vol. 30 (1970), pp. 1806–1811.

[11] P. S. HENSHAW and H. L. MEYER, "Further studies on urethane-induced pulmonary tumors," *J. Nat. Cancer Inst.*, Vol. 5 (1945), pp. 415–417.

[12] H. JEFFAY and J. ALVAREZ, "Liquid scintillation counting of carbon-14. Use of ethanol-amine-ethylene glycol monomethyl ether-toluene," *Anal. Chem.*, Vol. 33 (1961), pp. 612–615.

[13] A. M. KAYE, "Urethan carcinogenesis and nucleic acid metabolism: *In vitro* interactions with enzymes," *Cancer Res.*, Vol. 28 (1968), pp. 1041–1046.

[14] ———, "A study of the relationship between the rate of ethyl carbamate (urethan) catabolism and urethan carcinogenesis," *Cancer Res.*, Vol. 20 (1960), pp. 237–241.

[15] S. S. MIRVISH, "The metabolism of N-hydroxyurethane in relation to its carcinogenic action: conversion into urethane and an N-hydroxyurethane glucuronide," *Biochim. Biophys. Acta*, Vol. 117 (1966), pp. 1–12.

[16] S. MIRVISH, G. CIVIDALLI, and I. BERENBLUM, "Slow elimination of urethan in relation to its high carcinogenicity in newborn mice," *Proc. Soc. Exp. Biol. and Med.*, Vol. 116 (1964), pp. 265–268.

[17] R. NERY, "Some aspects of the metabolism of urethane and N-hydroxyurethane in rodents," *Biochem. J.*, Vol. 106 (1968), pp. 1–13.

[18] J. NEYMAN and E. L. SCOTT, "Statistical aspect of the problem of carcinogenesis," *Proceedings of the Fifth Berkeley Symposium on Mathematical Statistics and Probability*, Berkeley and Los Angeles, University of California Press, 1967, Vol. 4, pp. 745–776.

[19] G. PRODI, P. ROCCHI, and S. GRILLI, "*In vivo* interaction of urethan with nucleic acids and proteins," *Cancer Res.*, Vol. 30 (1970), pp. 2887–2892.

[20] M. B. SHIMKIN, T. SASAKI, M. McDONOUGH, R. BASERGA, D. THATCHER, and R. WIEDER, "Relation of thymidine index to pulmonary tumor response in mice receiving urethan and other carcinogens," *Cancer Res.*, Vol. 29 (1969), pp. 994–998.

[21] M. B. SHIMKIN, R. WIEDER, D. MARZI, N. GUBAREFF, and V. SUNTZEFF, "Lung tumors in mice receiving different schedules of urethane," *Proceedings of the Fifth Berkeley Symposium on Mathematical Statistics and Probability*, Berkeley and Los Angeles, University of California Press, 1967, Vol. 4, pp. 707–719.

[22] H. E. SKIPPER, L. L. BENNETT, JR., C. E. BRYAN, L. WHITE, JR., M. A. NEWTON, and L. SIMPSON, "Carbamates in the chemotherapy of leukemia. VIII. Over-all tracer studies on carbonyl-labeled urethan, methylene-labeled urethan, and methylene-labeled ethyl alcohol," *Cancer Res.*, Vol. 11 (1951), pp. 46–51.

[23] B. M. Tolbert, M. Kirk, and E. M. Baker, "Continuous $C^{14}O_2$ and CO_2 excretion studies in experimental animals," *Amer. J. Physiol.*, Vol. 185 (1956), pp. 269–273.

[24] M. White, A. Grendon, and H. B. Jones, "Effects of urethane dose and time patterns on tumor formation," *Proceedings of the Fifth Berkeley Symposium on Mathematical Statistics and Probability*, Berkeley and Los Angeles, University of California Press, 1967, Vol. 4, pp. 721–743.

[25] ———, "Tumor incidence and cellularity in lungs of mice given various dose schedules of urethan," *Cancer Res.*, Vol. 30 (1970), pp. 1030–1036.

[26] M. R. White, unpublished data.

EVALUATION OF THE INTERNAL EXPOSURE DUE TO VARIOUS ADMINISTERED DOSAGES OF URETHANE TO MICE

CLAUDE L. GUILLIER
UNIVERSITY OF CALIFORNIA, BERKELEY

1. Introduction

This is a companion paper to that of Margaret R. White [1]. Using Miss White's data, the purpose is to develop the methodology needed to evaluate internal exposure to urethane following the injection of this chemical into mice, administered in varying doses measured in milligrams of urethane per gram of body weight (mg/g). Experimental details, including the use of urethane labeled in two ways, ethyl (1-^{14}C) carbamate and ethyl carbamate (carbonyl-^{14}C), denoted E and C labeled, respectively, will be found in Miss White's paper. Here a brief description illustrated by Figure 1 must suffice.

2. Experimental setup

Each of the 70 separate experiments (or runs) performed by Miss White consisted of: (1) injecting a randomly selected group of four mice with the same dose D of ^{14}C labeled urethane (D measured in mg/g); (2) placing the mice in the metabolism cage I (see Figure 1); (3) establishing a flow of fresh air, at a constant rate F, through chamber I, then through chambers II and III; and (4) measuring the radioactivity in the ionization chamber III. These measurements, made every 20 seconds, were automatically recorded giving the values that will be called $Y_3(t)$. This quantity is supposed to be proportional to the number of atoms of the radioactive carbon ^{14}C present in chamber III at time t. Chamber II in Figure 1 was filled with water absorber.

The arrangement of the experiments was based on the premise that, after being injected into mice, the urethane molecules are catabolized into at least two daughter molecules. Further catabolism results in practically all the labeled ^{14}C atoms being incorporated into CO_2 molecules which are gradually exhaled. Calculations performed at the Donner Laboratory (University of California,

This investigation was partially supported by USPHS Research Grant No. GM-10525-08, National Institutes of Health, Public Health Service.

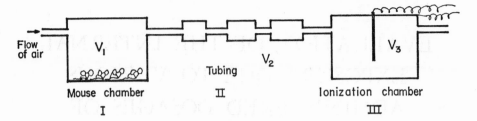

FIGURE 1

Experimental setup.

Berkeley) determined the quantities $X(0, D)$ proportional to the numbers of radioactive ^{14}C atoms injected in dose D of urethane. After the lapse of time t, a certain part of the original $X(0, D)$ is exhaled leaving the quantity $X(t, D)$ still unexhaled, possibly remaining in the bodies of the mice, but possibly partly eliminated in urine and feces. For simplicity of notation, we shall write $X(t)$ for $X(t, D)$.

Let V_1, V_2, V_3 denote the volume of air in chambers I, II, and III. Also, let F stand for the known constant rate of flow of fresh air through the whole apparatus. Finally, let $Y_1(t)$, $Y_2(t)$, and $Y_3(t)$ be the measures of the numbers of molecules of ^{14}C present at time t in chambers I, II, and III.

The purposes of the calculations performed are: (1) to estimate $X(t)$ for $t > 0$; and (2) to calculate what is termed the internal exposure over a period T, due to the injection of D mg/g, that is,

$$(1) \qquad E(T, D) = \int_0^T X(t) \, dt.$$

3. Method of estimating X(t)

The calculations were performed on a deterministic model, involving the following differential equations:

$$(2) \qquad \begin{aligned} Y_1' &= -X' - c_1 Y_1, \\ Y_2' &= c_1 Y_1 - c_2 Y_2, \\ Y_3' &= c_2 Y_2 - c_3 Y_3, \end{aligned}$$

where the primes indicate derivatives with respect to t and where $c_i = F/V_i$.

Easy manipulations yield

$$(3) \qquad X' = -c_3 Y_3 - \frac{c_1 c_2 + c_2 c_3 + c_3 c_1}{c_1 c_2} Y_3' - \frac{c_1 + c_2 + c_3}{c_1 c_2} Y_3'' - \frac{1}{c_1 c_2} Y_3''',$$

which implies

$$(4) \qquad X(t) = X(0) - c_3 \int_0^t Y_3(x) \, dx - \frac{c_1 c_2 + c_2 c_3 + c_3 c_1}{c_1 c_2} [Y(t) - Y(0)]$$

$$- \frac{c_1 + c_2 + c_3}{c_1 c_2} [Y_3'(t) - Y_3'(0)] - \frac{1}{c_1 c_2} [Y_3''(t) - Y_3''(0)].$$

Since the actual measurements refer to radioactivity of the dose injected and of the air in chamber III, it is convenient to express all the variables as percentages of the dose injected $X(0)$. At time $t = 0$, the value of Y_3 must be zero. Whether the values of the first and the higher derivations of Y_3 must vanish at $t = 0$, is not clear *a priori*, but they were assumed to be zero.

4. Validation of the theory behind formula (4)

In order to obtain some idea of the relationship between formula (4) and the actual phenomena, Miss White performed ten experiments, or runs, conducted so that both the quantities $X(0)$ and $X(t)$ could be measured by a particular, say direct, method, while the radioactivity $Y_3(t)$, in chamber III, was measured by exactly the same procedure as was done with the runs with injected mice. Then the use of formula (4), and also the result of integration to obtain the quantity defined by (1), provided "theoretical" counterparts to be compared with independently obtained "direct" measurements of the same quantities.

These validating experiments consisted of replacing the radioactivity exhaled by experimental mice by a steady flow of radioactive CO_2 through the whole apparatus, at an approximately known rate K per unit of time. Such flow was maintained over a known period of time T. Then (and here was an experimental difficulty) the flow of radioactive CO_2 was interrupted and replaced by the flow of fresh air, intended to be at the same constant rate K. In some of such runs noninjected mice were placed in chamber I, but not in all of the runs. The measurements of Y_3 in the ionization chamber III continued up to such time as the readings were essentially zero.

It will be realized, that in the validating experiment, the presumed known rate K of flow of labeled CO_2 corresponds to the derivative

$$(5) \qquad\qquad X'(t) = -K \qquad \text{for } t < T.$$

For values of $t > T$, we have $X'(t) = 0$. Thus,

$$(6) \qquad\qquad X(0) - X(t) = \begin{cases} Kt & \text{for } t < T, \\ KT & \text{for } t \geq T, \end{cases}$$

and the integration yields

$$(7) \qquad \int_0^t [X(0) - X(x)]\, dx = \begin{cases} Kt^2/2 & \text{for } t < T, \\ KT(t - T/2) & \text{for } t > T. \end{cases}$$

The difference $X(0) - X(T)$ will be called *activity loss*. For values of t at which the $Y_3(t)$ was essentially zero, the integral in (7) will be called the *exposure loss*. The values of these quantities obtained from the presumed known T, K, and t will be described as *direct measurements*. The values of the same quantities obtained through measurements of $Y_3(x)$ and the use of the formula (4) will be called *theoretical values*.

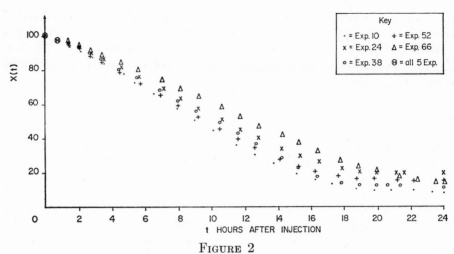

FIGURE 2

C labeled urethane, dose 1.00 mg/g.

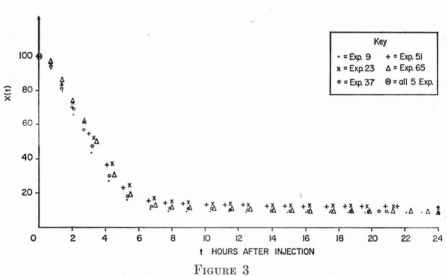

FIGURE 3

C labeled urethane, dose 0.125 mg/g.

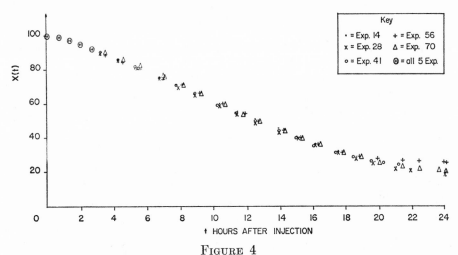

FIGURE 4

E labeled urethane, dose 1.00 mg/g.

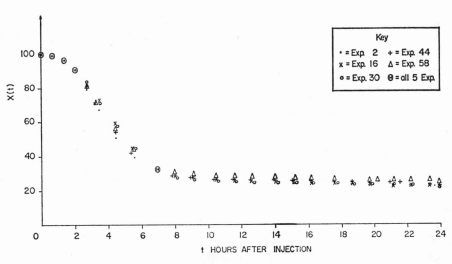

FIGURE 5

E labeled urethane, dose 0.125 mg/g.

TABLE I

RESULTS OF TEN VALIDATING RUNS

	Measurements of activity loss			Measurements of exposure loss		
Run	Direct = KT	Theory	Per cent difference	Direct $KT(t - T/2)$	Theory	Per cent difference
1	3.12	3.08	1.51	3.06	2.72	11.74
2	2.82	2.74	2.58	1.93	1.64	16.30
3	4.58	4.75	−3.61	5.18	4.83	7.01
4	3.46	3.42	1.21	2.37	2.54	−7.02
5	2.65	2.80	−5.52	3.01	2.93	2.67
6	5.38	5.31	1.19	5.78	5.24	9.85
7	2.84	2.91	−2.31	3.05	2.86	6.38
8	1.79	1.83	−1.94	1.20	1.33	−9.92
9	1.77	1.76	0.54	1.21	1.08	11.42
10	2.40	2.53	−5.28	3.00	2.93	2.37

Table I summarizes the results of ten validating runs performed by Miss White.

It is seen that the comparison of the direct and theoretical measurements of activity loss is satisfactory. For the exposure loss, however, the situation is not that good. The suspected sources of errors include the difficulty of maintaining a really constant rate of flow of labeled CO_2 and the sudden interruption of that flow, supposed to be immediately followed by an equal flow of fresh air. Since the real experiments with mice did not involve sudden changes in the procedure and used more precise flow regulators, it is hoped that the values of internal exposure obtained through the use of formula (4) and then of formula (1) will be more accurate than the data of Table I might suggest.

5. Estimates of X(t) and of E(T, D)

As described by Miss White, her experiments covered a substantial range of urethane doses $D = 0.125, 0.25, 0.50, 0.75, 1.00, 1.20,$ and 1.40, all measured in mg/g. Because quite a few mice did not survive the injections of urethane doses in excess of 1.00 mg/g, the numbers of experiments completed with the two largest doses 1.2 and 1.4 mg/g are small. It is plausible that the mice surviving the large doses of urethane are somehow more resistant than those that died. For this reason, the applicability to the whole population of mice of the results of the completed experiments with the two largest doses injected is subject to doubt.

For doses up to 1.00 mg/g, the results of calculation of $X(t)$ proved unexpectedly consistent. Figures 2 and 3 give graphs of calculated $X(t)$ for C labeled urethane and Figures 4 and 5 for E labeled urethane. The graphs in Figures 2 and 4 correspond to the highest dose of urethane, 1.00 mg/g, and those in Figures 3 and 5 to the smallest dose, 0.125 mg/g.

In each figure, there are five sequences of different symbols, each sequence corresponding to a particular experiment with four mice. The ordinate of each symbol gives the value of formula (4) calculated for the given value of t. Here

$X(0)$ was replaced by a conventional 100 and all amounts of radioactivity Y_3, and so on, were expressed as percentages of the injected $X(0)$. For technical reasons, in performing the experiments, the values of t for which $X(t)$ was calculated for one experiment do not coincide with those for others.

With the possible exception of dose 1.00 mg/g of C labeled urethane (Figure 2), the $X(t)$ curves computed for five replicates of an experiment are remarkably consistent with each other.

6. Conclusions suggested by the graphs of X(t)

(i) The comparison of Figure 2 with 3 and Figure 4 with 5 leaves no room for doubt that the speed of elimination of ^{14}C atoms from the bodies of mice through exhaling depends very much on the dose injected, and this whether the urethane is C or E labeled. With the larger doses, twelve hours after the injection, the exhaled ^{14}C amounts to about 50 per cent of the injected quantity. With the minimal dose of 0.125 mg/g, the amount exhaled during the same period is something between 70 and 90 per cent.

(ii) All the curves $X(t)$ appear to approach a horizontal asymptote. For E labeled urethane this asymptote is higher than for that C labeled. In each case, the height of the asymptote indicates the percentage of the injected ^{14}C atoms that are "not exhalable" over the period studied. A part of these "unexhalable" atoms must be involved in some molecules eliminated through urine or feces. However, there may be a part of them remaining in the bodies of mice more or less indefinitely.

7. Values of internal exposure

The calculated values of the internal exposure E, over 24 and 48 hours are reported in Miss White's paper [1]. As the dose D in mg/g grows, the value of E increases somewhat faster than D. For $D \leq 1.00$ mg/g, the average number of lung tumors per mouse is very nearly proportional to E. This suggests that, for not too large doses of D injected, the number of initial events of carcinogenesis is proportional to E rather than to D. For higher values of D, the average number of tumors increases at a rate somewhat slower than that of E. This may be an indication of the anesthetic effect of urethane which slows down the functioning of the various organs, including the exhaling of the accumulated CO_2.

Closer analysis of Miss White's experimental data is clearly indicated.

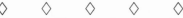

I want to thank Professor J. Neyman for proposing this research and for suggestions regarding the model. I thank Mrs. Margaret Darland, Mr. Richard Green, and Mrs. J. L. Lovasich for their help in digitizing the values of Y_3 and in computer programming.

REFERENCE

[1] M. WHITE, "Studies of the mechanism of induction of pulmonary adenomas in mice," *Proceedings of the Sixth Berkeley Symposium on Mathematical Statistics and Probability,* University of California Press, Berkeley and Los Angeles, 1972, Vol. 4, pp. 287–307.

SOURCE OF EVALUATIONS REFORMULATED AND ANALYZED

I. RICHARD SAVAGE

CENTER FOR ADVANCED STUDY IN THE BEHAVIORAL SCIENCES

and

MURRAY WEBSTER, JR.

THE JOHNS HOPKINS UNIVERSITY

1. Introduction

Webster [8] has published a theory of the source of evaluations and expectations for performance (which we will henceforth refer to as the *source theory*), along with results of experiments intended to test derivations from the theory. The empirical results were interpreted as being in accord with the derivations, and thus, as supportive of the theory. Study of the theory and the *derivations* indicates there are logical problems with the assumptions, and that as a result, the derivations are *not* logical consequences of the assumptions. Therefore, the results of the experiments are indeterminate with respect to the theory Webster presented.

We begin the analysis with a description of the substantive ideas of the source theory, along with the original statement of the theory. Next, we present a simple formalization of the theory, using ideas from probability theory to restate the propositions.

The source theory is strengthened, qualitative inequalities on probabilities of being influenced are replaced by expressions with estimatible parameters.

2. The source theory

The source theory was an attempt to state explicitly some ideas deriving from two theoretical traditions. The first, which might be called the *looking glass self*, derives from the Cooley [5] and Mead [6] ideas regarding the individual's sources of selfconcept. According to this tradition, the individual's ideas regarding himself, including particularly his selfevaluation, come from the opinions of others. Moreover, these others are not all expected to be equally important in

The research of I. R. Savage was done while a Senior Post Doctoral Fellow of the National Science Foundation and with the assistance of the Army, Navy and Air Force under Office of Naval Research Contract number N00014-67-A-0235-0006. Current address is Florida State University, Department of Statistics, Tallahassee, Florida.

The research of M. Webster was supported by U.S. Office of Education Grant OEG-3-71-0122 to Doris R. Entwisle and Murray Webster, Jr.

determining the selfevaluation. Evaluations from a *significant other*, to use Sullivan's term [7], are predicted to be accepted by the individual, while opinions from other people (of unspecified characteristics) are likely to be ignored. Incorporation of these ideas into Webster's theory involved both an explicit statement of the idea that one's own ideas regarding himself come from others, and an explicit statement that what makes an other a significant other is the belief that the other possess high ability at whatever task is being performed and evaluated.

The second theoretical tradition is that of expectation theory, deriving from the work of Joseph Berger and associates [1], [2], [3]. According to this tradition, many regularly reported observable behaviors among the members of problem solving groups, such as unequal number of chances to perform, evaluations of performances, likelihood of performing, and rejection of influence, may be explained if one postulates the existence of *expectation states*, or cognitive beliefs about the ability of each member of the group. The construct *expectation state* was used in the source theory as being roughly equivalent to selfevaluation, though with some slight—and for our purposes, unimportant—differences. The source theory and the derivations are given in Charts I and II. Combining the looking glass self tradition and expectation theory yields such assertions as: an

CHART I

THE ORIGINAL VERSION OF THE THEORY
(taken from Webster, 1969)

Definition 1. A situation is a *task situation* S if and only if it contains:
    (a) at least two actors p and o making performance outputs;
    (b) an actor E making unit evaluations of those performance outputs;
    (c) no previous expectations held by p and o of their own or each other's abilities at the task;
    (d) task orientation of all actors;
    (e) collective orientation of all actors.
Definition 2. E is a *source* for p in task situation S if and only if p believes that E is more capable of evaluating performances than p is.
Assumption 1. In task situation S, if E is a source for p, then p will agree with E's unit evaluations of any actor's performance.
Assumption 2. In task situation S, if p evaluates a series of performances of any actor, then he will come to hold an expectation state for that actor which is in accord with those evaluations.
Assumption 3. In task situation S, if p holds high expectations for any actor o_1, then as compared to a second actor o_2 for whom p holds low expectations:
    (a) p will give o_1 more action opportunities than o_2;
    (b) p will be more likely to evaluate positively the future performance outputs of o_1 than those of o_2;
    (c) in case of disagreement between o_1 and o_2, p will be more likely to agree with o_1;
    (d) p will be more likely to accept o_1 than o_2 as a source.
Assumption 4. In task situation S, if an actor p_1 holds high expectations for himself and low for o, then as compared to a second actor p_2 who holds low expectations for himself and high for o:
    (a) p_1 will be more likely to accept a given action opportunity and make a performance output;
    (b) in case of disagreement with o, p_2 will be more likely to accept influence than p_1.

CHART II

THE ORIGINAL DERIVATIONS
(taken from Webster, 1969)

Derivation 1. In case of disagreement with *o*, the probability of *p* accepting influence is less in the $HE(+ -)$ case than in the $HE(- +)$ case.

Derivation 2. In case of disagreement with *o*, the probability of *p* accepting influence is less in the $LE(+ -)$ case than in the $LE(- +)$ case.

Derivation 3. In case of disagreement with *o*, the probability of *p* accepting influence is less in the $HE(+ -)$ case than in the $LE(+ -)$ case.

Derivation 4. In case of disagreement with *o*, the probability of *p* accepting influence is *greater* in the $HE(- +)$ case than in the $LE(- +)$ case.

Derivation 5. In case of disagreement between *p* and *o*, the probabilities of *p* accepting influence will be in the following order: $HE(- +) > LE(- +) > LE(+ -) > HE(+ -)$.

individual who is evaluated by a high ability evaluator (the *HE* in Chart II) will often believe him and form an expectation state based on those evaluations, while an individual evaluated by a low ability evaluator (the *LE* in Chart II) will usually ignore him; and an individual who holds high selfexpectations (the $(+ -)$ conditions in Chart II) will be more likely to reject influence than an individual who holds low selfexpectations (the $(- +)$ conditions in Chart II).

Although the source theory is quite abstract and formal, the presentation does not allow a precise analysis of how the derivations follow from the theory. The primary objective of this paper is to formalize the theory so that the method of deduction of the derivations will be explicit. The resulting formalization also may have other advantages, such as: (1) giving an alternative view of the source theory, (2) showing places where it might be desirable to modify the source theory, and (3) helping to generalize the source theory to make it useful in new experimental conditions.

The derivations in Chart II were tested in a two phase experiment with four conditions. Subjects were told that the study was concerned with measuring their ability to judge which of a pair of patterns contained more white area. The patterns resemble very complex checkerboards, and all contain exactly 50 per cent white area; thus, there is no objective basis upon which to judge the answer. More important for the theory, extensive pretesting has established that the empirical probability of choosing either alternative is close to 0.50. This means that there is no subjective basis for evaluating choices as correct in the situation, except for the communicated opinions of another individual, the potential *source of evaluations*. Subjects are requested to do the best job they possibly can at judging the patterns, in the attempt to produce the *task orientation* condition (Definition 1(d) in Chart I). Experience with related experiments has shown that these instructions are generally successful at inducing task orientation.

In all conditions, pairs of subjects received evaluations of their performances from an evaluator—the potential *source*—in phase I. In phase II each pair of subjects worked on a second set of problems, and they were instructed to come to a joint, or *team* decision about them. This is the *collective orientation* of Definition 1(e) in Chart I. Initial choice disagreements were experimentally introduced, and subjects restudied each slide before making a private final decision. The proportion of times that subjects changed their own initial choices under disagreement—the *acceptance of influence* in the derivations—was computed as the main statistic for testing the theory. The observed ordering of experimental conditions by this statistic, $HE(-+) > LE(-+) > LE(+-) > HE(+-)$, was the same as that stated in the derivations. The following analysis will be confined to derivations relating directly to this particular experiment.

3. Parametric formalization

The following notation will be needed:
   (i) *universal event:* Ω; in the following each event is a subset of Ω;
   (ii) *experimental conditions:* H_-, H_+, L_-, L_+;
   (iii) *performer accepts source:* A;
   (iv) *performer's expectation state:* E_-, $E_=$, E_+;
   (v) *performer disagrees:* D;
   (vi) *performer accepts influence:* I.

All probabilities will be written in the form $P\{M|N\}$, unless it is clear that $N = \Omega$, in which case we write $P\{M\}$. Whenever $P\{M|N\}$ appears, either we should verify that $P\{N\} > 0$, or that the term is explicitly multiplied by 0. In statements of assumptions and theorems (Sections 4 and 5), all probabilities which appear are implicitly assumed to have been defined properly.

The assumptions of the parametric theory follow.

ASSUMPTION 3.1.   *Assume*

$$(3.1) \qquad\qquad P\{E_=|\overline{A}\} = 1,$$

where, generally, $\overline{N}$ *is the complement of N. Assume*

$$(3.2) \qquad\qquad P\{E_+|AH_+\} = P\{E_+|AL_+\} = 1$$

and

$$(3.3) \qquad\qquad P\{E_-|AH_-\} = P\{E_-|AL_-\} = 1.$$

ASSUMPTION 3.2.   *Assume*

$$(3.4) \qquad\qquad P\{A|H_+\} = P\{A|H_-\},$$

and let H denote the common probability of accepting H_+ or H_- as a source. Assume

$$(3.5) \qquad\qquad P\{A|L_+\} = P\{A|L_-\},$$

and let L denote the common probability of accepting L_+ or L_- as a source. Assume

$$(3.6) \qquad\qquad 0 \leq L < H \leq 1.$$

ASSUMPTION 3.3.   *If M can be specified in terms of A, H_+, H_-, L_+, L_-, E_+, $E_=$, E_- and without the use of I or D, then the value of $P\{D|M\}$ does not depend on M.*

ASSUMPTION 3.4. *Assume*

(3.7) $P\{I|DE_=H_+\} = P\{I|DE_=H_-\} = P\{I|DE_=L_+\} = P\{I|DE_=L_-\}$

and denote the common value by R. Assume

(3.8) $P\{I|DH_+E_+\} = P\{I|DL_+E_+\}$

and denote the common value by E. Assume

(3.9) $P\{I|DH_-E_-\} = P\{I|DL_-E_-\}$

and denote the common value by e. And finally, assume

(3.10) $0 \leqq E < R < e \leqq 1.$

This completes the description of the theory, or as we will often say, the *model*. It appears incomplete in that terms like $P(D|\bar{I})$ have never been mentioned, but they have no substantive interpretation in the experiment and will never be mentioned in the derivations. Also there is no term for the performer's evaluation by source, since in the theory and the experiment the evaluations either were ignored (and consequently irrelevant) or they were equivalent to performer's expectation state for self (iv).

The source theory speaks of a situation containing at least three actors, p, o, and E. Two of these, p and o, both perform and evaluate; E only evaluates. However in the experiment, p and o never actually interact, and E is not even an actor (a tape recorded voice was used). Thus, the theory, when applied to the experimental situation, refers to one human being who is always present, and consequently, there is no need specifically to include symbols for individuals in the notation.

The source theory contains some appearances of a dynamic model, especially in Assumption 2 of Chart I. However, the dynamics appear relatively unimportant to the main theoretical interest in the source. In any case, there is no discussion of the acceptance *process*, and the data of the experiment are collected after the active introduction of all the theoretical variables. The dynamic aspects do not appear in the probability version.

There is also at least one elaboration: the case $E_=$ was excluded from consideration in the source theory. For the probability analysis, its inclusion was necessary for making some of the derivations.

Typically, if $P\{N\} > 0$, then we must make assumptions about $P\{M|N\}$. Thus, contrast (3.1) with Definition 1(c) of Chart I. In the theory, *no previous expectations* apparently was intended to mean that there are two states E_+ and E_- such that $\Omega = E_+ + E_-$ and no assumption is made about $P\{E_+|\bar{A}\}$. We now interpret no previous expectation as meaning there are three disjoint states, $E_=$, E_-, E_+ such that $\Omega = E_- + E_+ + E_=$ and $P\{E_+|\bar{A}\} = P\{E_-|\bar{A}\} = 1 - P\{E_=|\bar{A}\} = 0$. Since the theory does not exclude the possibility of $\bar{A}$ at the time data are collected and we cannot directly tell if a person is A or $\bar{A}$, we make assumptions for the $\bar{A}$ case as well as the A case.

Finally, this analysis is somewhat more complicated than the minimal statement necessary for our purposes. In the interests of preserving comparability to the source theory, variables unnecessary to this analysis were introduced which had an uninteresting probability structure; for example, $AH_+ \to E_+$, $AH_- \to E_-$, $AL_+ \to E_+$, $AL_- \to E_-$, $\overline{A} \to E_=$, where $N \to M$ means $P\{M|N\} = 1$. If (3.8) and (3.9) had been expanded in terms of H_+, H_-, L_+, L_- instead of E_+, E_-, the analysis would be easier. On the other hand, the theory might be enriched if (3.2) and (3.3) were weakened to $P\{E_+|AH_+\} = P\{E_+|AL_+\}$ and $P\{E_-|AH_-\} = P\{E_-|AL_-\}$. To do this one must check to see what other changes would be appropriate to modify the proofs of Section 5, and see what experimental evidence or arrangements could discriminate between (3.2) and (3.3) and their modification.

The E of Definition 1(c) of Chart I fixes the experimental conditions as described in (ii). Definitions 1(d) and 1(e) are not explicitly used in the source theory and are not incorporated into the probability formalization. Formulas (3.1) and (3.7) express the idea that the experimental conditions have no effect without acceptance, and formulas (3.2), (3.3) and (3.10) show the effects of acceptance; this captures Definition 2 of Chart I.

Assumptions and formulas of Chart I are paired with those presented in this section as follows.

Assumptions 1 and 2 of Chart I are paired with (3.2) and (3.3) and the last sentence in the paragraph following (3.10).

Assumption 3(d) of Chart I is paired with (3.4), (3.5), and (3.6).

Assumption 4(b) is paired with (3.8), (3.9), and (3.10).

Assumptions 3(a), 3(b), 3(c), and 4(a) are not relevant to the current theory and the experiment.

A critical new assumption in the model is the intermediate value R, the common value of (3.7). This assumption was not implicit in the source theory. Although the theorem of Section 5 can be proved without the full strength of (3.7), (3.8), and (3.9), the intermediate value property (3.10) is essential (see Note 6.1).

4. Probability theory

The following are some standard results needed later:

$$(4.1) \quad 0 \leq P\{M|N\} \leq 1, \qquad P\{N|N\} = 1, \qquad P\{M|N\} + P\{\overline{M}|N\} = 1;$$

$$(4.2) \quad P\{M_1M_2|N\} \leq \min\,[P\{M_1|N\}, P\{M_2|N\}]$$
$$\leq \max\,[P\{M_1|N\}, P\{M_2|N\}]$$
$$\leq P\{M_1 \text{ or } M_2|N\}$$
$$= P\{M_1|N\} + P\{M_2|N\} - P\{M_1M_2|N\}$$
$$\leq P\{M_1|N\} + P\{M_2|N\};$$

$$(4.3) \quad P\{M_1M_2|N\} = P\{M_1|N\}\,P\{M_2|NM_1\};$$

$$(4.4) \quad P\{M|N\} = P\{MQ|N\} + P\{M\overline{Q}|N\}.$$

The next results are elementary but not standard.

LEMMA 4.1. *If $P\{M|N_1\} = 1$, then $P\{M|N_1N_2\} = 1$. If $P\{M|N_1\} = 0$, then $P\{M|N_1N_2\} = 0$.*

PROOF. We prove the second of these equivalent statements: $P\{M|N_1\} = 0$ implies $P\{MN_1\} = 0$, which implies $P\{MN_1N_2\} = 0$, which implies the conclusion $P\{M|N_1N_2\} = 0$.

LEMMA 4.2. *If $P\{N_2|N_1\overline{N}_3\} = 0$, then $P\{M|N_1N_2\} = P\{M|N_1N_2N_3\}$.*

PROOF. The following computation yields the desired result:

$$(4.5) \qquad P\{M|N_1N_2\} = \frac{P\{MN_1N_2\}}{P\{N_1N_2\}}$$

$$= \frac{P\{MN_1N_2N_3\} + P\{MN_1N_2\overline{N}_3\}}{P\{N_1N_2N_3\} + P\{N_1N_2\overline{N}_3\}}$$

$$= \frac{P\{MN_1N_2N_3\}}{P\{N_1N_2N_3\}} = P\{M|N_1N_2N_3\}.$$

LEMMA 4.3. *Let Γ be a collection of events. Assume $P\{D|Q\} = p$ for each $Q \in \Gamma$, then $P\{M|N\} = P\{M|DN\}$ if MN and N are in Γ.*

PROOF. We compute

$$(4.6) \qquad P\{M|DN\} = \frac{P\{DMN\}}{P\{DN\}} = \frac{P\{MN\}\,P\{D|MN\}}{P\{N\}\,P\{D|N\}}$$

$$= \frac{P\{MN\}}{P\{N\}} = P\{M|N\}.$$

5. Derivation of the source theory

For later reference, we introduce some additional notation and give the basic experimental results from Webster ([8], Table 1):

$$(5.1) \qquad\qquad a = P\{I|DH_+\} = 0.20;$$

$$(5.2) \qquad\qquad b = P\{I|DH_-\} = 0.52;$$

$$(5.3) \qquad\qquad c = P\{I|DL_+\} = 0.35;$$

$$(5.4) \qquad\qquad d = P\{I|DL_-\} = 0.42.$$

Theorem 5.1, below, will be proved at the end of this section.

THEOREM 5.1. *With the assumptions and notation of Section 3:*

$$(5.5) \qquad\qquad a = R + H(E - R);$$

$$(5.6) \qquad\qquad b = R + H(e - R);$$

$$(5.7) \qquad\qquad c = R + L(E - R);$$

and

$$(5.8) \qquad\qquad d = R + L(e - R).$$

Corollary 5.1, below, is equivalent to the derivations of Webster [8].

COROLLARY 5.1. *With the assumptions and notation of Section 3:*

(5.9) $$b > d;$$

(5.10) $$d > c;$$

and

(5.11) $$c > a.$$

PROOF. From (5.6) and (5.8), inequality (5.9) is equivalent to the inequality $R + H(e - R) > R + L(e - R)$, which is equivalent to $(H - L)(e - R) > 0$, which is true since $H - L > 0$ from (3.6) and $e - R > 0$ from (3.10).

From (5.8) and (5.7), inequality (5.10) is equivalent to $R + L(e - R) > R + L(E - R)$, which is equivalent to the assumed $e > E$ from (3.10).

From (5.7) and (5.5), inequality (5.11) is equivalent to $R + L(E - R) > R + H(E - R)$, which is equivalent to $(L - H)(E - R) > 0$, which is true since $L - H < 0$ from (3.6) and $E - R < 0$ from (3.10).   Q.E.D.

NOTE 5.1. The empirical values (5.1) through (5.4) agree with Webster's derivations (5.9) through (5.11). Each of those relative frequencies is based on 20 trials involving between 18 and 20 subjects. An examination of Webster's unpublished data indicates a component of variance between individuals for H_- and L_- conditions. We will not, however, consider the statistical analysis of this data. We will work with the relative frequencies in (5.1) through (5.4) as if they were parameter values.

COROLLARY 5.2. *With the assumptions and notations of Section 3:*

(5.12) $$R = \frac{ad - bc}{a + d - b - c};$$

(5.13) $$H = \frac{L(a - R)}{c - R};$$

(5.14) $$E - R = \frac{c - R}{L};$$

(5.15) $$e - R = \frac{d - R}{L};$$

(5.16) $$c < R < d;$$

(5.17) $$1 < \frac{a - R}{c - R};$$

and

(5.18) $$\max \left[0, \frac{R - c}{R}, \frac{d - R}{1 - R} \right] < L < \frac{c - R}{a - R}.$$

PROOF. Verify (5.12) by using the formulas in Theorem 5.1. The other results readily follow.

NOTE 5.2. The model contains five parameters, H, L, E, R, e and four equations (5.5) through (5.8), so that we cannot evaluate the parameters even if the numerical values in (5.1) through (5.4) were free of sampling errors. However, various inequalities, such as (5.16), (5.17), and (5.18), must be satisfied. From (5.1) through (5.4) we obtain $R = 0.392$ and $21/196 < L < 42/192$. In particular, if we assign the value of 0.15 to L, we find $H = 0.69$, $E = 0.112$, and $e = 0.579$.

Now we present the proof of Theorem 5.1.

PROOF OF THEOREM 5.1. The four parts of the theorem are proved in the same manner, and thus, we shall show only the proof of $P\{I|DH_+\} = R + H(E - R)$, which is equivalent to (5.5). We begin with the identity

$$(5.19) \qquad P\{I|DH_+\} = A_+ + A_- + A_= + \overline{A}_+ + \overline{A}_- + \overline{A}_=,$$

where $A_+ = P\{IAE_+|DH_+\}$, $A_- = P\{IAE_-|DH_+\}$, $A_= = P\{IAE_=|DH_+\}$, $\overline{A}_+ = P\{I\overline{A}E_+|DH_+\}$, $\overline{A}_- = P\{I\overline{A}E_-|DH_+\}$, $\overline{A}_= = P\{I\overline{A}E_=|DH_+\}$.

Now (3.1) implies $P\{E_+|\overline{A}\} = P\{E_-|\overline{A}\} = 0$. Then Lemma 4.1 implies $\overline{A}_+ = \overline{A}_- = 0$. Also (3.2) implies $P\{E_-|AH_+\} = P\{E_=|AH_+\} = 0$, so that $A_- = A_= = 0$. Now we have

$$(5.20) \qquad P\{I|DH_+\} = A_+ + \overline{A}_=.$$

We compute

$$(5.21) \quad \overline{A}_= = P\{I\overline{A}E_=|DH_+\} = P\{\overline{A}|DH_+\} \, P\{E_=|DH_+\overline{A}\} \, P\{I|DH_+\overline{A}E_=\},$$

where we have used (4.3) several times. By using Lemma 4.3 and equation (3.4), we obtain

$$(5.22) \qquad P\{\overline{A}|DH_+\} = P\{\overline{A}|H_+\} = 1 - H.$$

By using Lemma 4.2, we have $P\{E_=|DH_+\overline{A}\} = P\{E_=|H_+\overline{A}\}$. Now with (3.1) and Lemma 4.1, we obtain $P\{E_=|H_+\overline{A}\} = P\{E_=|\overline{A}\} = 1$ or

$$(5.23) \qquad P\{E_=|DH_+\overline{A}\} = 1.$$

Next we obtain

$$(5.24) \qquad P\{I|DH_+\overline{A}E_=\} = P\{I|DH_+E_=\} = R,$$

by using Lemma 4.2 with $M = I$, $N_1 = DH_+$, $N_2 = E_=$, $N_3 = \overline{A}$, and $P\{N_2|N_1\overline{N}_3\} = 0$ from (3.2) and Lemma 4.1; also (3.7) is used. Combining (5.22), (5.23) and (5.24) in (5.21) yields

$$(5.25) \qquad \overline{A}_= = R(1 - H).$$

We compute

$$(5.26) \quad A_+ = P\{IAE_+|DH_+\} = P\{A|DH_+\} \, P\{E_+|DH_+A\} \, P\{I|DH_+AE_+\}.$$

From Lemma 4.3 and equation (3.4), we obtain

$$(5.27) \qquad P\{A|DH_+\} = H.$$

From Lemma 4.2 and equation (3.2), we obtain

$$(5.28) \qquad P\{E_+|DH_+A\} = 1.$$

Next, we obtain

$$(5.29) \qquad P\{I|DH_+AE_+\} = P\{I|DH_+E_+\} = E,$$

by using Lemma 4.2 with $M = I$, $N_1 = DH_+$, $N_2 = E_+$, $N_3 = A$, and $P\{N_2|N_1\overline{N}_3\} = 0$ from (3.1) and Lemma 4.1; also (3.8) is used. Combining (5.27), (5.28) and (5.29) in (5.26) yields

$$(5.30) \qquad\qquad A_+ = HE.$$

Finally, using (5.25) and (5.30) in (5.20) yields

$$(5.31) \qquad a = P\{I|DH_+\} = HE + (1 - H)R = R + H(E - R). \qquad Q.E.D.$$

6. Additional notes

NOTE 6.1.   In reading Webster [8], a possible value of R appears to be 0. Then instead of (5.11), we obtain

$$(6.1) \qquad\qquad \begin{aligned} P\{I|DH_+\} &= HE \\ &> LE = P\{I|DL_+\}. \end{aligned}$$

And if $R = 1$, we obtain

$$(6.2) \qquad\qquad \begin{aligned} P\{I|DL_-\} &= 1 + L(e - 1) \\ &> 1 + H(e - 1) = P\{I|DH_-\}. \end{aligned}$$

These counter intuitive results bolster our assumption that the probability of being influenced prior to accepting a source should be intermediate between the extreme probabilities that will prevail after a source is accepted (3.10).

NOTE 6.2.   The present theory (Section 3) has the following advantages when compared to the source theory of Webster [8]:

(1) the theory is complete in the sense that the desired conclusions are derived by standard logical methods;

(2) the theory is simple and appears not to have unnecessary assumptions;

(3) the theory generates quantitative results (numerical parameters) instead of only qualitative results (ordinal inequalities);

(4) the theory is explicit and hence easily discussed.

NOTE 6.3.   The theory (Section 3) is fragmentary. It would be important to extend the theory to cover other experimental situations. The extensions should preserve the good properties mentioned in Note 6.2. Modest extensions would include more than two of each of the following: (1) types of sources; (2) types of evaluations or expectation states; and (3) individuals in the task group.

NOTE 6.4.   It would be desirable to develop statistical theory for the estimation of the parameters. The theory will become more binding when the number of equations is at least as large as the number of parameters.

NOTE 6.5.   The theory (Section 3) is not the only *type* of model which could be constructed for this particular experimental situation. It is basically an information processing model, and assumes that the observable behavior, which we call $P\{I|D\}$ is a function of the subject's judgment of the accuracy of his own initial choice. Another sort of model, one based upon exchange ideas, has been constructed by Camilleri and Berger [4], and assumes that the observable behavior is determined by the subject's desire to avoid losses in selfesteem and approval from others. We do not wish to comment here upon the relative merits of exchange and information processing models for this experiment; we merely note that we have chosen to deal with only one of many possible approaches to the situation.

NOTE 6.6. The assumption $P\{E_+|AL_-\} > 0$ (contrary to (3.3)) corresponds to the subject accepting the source but "believing" either the source is dishonest in his evaluations or that the source is more likely wrong than correct. The realization of this assumption is plausible and future experiments might explore its consequences.

NOTE 6.7. The extension of this theory to include the acceptance process and other dynamic aspects would increase the mathematical interest and be of substantive value.

$$\Diamond \quad \Diamond \quad \Diamond \quad \Diamond \quad \Diamond$$

We thank R. H. Conviser and I. Olkin for constructive readings of earlier versions of this manuscript.

REFERENCES

[1] J. BERGER, B. P. COHEN, T. L. CONNER, and M. ZELDITCH, JR., "Status characteristics and expectations states: a process model," *Sociological Theories in Progress* (edited by J. Berger, M. Zelditch, Jr., and B. Anderson), Boston, Houghton-Mifflin, 1966. Vol. 1, pp. 47–73.

[2] J. BERGER and T. L. CONNER, "Performance expectations and behavior in small groups," *ACTA Sociologica*, Vol. 12 (1969), pp. 186–198.

[3] J. BERGER and M. H. FISEK, "Consistent and inconsistent status characteristics and the determination of power and prestige order," *Sociometry*, Vol. 33 (1970), pp. 327–347.

[4] S. CAMILLERI and J. BERGER, "Decision making and social influence: A model and an experimental test," *Sociometry*, Vol. 30 (1967), pp. 365–378.

[5] C. H. COOLEY, *Human Nature and the Social Order*, New York, Charles Scribner's Sons, 1902.

[6] G. H. MEAD, *Mind, Self, and Society*. Chicago, University of Chicago Press, 1934.

[7] H. S. SULLIVAN, *Conception of Modern Psychiatry*, Washington, D.C., The William Alanson White Psychiatric Foundation, 1947.

[8] M. WEBSTER, "Source of evaluations and expectations for performance," *Sociometry*, Vol. 32 (1969), pp. 243–258.

SELF-SELECTION—A MAJOR PROBLEM IN OBSERVATIONAL STUDIES

J. YERUSHALMY

CHILD HEALTH AND DEVELOPMENT STUDY
SCHOOL OF PUBLIC HEALTH
UNIVERSITY OF CALIFORNIA, BERKELEY

1. Introduction

I am pleased to have been asked to participate in the Sixth Berkeley Symposium on Mathematical Statistics. It provides an opportunity for an exchange of information and ideas on some methodologic problems encountered in observational studies of etiologic factors in chronic diseases. These problems present different aspects than those ordinarily involved in experimental studies usually encountered in statistical investigations. In the latter, especially in those on inferences derived from comparisons of two samples, there is a tacit assumption that the samples have been equalized usually through a procedure of randomization.

In studies on human beings, experimentations are difficult, if not impossible. In attempts to determine the roles of environmental factors in development of disease, one must depend on observation of phenomena as they occur in nature. Often factors such as emotional stress, physical conditions, certain components in the diet, cigarette smoking, sedentary occupations, and other characteristics require prolonged periods of observation between the exposure to the environmental factor and the development of disease. In many cases the period is measured in years and sometimes decades. Consequently, a manipulative study would involve major changes in modes of life of large groups of people over prolonged periods of time. Such experimentations are impractical, if not impossible. Of necessity, therefore, the main methods are those of observations of associations between prevalence of a given disease or condition and environmental factors as they occur in nature without interference on the part of the investigator.

The most elementary and least desirable of these observational studies are the so-called "indirect studies." In these, the unit of investigation is the group rather than the individual. Often mortality or morbidity data derived from vital statistics are compared with indices of suspected environmental characteristics. Such studies are useful to provide leads for further investigations. They have,

Supported by Grant No. HD 7256 of the National Institutes of Health.

however, great weaknesses in that the groups differ along many other characteristics in addition to the variables of discourse.

More desirable are studies which focus on the individual. These are mainly
of two types: retrospective and prospective. The former start with a group of
individuals, each of whom experienced a certain disease or condition and a selected group of controls, matched on a number of pertinent characteristics. The
two groups are then compared for a number of variables. The prospective study
starts with the selection of a sample of the population in which individuals are
identified as those possessing and those not possessing the suspected environmental variable. The two groups are followed for a length of time sufficient to
detect differences in incidences of the disease or condition.

It is clear that these methods are also not free from the major difficulty of
lack of group comparability since the groups have been self-selected. They therefore do not satisfy the basic rule for valid scientific inference—that, *a priori*,
groups being compared be alike in all pertinent characteristics. Unfortunately,
the inherent weaknesses of the methods are often escalated by deficiencies and
carelessness in study design.

Before proceeding to discuss the major problem of self-selection, it is desirable
to illustrate some of the more simple pitfalls in investigations of etiologic factors
in chronic diseases. These errors are relatively simple and should not have to be
mentioned. They are, however, important because of the frequency with which
they are encountered in the literature. Examples are the recent studies which
attempt to correlate radiation effects with the infant mortality rates [1], [2].
These suffer not only from noncomparabilities of the groups, but the method
employed has the additional weakness that the comparisons are made not with
current and past trend of the infant mortality rates, but with hypothetical rates
derived from extrapolation of current and past rates into the future; a procedure
based on the speculative assumption that if it were not for the radiation effect
the past trend would continue into the future with the absurd consequence that
a zero rate would have been reached.

Another important error often encountered in the literature is the fallacy of
utilizing evidence supporting a given hypothesis and neglecting evidence con-
tradicting it. An illustration is shown in Figure 1. In this case, the investigator
selected six countries and correlated the per cent of fat in the diet with the
mortality of coronary heart disease in these six countries [3]. On the face of it,
the correlation appears very striking and indeed the author in reviewing the
data in Figure 1 makes the following strong statement: "The analysis of international vital statistics shows a striking feature when the national food consumption statistics are studied in parallel. Then it appears that for men aged
40 to 60 or 70, that is, at the ages when the fatal result of atherosclerosis are
most prominent, there is a remarkable relationship between the death rate from
degenerative heart disease and the proportion of fat calories in the national diet.
A regular progression exists from Japan through Italy, Sweden, England and
Wales, Canada, and Australia to the United States. No other variable in the

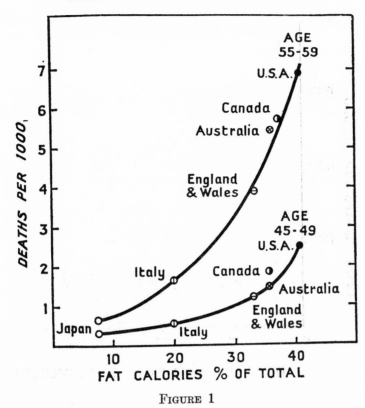

FIGURE 1

Mortality from degenerative heart disease (1948–1949, men).
National vital statistics from official sources. Fat calories as percentage of total
calories calculated from national food balance data for 1949 supplied by the
Nutrition Division, Food and Agriculture Organization of the United Nations.
(After A. Keys [3].)

mode of life besides the fat calories in the diet is known which shows anything
like such a consistent relationship to the mortality rate from coronary or degenerative heart disease."

The question arises how were these six countries selected. Further investigation reveals that these six countries are not representative of all countries for
which the data are available. For example, it is easy enough to select six other
countries which differ greatly in their dietary fat consumptions, but have nearly
equal death rates from coronary heart disease (Figure 2). Similarly, six other
countries were easily selected which consumed nearly equal proportions of dietary fat, but which differed widely in their death rates from coronary heart
disease (Figure 3). This tendency of selecting evidence biased for a favorable
hypothesis is very common. For example, investigations among the Bantu in
Africa are often mentioned in support of the dietary fat hypothesis of coronary

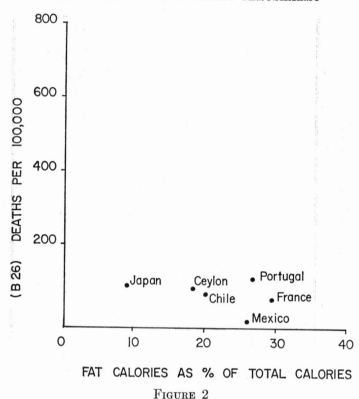

FIGURE 2

Six countries selected for equality in mortality from coronary heart disease, but differing greatly in consumption of fat calories in per cent of total calories.

heart disease, while observations on other African tribes, Eskimos, and other groups which do not support the hypothesis are generally ignored.

However, even when these errors are avoided and the studies are well conducted, the conclusions which may be derived from observational studies have great limitations stemming primarily from noncomparability of the self-formed groups. The phenomenon of self-selection is the root of many of the difficulties. Were all other complications eliminated, the inequalities between groups which result from self-selection would still leave in doubt inferences on causality. For example, in the study of the relationship of cigarette smoking to health, if we assume well conducted investigations in which (a) large random samples of the population have been selected and the individuals correctly identified as smokers, nonsmokers, or past smokers, (b) the problem of nonresponse did not exist, (c) the population had been followed long enough to identify all cases of the disease in question, (d) no problems of misdiagnosis and misclassification existed, (e) and no one in the population had been lost from observation, then even under these ideal conditions, the inferences that may be drawn from

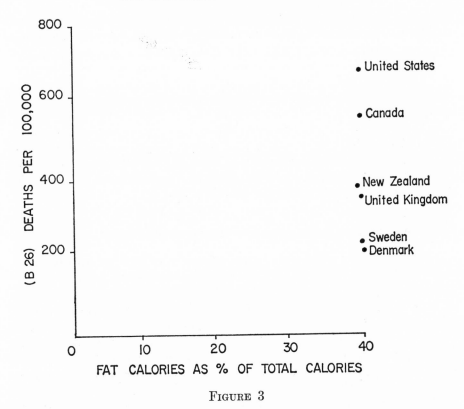

FIGURE 3

Six countries selected for equality in consumption of fat calories in per cent of total calories, but differing greatly in mortality from coronary heart disease.

the study are limited because the individuals being observed, rather than the investigator, made for themselves the crucial choice: smoker, nonsmoker, or past smoker.

Faced with these difficulties, it becomes necessary to develop auxiliary and supplementary methods of study which would help overcome their built-in limitations, and increase the probability of arriving at correct conclusions. This, unfortunately, has so far not been seriously tackled. To date, epidemiologists and statisticians have not responded fully to this challenge. We have made only a meager beginning in refining the tools and redefining the standards that would aid the process of inferring causation from observed associations.

A helpful first step is to determine whether the observed association is *specific* to the disease under study. For it is intuitively recognized that if the association is specific there is a greater likelihood of an etiologic relationship than when it is not. An association which is nonspecific, diffuse, manifesting itself in a large and varied number of diseases, increases the probability that the observed differences may be due to extraneous factors which differentiate the self-formed subgroups.

Another important activity in evaluating the significance of observed associations is to investigate whether the findings fit with other known phenomena. For, again, it is intuitively apparent that if the observed association contradicts other aspects of an overall phenomenon, doubts are raised concerning the causation hypothesis, and it becomes necessary to dig and explore further in an attempt to derive at a more reasonable evaluation of the meaning of the observed association.

In the following, I will attempt to demonstrate the usefulness of exploring additional leads in order to arrive at a sharper judgment and evaluation of whether an observed association may be interpreted as indicating a cause and effect relationship. I will use for this exercise two recent studies on the association of cigarette smoking and premature birth [4], [5].

2. Cigarette smoking during pregnancy and "premature birth"

A large number of investigators have demonstrated that women who smoke cigarettes during pregnancy have a larger proportion of "premature births," than women who do not smoke [5]–[37]. Prematurity in this case is defined by the birth weight criterion and refers to low birth weight infants (weighing 2,500 grams or less). In our Child Health and Development Studies, we also investigated this problem in 1964 and found the same phenomenon. Women who smoked cigarettes have nearly twice as many low birth weight infants as women who do not smoke. An increase in low birth weight infants has very serious implications, for the neonatal mortality rate (the risk of dying in the first month of life) is more than 20 times higher than the neonatal mortality rate of heavier infants [38]. The expectation is, therefore, that the perinatal mortality rate should be considerably higher for infants of smoking than for those of non-smoking mothers. (The perinatal mortality rate is the number of stillborn infants of at least 28 weeks gestation and liveborn infants who died within seven days after birth per 1,000 total births.) However, we found that the mortality rate was nearly identical for infants of smokers and nonsmokers. Thus, the findings from this observational study did not fit with other known phenomena.

The next step therefore was to consider the mortality of the low birth weight infants. The surprising finding was that the neonatal mortality rate of low birth weight infants of smoking mothers was substantially and significantly lower than that of low birth weight infants of nonsmoking mothers. Our findings were later corroborated by several other investigators [35], [36].

To date, there are some 33 studies on the subject. Fifteen of these did not investigate mortality [6]–[20], fourteen others were based on relatively small samples of approximately 2,000 births. Of these, seven found no increase in mortality [21]–[27], and seven found some increase [28]–[34]. But even the increase in most of the latter were of relatively small magnitude. Moreover, it can be shown that if the perinatal mortality rate of infants of smoking mothers is indeed greater by 35 per cent than that of nonsmoking mothers, (the figure 35 per cent was selected because such an increase is to be expected from a doubling of the incidence of low birth weight infants) then the probability that seven of fourteen such studies should fail to detect such increases is very small ($p < 0.005$). More important is the fact that there are several studies based on large samples. In addition to our 1964 studies, which we recently enlarged [5], there appeared three other studies based on relatively large samples (Table I) [35]–[37]. The

TABLE I

PERINATAL MORTALITY AMONG ALL INFANTS AND AMONG LOW BIRTH WEIGHT INFANTS BY MOTHER'S SMOKING STATUS IN FIVE LARGE STUDIES

Numbers 1 and 5 refer to neonatal mortality only.

| | | Perinatal mortality per 1,000 | | | |
| | | Total | | ≤ 2,500 grams | |
Investigator	Number of births	Nonsmoker	Smoker	Nonsmoker	Smoker
1. Yerushalmy 1964 White	5,381	12.4	13.9	232.1	137.7
Black	1,419	23.4	22.9	260.9	109.4
2. Underwood, et al. 1967	48,505	19.7	20.8	269.0	187.0
3. Rantakallio 1969	11,931	23.2	23.4	343.6	287.6
4. Butler, et al. 1969	16,994	32.4	44.8	284.5	268.5
5. Yerushalmy 1971 White	9,793	11.0	11.3	218.3	113.9
Black	3,290	17.1	21.5	201.6	113.6

study by Underwood is based on 48,000 births, by Rantakallio on 12,000 and by Butler on some 17,000 births. Butler's study was retrospective, the others were prospective. Only Butler's study showed an increase in perinatal mortality. The others did not. It is of great interest that the large prospective studies confirmed our interesting findings that the perinatal mortality rate of low birth weight infants of smokers was substantially and significantly lower than that of infants of nonsmoking mothers.

In addition, in an extensive study on etiological factors in prematurity, Jansson [27] considered also the question of smoking. He states: "Recently Yerushalmy (1964) in an extensive prospective study found the same relationship, but he was unable to confirm a higher perinatal mortality in infants of smoking mothers. On the contrary he made the surprising observation that in single live births, which fulfilled both criteria of prematurity, i.e. birthweight 2,500 g or less and gestational age less than 37 weeks, the neonatal mortality was significantly lower in infants of smoking than of nonsmoking mothers. Yerushalmy could not explain the apparently higher survival rate for those prematures whose mothers were smoking during pregnancy.

"In our series we made observations of a similar kind. If the malformed infants are not included, the perinatal mortality in premature infants of nonsmoking mothers was 29 per cent, while the corresponding figure for infants of smoking mothers was 8 per cent. . . .

"Another observation in our series was that the number of smoking mothers of premature infants was higher in social class III than in classes I and II. It is a well established fact that premature birth is considerably more common in the lower social classes. Thus, the relationship of smoking to prematurity may be indirect. As Yerushalmy points out, it may be the smoker, not the smoking in itself, which offers an explanation of the differences observed."

It is thus abundantly clear that we are presented with phenomena which do not fit and contradict each other. The proportion of low birth weight infants born to smoking mothers is much higher than that of infants of nonsmokers, but the perinatal mortality of infants of smokers is not higher. Especially surprising is the fact that low birth weight infants of smokers have substantially lower perinatal mortality rates than infants of nonsmoking mothers. Other paradoxical phenomena were noted in our more detailed study. A number of variables such as parity, age of mother, length of pregnancy, and other factors were investigated and none of them could offer a reasonable explanation for the paradoxical findings [5].

It was next necessary to investigate differences between smokers and nonsmokers. A number of investigators demonstrated great differences in smokers and nonsmokers in many characteristics. For example, smokers were found to be significantly different from nonsmokers in morphologic dimensions and proportions [39]. Smokers were found to be more neurotic and changed jobs and spouses more often than nonsmokers [40]-[43]. When we investigated and compared our smokers and nonsmokers, we found striking differences in mode of life characteristics between the two groups. Smokers were less likely to use contraceptive methods than nonsmokers. They were less likely to plan the pregnancy. They were more likely to drink hard liquor, beer, and coffee, while nonsmokers were more likely to drink tea, milk, and wine. The smoker was more likely to indulge in these habits to a greater extreme than the nonsmoker. We also found some differences in biologic characteristics. For example, the age of menarche was significantly lower for women who subsequently became smokers than for nonsmokers. These differences bring into sharp focus the fact that inferences concerning etiology from observational studies are derived from comparison of groups which violate the principle of group comparability.

These findings raised doubts and argued against the proposition that cigarette smoking acts as an exogenous factor which interferes with the intrauterine growth and development of the fetus. It appears that these findings give support also to the hypothesis that smokers may represent a group of people whose reproductive experience would have duplicated the observed pattern whether or not they smoked. Smoking may be considered an index which characterizes the smoker, but smoking *per se* is only incidental as a causal factor in the observed phenomena. The difference in incidence of low birth weight may be due to the *smoker* not the *smoking*.

We explored this suggestion in two ways, one indirectly, namely, we investigated whether it would be possible to duplicate some of the findings between smokers and nonsmokers in groups of women who were differentiated along a selected biologic characteristic. The height variable was selected because it is known that infants of short women are, on the average, smaller than those of tall women. We found that short and tall women showed differences in incidence and mortality of low birth weight infants very similar to those of smoking and nonsmoking women. Thus, short women have higher proportion of low birth weight infants, but these low birth weight infants of short women had lower neonatal mortality rates than low birth weight infants of tall women (Figure 4).

In a recent paper [44], we investigated this problem more directly. In our Child Health and Development Studies, we obtained detailed information about the women's previous births, including the birth weight. Much later in the interview, we obtained from the woman a history of her smoking habits, including the age at which she started to smoke. We tested the reliability of the answers to these questions and found that they were reliable and not biased one by the other. From this information, we were able to divide the women into four groups: (1) women who never smoked, (2) women all of whose previous children were born under smoking conditions, (3) women who subsequently became smokers but who produced infants during the period before they acquired the smoking habit, and (4) women who quit smoking but who produced liveborn infants before they quit. It is therefore possible to investigate the reproductive performance of the women in group 3 during their nonsmoking periods and women in group 4 during periods of smoking.

If it is the *smoking* that *causes* the increase in low birth weight, then women in group 3 should have had relatively few infants of low birth weight during the period before they started to smoke. On the other hand, if it is the *smoker* not the smoking, then we would expect that women who eventually became smokers should have already a high incidence of low birth weight infants even in the period before they started to smoke. Similarly, the data may be used to test the proposition that women who quit smoking are basically nonsmokers, and thus, should have relatively low incidence of low birth weights even before they quit smoking. In order to narrow the age gap between the women in the four groups, the incidence of low birth weight infants is compared only for those born when the women were 25 years of age or younger.

Figure 5 shows that the reproductive performance of smokers before they started to smoke was much like that of smokers, and that of past smokers before they quit smoking was much like that of nonsmokers. The differences are statistically significant in both groups. The evidence appears, therefore, to support the proposition that the incidence of low birth weight infants is due to the *smoker* and not the *smoking*.

3. Comment

While the results of this study have inherent value in themselves and are very suggestive, it is, nevertheless, only a single study and the results must be

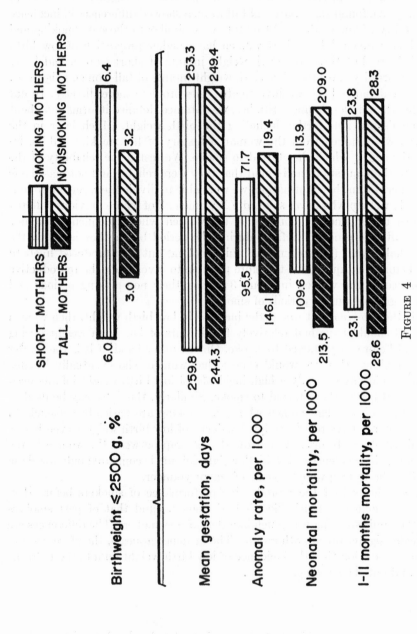

FIGURE 4

Reproductive performance of nonsmoking and smoking gravidas contrasted with that of tall and short gravidas.

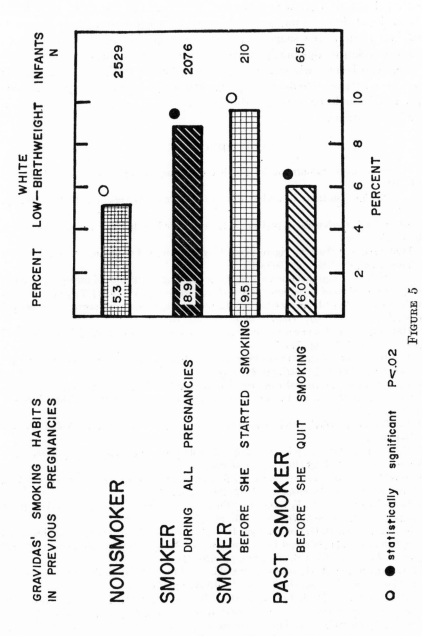

FIGURE 5

Per cent of low birth weight infants by smoking status of their mothers.

considered tentative until confirmed by more studies based on larger samples in other population groups. The study, however, makes a strong point that observational studies have a number of weaknesses and the results of studies must be explored along a number of additional areas before they can be accepted.

Most important is the suggestion that the profession must devote serious study and develop methodologies which are especially applicable to investigations on human beings, where the basic assumption of statistical inferences do not hold. It is necessary to develop supplementary and complimentary methods of study which would be helpful in the difficult area of inferring causation from observed associations.

REFERENCES

[1] E. J. STERNGLASS, "Controversial prophet of doom," *Science*, Vol. 166 (1969), pp. 195–200.

[2] ———, "Infant mortality in nuclear tests," *Bull. Atomic Scientists*, Vol. 25 (1969), pp. 18–20.

[3] A. KEYS, "Atherosclerosis—a problem in newer public health," *J. Mt. Sinai Hosp.*, Vol. 20 (1953), p. 134.

[4] J. YERUSHALMY, "Mothers' cigarette smoking and survival of infant," *Amer. J. Obstet. & Gynec.*, Vol. 88 (1964), pp. 505–518.

[5] ———, "The relationship of parents' cigarette smoking to outcome of pregnancy—implications to problem of causation," *Amer. J. Epidemiology*, Vol. 93 (1971), pp. 443–456.

[6] W. J. SIMPSON, "A preliminary report on cigarette smoking and incidence of prematurity," *Amer. J. Obstet. & Gynec.*, Vol. 73 (1957), pp. 808–815.

[7] A. HERRIOT, W. Z. BILLEWICZ, and F. E. HYTTEN, "Cigarette smoking in pregnancy," *Lancet*, Vol. 1 (1962), pp. 771–773.

[8] A. L. VILLUMSEN, "Cigarette smoking and low birth weights. A preliminary report," *Ugeskr. Laeg.*, Vol. 124 (1962), pp. 630–631.

[9] J. YERUSHALMY, "Statistical consideration and evaluation of epidemiologic evidence," *Tobacco and Health* (edited by James George and T. Rosenthal), Springfield, Charles C Thomas, 1962.

[10] D. E. MURDOCK, "Birth weight and smoking," *Nebraska State Med. J.*, Vol. 48 (1963), pp. 604–606.

[11] C. D. MANTELL, "Smoking in pregnancy: the role played by carbonic anhydrase," *New Zealand Med. J.*, Vol. 63 (1964), pp. 601–603.

[12] B. MACMAHON, M. ALPERT, and E. J. SALBER, "Infant weight and parental smoking habits," *Amer. J. Epidemiology*, Vol. 82 (1965), pp. 247–261.

[13] R. L. MCDONALD and C. F. LANFORD, "Effects of smoking on selected clinical obstetric factors," *Obstet. & Gynec.*, Vol. 26 (1965), pp. 470–475.

[14] J. R. ABERNATHY, B. G. GREENBURG, H. B. WELLS, and T. FRAZIER, "Smoking as an independent variable in a multiple regression analysis upon birthweight and gestation," *Amer. J. Public Health*, Vol. 56 (1966), pp. 626–633.

[15] W. A. REINKE and M. HENDERSON, "Smoking and prematurity in the presence of other variables," *Arch. Environ. Health*, Vol. 12 (1966), pp. 600–606.

[16] R. T. RAVENHOLT, M. J. LEVINSKI, D. J. NELLIST, and M. TAKENAGA, "Effects of smoking on reproduction," *Amer. J. Obstet. & Gynec.*, Vol. 96 (1966), pp. 267–281.

[17] S. KIZER, "Influencia del Habito de Fumar Sobre el Embarazo, Parto y recien Nacido," *Rev. Obst. Gin. Vanezuela*, Vol. 27 (1967), pp. 595–643.

[18] M. TERRIS and E. GOLD, "An epidemiologic study of prematurity," *Amer. J. Obstet. & Gynec.*, Vol. 103 (1969), pp. 358–370.

[19] C. R. BUNCHER, "Cigarette smoking and duration of pregnancy," *Amer. J. Obstet. & Gynec.*, Vol. 103 (1969), pp. 943–946.

[20] R. MULCAHY, J. MURPHY, and F. MARTIN, "Placental changes and maternal weight in smoking and nonsmoking mothers," *Amer. J. Obstet. & Gynec.*, Vol. 106 (1970), pp. 703–704.

[21] L. SAVEL and E. ROTH, "Effects of smoking in pregnancy: a continuing retrospective study," *Obstet. & Gynec.*, Vol. 20 (1962), pp. 313–316.

[22] J. M. O'LANE, "Some fetal effects of maternal cigarette smoking," *Obstet. & Gynec.*, Vol. 22 (1963), pp. 181–184.

[23] P. B. UNDERWOOD, L. L. HESTER, T. LAFITTE, JR., and J. V. GREGG, "The relationship of smoking to the outcome of pregnancy," *Amer. J. Obstet. & Gynec.*, Vol. 91 (1965), pp. 270–276.

[24] W. F. PETERSON, K. N. MORISE, and D. F. KALTREIDER, "Smoking and prematurity. A preliminary report based on study of 7,740 caucasians," *Obstet. & Gynec.*, Vol. 26 (1965), pp. 775–779.

[25] G. C. DOWNING and W. E. CHAPMAN, "Smoking and pregnancy—A statistical study of 5,659 patients," *Calif. Med.*, Vol. 104 (1966), p. 187.

[26] P. ROBINSON, "Smoking of Burmese women during pregnancy and its influence on mother, fetus and newborn," *Harefuah*, Vol. 69 (1965), pp. 37–39.

[27] I. JANSSON, "Aetiological factors in prematurity," *Acta Obstet. et Gynec., Scandinav.*, Vol. 45 (1966), pp. 279–300.

[28] C. R. LOWE, "Effect of mothers' smoking habits on birthweight of their children," *Brit. Med. J.*, Vol. 2 (1959), pp. 673–676.

[29] T. M. FRAZIER, G. H. DAVIS, H. GOLDSTEIN, and I. D. GOLDBERG, "Cigarette smoking and prematurity: a prospective study," *Amer. J. Obstet. & Gynec.*, Vol. 81 (1961), pp. 988–996.

[30] J. F. ZABRISKIE, "Effect of cigarette smoking during pregnancy, study of 2,000 cases," *Obstet. & Gynec.*, Vol. 21 (1963), pp. 405–411.

[31] C. S. RUSSELL, R. TAYLOR, and R. N. MADDISON, "Some effects of smoking in pregnancy," *J. Obstet. Gynec. Brit. Cwlth.*, Vol. 73 (1966), pp. 742–746.

[32] G. W. COMSTOCK and F. E. LUDIN, "Parental smoking and perinatal mortality," *Amer. J. Obstet. & Gynec.*, Vol. 98 (1967), pp. 708–718.

[33] R. MULCAHY and J. F. KNAGGS, "Effect of age, parity and cigarette smoking on outcome of pregnancy," *Amer. J. Obstet. & Gynec.*, Vol. 101 (1968), pp. 844–849.

[34] S. KULLANDER and B. KALLEN, "A prospective study of smoking and pregnancy," *Acta Obstet. et Gynec. Scand.*, Vol. 50 (1971), pp. 83–94.

[35] P. B. UNDERWOOD, C. F. KESLER, J. M. O'LANE, and D. A. CALLAGAN, "Parental smoking empirically related to pregnancy outcome," *Obstet. & Gynec.*, Vol. 29 (1967), pp. 1–8.

[36] P. RANTAKALLIO, "Groups at risk in low birth weight infants and perinatal mortality," *Acta Paeditricia Scand.*, Vol. 193 (1969) Suppl., p. 193.

[37] N. R. BUTLER and E. D. ALBERMAN (editors), "The second report of the 1958 British perinatal mortality survey," *Perinatal Mortality*, Edinburgh, B. & S. Livingston Ltd., 1969.

[38] S. SHAPIRO, E. R. SCHLESINGER, and R. E. L. NESBITT, JR., "Infant, perinatal maternal and childhood mortality in the United States," Cambridge, Harvard University Press, 1968, p. 51.

[39] C. C. SELTZER, "Morphologic constitution and smoking," *J. Amer. Med. Assoc.*, Vol. 183 (1963), pp. 639–645.

[40] A. M. LILIENFELD, "Emotional and other selected characteristics of cigarette smokers and nonsmokers as related to epidemiologic study of lung cancer and other diseases," *J. Nat. Cancer Inst.*, Vol. 22 (1959), pp. 259–282.

[41] H. J. EYSENCK, M. TARRANT, M. WOOLF, and L. ENGLAND, "Smoking and personality,"
     Brit. Med. J., Vol. 1 (1960), pp. 1456–1460.
[42] C. W. HEATH, "Differences between smokers and nonsmokers," Arch. Intern. Med.
     (Chicago), Vol. 101 (1958), pp. 377–388.
[43] C. V. THOMAS, "Characteristics of smokers compared with nonsmokers in a population
     of healthy young adults, including observations on family history, blood pressure, heart
     rate, body weight, cholesterol and certain psychologic traits," Ann. Intern. Med., Vol. 53
     (1960), pp. 697–718.
[44] J. YERUSHALMY, "Low-birth-weight infants born before their mothers started to smoke
     cigarettes," Amer. J. Obstet. & Gynec., Vol. 112 (1972), pp. 277–284.

Allard	Patterns of Molecular Variation	Vol. V
with Kahler		
Ambartsumian	Random Mosaics on a Plane	Vol. III
Anderson	Regression in Time Series	Vol. I
Ayala	Natural Populations of *Drosophila*	Vol. V
Azencott	Random Walks on Groups	Vol. III
with Cartier		
Bahadur	Likelihood Ratios	Vol. I
with Raghavachari		
Barlow	Air Pollution Concentrations	Vol. VI
Barlow	Isotonic Tests	Vol. I
with Doksum		
Behar	Computer Simulation Techniques	Vol. VI
Bellman	Hierarchies of Control Processes	Vol. V
Belyayev	First Passage	Vol. III
Beran	Minimax Procedures	Vol. I
Bhattacharya	Central Limit Theorem	Vol. II
Bickel	Wiener Process Sequential Testing	Vol. I
with Yahav		
Birnbaum	Distribution Free Statistics	Vol. I
Blumenthal	Collections of Measures	Vol. II
with Corson		
Blyth	Inequalities of Cramér-Rao Type	Vol. I
with Roberts		
Bodmer	Fitness and Molecular Evolution	Vol. V
with Cavalli-Sforza		
Borovkov	Random Walks with Boundaries	Vol. III
Brillinger	Interval Functions	Vol. I
Brown	Statistical Aspects of Clinical Trials	Vol. IV
Bucy	Riccati Equation	Vol. III
Bühler	Generations in Branching Processes	Vol. III
Bühlmann	Credibility	Vol. I
Burkholder	Operators on Martingales	Vol. II
with Davis and Gundy		
Burton	CHESS, Surveillance System	Vol. VI
with Finklea, Hammer, Hasselblad, Riggan, Sharp, and Shy		

343

Cartier with Azencott	Random Walks on Groups	Vol. III
Cavalli-Sforza with Bodmer	Fitness and Molecular Evolution	Vol. V
Chernoff	Cluster Analysis	Vol. I
Chiang	An Equality in Stochastic Processes	Vol. IV
Chiang with Yang	Time Dependent Epidemics	Vol. IV
Chibisov	Normal Approximation	Vol. I

Chiscon
  with Hoyer and
  Kohne
	Evolution of Mammalian DNA	Vol. V

Clark
  with Goodman and
  Wilson
	Mutation Monitoring	Vol. VI

Clifford	Survival of Bacteria after Irradiation	Vol. IV
Cochran	Errors in Measurement	Vol. I
Cogburn	Central Limit for Markov Processes	Vol. II
Collen with Friedman	Adverse Drug Reactions	Vol. VI
Collen with Kodlin	Automated Diagnosis	Vol. IV
Corson with Blumenthal	Collections of Measures	Vol. II
Cox with Lewis	Multivariate Point Processes	Vol. III

Cranmer
  with Finklea,
  Hammer, McCabe,
  Newill, and Shy
	Health Intelligence	Vol. VI

Crow	Darwinian and Non-Darwinian Evolution	Vol. V
Daniels	Polymer Chain Distributions	Vol. III
Darling	Fixed Number of Observations	Vol. IV

Das Gupta
  with Eaton, Olkin,
  Perlman, Savage,
  and Sobel
	Elliptically Contoured Distributions	Vol. II

David	Diversity	Vol. I
David	Diversity, II	Vol. IV
David	Neyman's $C(\alpha)$ Techniques	Vol. IV

Davis
  with Burkholder
  and Gundy
	Operators on Martingales	Vol. II

Debreu	Derivative of a Correspondence	Vol. II
with Schmeidler		
DeGroot	Low Level Radiation	Vol. VI
Doksum	Nonparametric Decision Theory	Vol. I
Doksum	Isotonic Tests	Vol. I
with Barlow		
Doob	Structure of Markov Chains	Vol. III
Doob	William Feller	Vol. II
Doubilet	Generating Function	Vol. II
with Rota and		
Stanley		
Dudley	Measurable Processes	Vol. II
Dvoretzky	Dependent Random Variables	Vol. II
Eaton	Elliptically Contoured Distributions	Vol. II
with Das Gupta,		
Olkin, Perlman,		
Savage, and Sobel		
Ewens	Statistical Aspects	Vol. V
Fearn	Galton-Watson Processes	Vol. IV
Feldman	Sets of Boundedness and Continuity	Vol. II
Ferguson	Double Your Fortune	Vol. III
Finklea	CHESS, Surveillance System	Vol. VI
with Burton,		
Hammer, Hasselblad,		
Riggan, Sharp, and		
Shy		
Finklea	Health Intelligence	Vol. VI
with Cranmer,		
Hammer, McCabe,		
Newill, and Shy		
Flehinger	Sequential Medical Trials	Vol. IV
with Louis		
Friedman	Adverse Drug Reactions	Vol. VI
with Collen		
Frolík	Projective Limits	Vol. II
Gaffey	Worsening Environmental Pollution	Vol. VI
Gani	First Emptiness Problems	Vol. III
Garsia	Continuity Properties	Vol. II
Gatlin	Evolutionary Indices	Vol. V
Getoor	Additive Functionals	Vol. III
Gill	Toxicity on Ecosystems	Vol. VI
Gleser	Regression with Unknown Covariance	Vol. I
with Olkin		

Gnedenko	Random Number of Variables	Vol. II
Gofman with Tamplin	Carcinogenesis by Ionizing Radiation	Vol. VI
Goldsmith	Environmental Epidemiology	Vol. VI
Goldsmith	Comprehensive Epidemiologic Study	Vol. VI
Goodman, D. with Clark and Wilson	Mutation Monitoring	Vol. VI
Goodman, L. A.	Cross Classified Data	Vol. I
Goulding	X-Ray Fluorescence	Vol. VI
Guillier	Internal Exposure of Urethane in Mice	Vol. IV
Gundy with Burkholder and Davis	Operators on Martingales	Vol. II
Hájek	Local Asymptotic Admissibility	Vol. I
Hamilton with Hoffman and Tompkins	Infant Mortality around Reactors	Vol. VI
Hammer with Burton, Finklea, Hasselblad, Riggan, Sharp, and Shy	CHESS, Surveillance System	Vol. VI
Hammer with Cranmer, Finklea, McCabe, Newill, and Shy	Health Intelligence	Vol. VI
Hammersley	Seedlings	Vol. I
Hasselblad with Burton, Finklea, Hammer, Riggan, Sharp, and Shy	CHESS, Surveillance System	Vol. VI
Hasselblad with Lowrimore and Nelson	Statistical Aspects of Surveillance	Vol. VI
Hexter	Study of Daily Mortality	Vol. VI
Hildenbrand	Spaces of Economic Agents	Vol. II
Hoel with Sobel	Comparisons of Sequential Procedures	Vol. IV
Hoem	Analytic Graduation	Vol. I
Hoffman with Hamilton and Tompkins	Infant Mortality around Reactors	Vol. VI
Holley	Helmholtz Free Energy	Vol. III

Holmquist   Foundations of Paleogenetics   Vol. V

Hook   Monitoring Human Birth Defects   Vol. VI

Hoyer   Evolution of Mammalian DNA   Vol. V
    with Chiscon and
    Kohne

Ionescu Tulcea   Liftings   Vol. II

Itô   Poisson and Markov Processes   Vol. III

Jain   Range of Random Walk   Vol. III
    with Pruitt

Johnson   Applications of Contiguity   Vol. I
    with Roussas

Jukes   Comparison of Polypeptide Sequences   Vol. V

Kac   Feller, *In Memoriam*   Vol. II

Kahler   Patterns of Molecular Variation   Vol. V
    with Allard

Kakutani   Strictly Ergodic Systems   Vol. II

Kallianpur   Supports of Gaussian Measures   Vol. II
    with Nadkarni

Karlin   Equilibria for Genetic Systems   Vol. IV
    with McGregor

Katz   Randomly Placed Rooks   Vol. III
    with Sobel

Keith   Mutagenesis and Carcinogenesis   Vol. VI

Kemperman   Moment Problems   Vol. II

Keyfitz   Mathematics of Sex and Marriage   Vol. IV

Kiefer   Iterated Logarithm Analogues   Vol. I

Kimura   Population Genetics   Vol. V
    with Ohta

King   Role of Mutation in Evolution   Vol. V

Kingman   Transition Probabilities   Vol. III

Klotz   Markov Chain Clustering of Births   Vol. IV

Kohne   Evolution of Mammalian DNA   Vol. V
    with Chiscon and
    Hoyer

Kodlin   Automated Diagnosis   Vol. IV
    with Collen

Krieger   Unique Ergodicity   Vol. II

Kushner   Stochastic Optimization   Vol. III

Landau   Radiation and Infant Mortality   Vol. VI

Le Cam   Limits of Experiments   Vol. I

Leadbetter   Point Process Theory   Vol. III

Lewis   Multivariate Point Processes   Vol. III
    with Cox

Lewontin   Comparative Evolution   Vol. V
  with Stebbins
Linnik   Sequential Estimation   Vol. I
  with Romanovsky
Liptser   Conditionally Gaussian Sequences   Vol. II
  with Shiryayev
Louis   Sequential Medical Trials   Vol. IV
  with Flehinger
Lowrimore   Statistical Aspects of Surveillance   Vol. VI
  with Hasselblad
  and Nelson
MacIntyre   Studies of Enzyme Evolution   Vol. V
Maharam   Extensions of Linear Functions   Vol. II
Marcus   Behavior of Gaussian Processes   Vol. II
  with Shepp
Marshall   Distributions in Replacement   Vol. I
  with Proschan
McCabe   Health Intelligence   Vol. VI
  with Cranmer,
  Finklea, Hammer,
  Newill, and Shy
McGregor   Equilibria for Genetic Systems   Vol. IV
  with Karlin
McShane   Stochastic Differential Equations   Vol. III
Messinger   Demographic Data   Vol. VI
Meyer   Markov Processes   Vol. III
  with Smythe and
  Walsh
Millar   Stochastic Integrals   Vol. III
Miller   Sequential Rank Tests   Vol. I
Mitra   Generalized Inverses   Vol. I
  with Rao
Mollison   Simple Epidemics   Vol. III
Müller   Randomness and Extrapolation   Vol. II
Nadkarni   Supports of Gaussian Measures   Vol. II
  with Kallianpur
Nelson   Statistical Aspects of Surveillance   Vol. VI
  with Hasselblad
  and Lowrimore
Newill   Health Intelligence   Vol. VI
  with Cranmer,
  Finklea, Hammer,
  McCabe, and Shy

Neyman	Epilogue	Vol. VI
Neyman	Statistical Health-Pollution Study	Vol. VI
O'Brien	Practical Problems in Clinical Trials	Vol. IV
with Taylor		
Ohta	Population Genetics	Vol. V
with Kimura		
Olkin	Elliptically Contoured Distributions	Vol. II
with Das Gupta, Eaton, Perlman, Savage, and Sobel		
Olkin	Regression with Unknown Covariance	Vol. I
with Gleser		
Olson	Eigenvalues of Random Matrices	Vol. III
with Uppuluri		
Oosterhoff	Likelihood Ratio Test	Vol. I
with Van Zwet		
Orchard	Missing Information	Vol. I
with Woodbury		
Orey	Growth Rate of Gaussian Processes	Vol. II
Ornstein	Root Problem	Vol. II
Patterson	Radiation and Risk	Vol. VI
with Thomas		
Perlman	Maximum Likelihood Estimators	Vol. I
Perlman	Elliptically Contoured Distributions	Vol. II
with Das Gupta, Eaton, Olkin, Savage, and Sobel		
Port	Logarithmic Potentials	Vol. III
with Stone		
Port	Potentials and Brownian Motion	Vol. III
with Stone		
Posner	Epsilon Entropy	Vol. III
with Rodemich		
Proschan	Distributions in Replacement	Vol. I
with Marshall		
Pruitt	Range of Random Walk	Vol. III
with Jain		
Puri	Integral Functionals	Vol. III
Puri	Quantal Response Assays	Vol. IV
with Senturia		
Pyke	Spacings	Vol. I
Raghavachari	Likelihood Ratios	Vol. I
with Bahadur		

Raman	Graphical Methods in Biometry	Vol. IV
with Tarter		
Rao	Generalized Inverses	Vol. I
with Mitra		
Reichert	Information Stored in Proteins	Vol. V
Riggan	CHESS, Surveillance System	Vol. VI
with Burton, Finklea,		
Hammer, Hasselblad,		
Sharp, and Shy		
Risebrough	Effects of Pollutants on Animals	Vol. VI
Roberts	Inequalities of Cramér-Rao Type	Vol. I
with Blyth		
Robbins	Iterated Logarithm	Vol. III
with Siegmund		
Robbins	Stopping Rules	Vol. IV
with Siegmund		
Rodemich	Epsilon Entropy	Vol. III
with Posner		
Romanovsky	Sequential Estimation	Vol. I
with Linnik		
Rosenblatt	Stationary Processes	Vol. II
Rosenthal, H. L.	Strontium 90 Accumulation	Vol. VI
Rosenthal, H. P.	Span of Random Variables	Vol. II
Rota	Generating Function	Vol. II
with Doubilet and		
Stanley		
Roussas	Applications of Contiguity	Vol. I
with Johnson		
Rubin	Large Sample Properties	Vol. I
Sailor	Exposure to Radiation	Vol. VI
Sato	Potential Operators	Vol. III
Savage, I. R.	Likelihood Ratio Based on Ranks	Vol. I
with Sethuraman		
Savage, I. R.	Source of Evaluations	Vol. IV
with Webster		
Savage, L. J.	Elliptically Contoured Distributions	Vol. II
with Das Gupta,		
Eaton, Olkin,		
Perlman, and Sobel		
Sazonov	Multidimensional Central Limit Theorem	Vol. II
Schmeidler	Derivative of a Correspondence	Vol. II
with Debreu		
Schmetterer	Poisson Laws	Vol. II
Schmetterer	Rényi, *In Memoriam*	Vol. II

Scott	Summary of Panel Discussion	Vol. VI
Senturia	Quantal Response Assays	Vol. IV
with Puri		
Sethuraman	Likelihood Ratio Based on Ranks	Vol. I
with Savage		
Sharp	CHESS, Surveillance System	Vol. VI
with Burton, Finklea, Hasselblad, Hammer, Riggan, and Shy		
Shepp	Behavior of Gaussian Processes	Vol. II
with Marcus		
Shiryayev	Conditionally Gaussian Sequences	Vol. II
with Liptser		
Shy	CHESS, Surveillance System	Vol. VI
with Burton, Finklea, Hammer, Hasselblad, Riggan, and Sharp		
Shy	Health Intelligence	Vol. VI
with Cranmer, Finklea, Hammer, McCabe, and Newill		
Siegmund	Iterated Logarithm	Vol. III
with Robbins		
Siegmund	Stopping Rules	Vol. IV
with Robbins		
Sirken	Survey Strategies	Vol. VI
Smythe	Markov Processes	Vol. III
with Meyer and Walsh		
Sobel	Elliptically Contoured Distributions	Vol. II
with Das Gupta, Eaton, Olkin, Perlman, and Savage		
Sobel	Comparisons of Sequential Procedures	Vol. IV
with Hoel		
Sobel	Randomly Placed Rooks	Vol. III
with Katz		
Sobel	Play the Winner Selection	Vol. I
with Weiss		
Solomon	Poisson Fields of Lines	Vol. III
with Wang		
Soloviev	First Passage in Birth and Death	Vol. III
Southward	Mean of a Random Binomial Parameter	Vol. IV
with Van Ryzin		

Stanley	Generating Function	Vol. II
with Doubilet and Rota		
Stebbins	Comparative Evolution	Vol. V
with Lewontin		
Stein	Error in Normal Approximation	Vol. II
Sterling	Herbicide Effect on Health	Vol. VI
Sternglass	Environmental Radiation	Vol. VI
Stone	Logarithmic Potentials	Vol. III
with Port		
Stone	Potentials and Brownian Motion	Vol. III
with Port		
Straf	Weak Convergence	Vol. II
Strawderman	Bayes Minimax Estimators	Vol. I
Stroock	Diffusion Processes	Vol. III
with Varadhan		
Stroock	Strong Maximum Principle	Vol. III
with Varadhan		
Switzer	Efficiency Robustness	Vol. I
Tamplin	Carcinogenesis by Ionizing Radiation	Vol. VI
with Gofman		
Tarter	Graphical Methods in Biometry	Vol. IV
with Raman		
Taylor	Practical Problems in Clinical Trials	Vol. IV
with O'Brien		
Thomas	Radiation and Risk	Vol. VI
with Patterson		
Tompkins	Infant Mortality around Reactors	Vol. VI
with Hamilton and Hoffman		
Totter	Research of AEC on Health and Pollution	Vol. VI
Uppuluri	Eigenvalues of Random Matrices	Vol. III
with Olson		
Ury	Health Effects of Air Pollution	Vol. VI
Van Ryzin	Mean of a Random Binomial Parameter	Vol. IV
with Southward		
Van Zwet	Likelihood Ratio Test	Vol. I
with Oosterhoff		
Varadhan	Diffusion Processes	Vol. III
with Stroock		
Varadhan	Strong Maximum Principle	Vol. III
with Stroock		
Varaiya	Differential Games	Vol. III
Vaughan	Ecological and Environmental Problems	Vol. VI

Vincze	Kolmogorov-Smirnov Type Statistics	Vol. I
Vogel	Analysis of Polarity Changes	Vol. V
Vogel	Polarity Relations in Globins	Vol. V
with Zuckerkandl		
Walsh	Markov Processes	Vol. III
with Meyer and		
Smythe		
Wang	Poisson Fields of Lines	Vol. III
with Solomon		
Waugh	Sojourn Time Series	Vol. III
Waugh	Synchronous Cellular Growth	Vol. IV
Webster	Source of Evaluations	Vol. IV
with Savage		
Weiner	Age Dependent Branching Processes	Vol. IV
Weiss	Play the Winner Selection	Vol. I
with Sobel		
White	Induction of Pulmonary Adenomas in Mice	Vol. IV
Wijsman	Bounded Stopping Time	Vol. I
Wilson	Mutation Monitoring	Vol. VI
with Clark and		
Goodman		
Winkelstein	Mortality Statistics in Air Pollution Studies	Vol. VI
Woodbury	Missing Information	Vol. I
with Orchard		
Yahav	Wiener Process Sequential Testing	Vol. I
with Bickel		
Yang	Time Dependent Epidemics	Vol. IV
with Chiang		
Yerushalmy	Self-selection—a Major Problem	Vol. IV
Zelen	Contingency Tables	Vol. I
Zuckerkandl	Polarity Relations in Globins	Vol. V
with Vogel		

2.9.73 — 20
415874

QA276
B513p
6th
v. 4